INTERVENTIONAL CARDIOLOGY CLINICS

www.interventional.theclinics.com

Editor-in-Chief

MATTHEW J. PRICE

Antiplatelet and Anticoagulation Therapy in PCI

January 2017 • Volume 6 • Number 1

Editors

DOMINICK J. ANGIOLILLO
MATTHEW J. PRICE

ELSEVIER

1600 John F. Kennedy Boulevard • Suite 1800 • Philadelphia, Pennsylvania, 19103-2899

http://www.theclinics.com

INTERVENTIONAL CARDIOLOGY CLINICS Volume 6, Number 1
January 2017 ISSN 2211-7458, ISBN-13: 978-0-323-48262-2

Editor: Lauren Boyle
Developmental Editor: Susan Showalter

Interventional Cardiology Clinics (ISSN 2211-7458) is published quarterly by Elsevier Inc., 360 Park Avenue South, New York, NY 10010-1710. Months of issue are January, April, July, and October. Subscription prices are USD 195 per year for US individuals, USD 449 for US institutions, USD 100 per year for US students, USD 195 per year for Canadian individuals, USD 536 for Canadian institutions, USD 150 per year for Canadian students, USD 295 per year for international individuals, USD 536 for international institutions, and USD 150 per year for international students. To receive student/resident rate, orders must be accompanied by name of affiliated institution, date of term, and the *signature* of program/residency coordinator on institution letterhead. Orders will be billed at individual rate until proof of status is received. Foreign air speed delivery is included in all *Clinics* subscription prices. All prices are subject to change without notice. **POSTMASTER:** Send address changes to *Interventional Cardiology Clinics*, Elsevier Health Sciences Division, Subscription Customer Service, 3251 Riverport Lane, Maryland Heights, MO 63043. **Customer Service: Telephone: 1-800-654-2452** (U.S. and Canada); **1-314-447-8871** (outside U.S. and Canada). **Fax: 1-314-447-8029. E-mail: journalscustomerservice-usa@elsevier.com (for print support); journalsonlinesupport-usa@elsevier.com (for online support).**

Reprints. For copies of 100 or more of articles in this publication, please contact the Commercial Reprints Department, Elsevier Inc., 360 Park Avenue South, New York, NY 10010-1710. Tel.: 212-633-3874; Fax: 212-633-3820; E-mail: reprints@elsevier.com.

CONTRIBUTORS

EDITOR-IN-CHIEF

MATTHEW J. PRICE, MD
Director, Cardiac Catheterization Laboratory,
Division of Cardiovascular Diseases, Scripps
Clinic, Assistant Professor, Scripps
Translational Science Institute, La Jolla,
California

EDITORS

DOMINICK J. ANGIOLILLO, MD, PhD
Professor of Medicine, Director,
Cardiovascular Research, Program Director,
Interventional Cardiology Fellowship, Division
of Cardiology, University of Florida College of
Medicine-Jacksonville, Jacksonville, Florida

MATTHEW J. PRICE, MD
Director, Cardiac Catheterization Laboratory,
Division of Cardiovascular Diseases, Scripps
Clinic, Assistant Professor, Scripps
Translational Science Institute, La Jolla,
California

AUTHORS

DOMINICK J. ANGIOLILLO, MD, PhD
Professor of Medicine, Director,
Cardiovascular Research, Program Director,
Interventional Cardiology Fellowship, Division
of Cardiology, University of Florida College of
Medicine-Jacksonville, Jacksonville, Florida

DEEPAK L. BHATT, MD, MPH
Heart & Vascular Center, Brigham and
Women's Hospital, Harvard Medical School,
Boston, Massachusetts

MARC P. BONACA, MD, MPH
TIMI Study Group, Division of Cardiovascular
Medicine, Brigham and Women's Hospital,
Harvard Medical School, Boston,
Massachusetts

LAWRENCE F. BRASS, MD, PhD
Professor of Medicine and Pharmacology,
Department of Medicine, Perelman School of
Medicine, University of Pennsylvania,
Philadelphia, Pennsylvania

RICHARD A. BROWN, MD
University of Birmingham Institute of
Cardiovascular Sciences, City Hospital,
Birmingham, West Midlands, United Kingdom

DAVIDE CAPODANNO, MD, PhD
Associate Professor, Cardio-Thoracic-Vascular
Department, Ferrarotto Hospital, University of
Catania, Catania, Italy

ILARIA CAVALLARI, MD
TIMI Study Group, Division of Cardiovascular
Medicine, Brigham and Women's Hospital,
Harvard Medical School, Boston,
Massachusetts

LARISA H. CAVALLARI, PharmD
Associate Professor, Department of
Pharmacotherapy and Translational Research,
Center for Pharmacogenomics, University of
Florida, Gainesville, Florida

MIKHAIL S. DZESHKA, MD
University of Birmingham Institute of
Cardiovascular Sciences, City Hospital,
Birmingham, West Midlands, United
Kingdom; Department of Internal Medicine I,
Grodno State Medical University, Grodno,
Belarus

FRANCESCO FRANCHI, MD
Assistant Professor, University of Florida
College of Medicine-Jacksonville,
Jacksonville, Florida

LISA GROSS, MD
Department of Cardiology,
Ludwig-Maximilians-Universität München
(LMU Munich), Munich, Germany

GREGORY Y.H. LIP, MD
Professor of Cardiovascular Medicine,
University of Birmingham Institute of
Cardiovascular Sciences, City Hospital,
Birmingham, West Midlands, United
Kingdom; Department of Clinical Medicine,
Aalborg Thrombosis Research Unit, Aalborg
University, Aalborg Hospital Science and
Innovation Center, Aalborg, Denmark

ARJUN MAJITHIA, MD
Landsman Heart and Vascular Center, Lahey
Hospital and Medical Center, Burlington,
Massachusetts

ANIWAA OWUSU OBENG, PharmD
Division of General Internal Medicine,
Department of Medicine, The Charles
Bronfman Institute for Personalized Medicine,
Icahn School of Medicine at Mount Sinai,
Department of Pharmacy, The Mount Sinai
Hospital, New York, New York

MATTHEW J. PRICE, MD
Director, Cardiac Catheterization Laboratory,
Division of Cardiovascular Diseases, Scripps
Clinic, Assistant Professor, Scripps
Translational Science Institute, La Jolla,
California

FABIANA ROLLINI, MD
Assistant Professor, University of Florida
College of Medicine-Jacksonville,
Jacksonville, Florida

DIRK SIBBING, MD, MHBA, FESC
Professor, Department of Cardiology,
Ludwig-Maximilians-Universität München
(LMU Munich), DZHK (German Center for
Cardiovascular Research), Partner Site Munich
Heart Alliance, Munich, Germany

TIMOTHY J. STALKER, PhD
Research Assistant Professor, Department of
Medicine, Perelman School of Medicine,
University of Pennsylvania, Philadelphia,
Pennsylvania

ROBERT F. STOREY, BM, DM, MRCP, FESC
Cardiology Professor, Department of
Infection, Immunity and Cardiovascular
Disease, University of Sheffield, Sheffield,
United Kingdom

WAEL SUMAYA, MD, MRCP
BHF Clinical research training fellow,
Department of Infection, Immunity and
Cardiovascular Disease, University of
Sheffield, Sheffield, United Kingdom

MAURIZIO TOMAIUOLO, PhD
Research Investigator, Senior, Department of
Medicine, Perelman School of Medicine,
University of Pennsylvania, Philadelphia,
Pennsylvania

PIERLUIGI TRICOCI, MD, MHS, PhD
Associate Professor of Medicine, Division of
Cardiology, Duke Clinical Research Institute,
Duke University Medical Center, Durham,
North Carolina

**FREEK W.A. VERHEUGT, MD, FACC,
FAHA, FESC**
Division of Cardiology, Onze Lieve Vrouwe
Gasthuis (OLVG), Amsterdam, Netherlands

CONTENTS

Hemostasis requires tightly regulated interaction of the coagulation system, platelets, blood cells, and vessel wall components at a site of vascular injury. Dysregulation of this response may result in excessive bleeding if the response is impaired, and pathologic thrombosis with vessel occlusion and tissue ischemia if the response is robust. Studies have elucidated the major molecular signaling pathways responsible for platelet activation and aggregation. Antithrombotic agents targeting these pathways are in clinical use. This review summarizes research examining mechanisms by which these multiple platelet signaling pathways are integrated at a site of vascular injury to produce an optimal hemostatic response.

Administering antiplatelet agents before coronary angiography to patients referred to elective or urgent percutaneous coronary intervention (PCI) requires a careful evaluation of advantages and disadvantages associated with platelet inhibition to avoid overtreatment on one side and undertreatment on the other. The delicate balance between ischemic protection and bleeding demands the ability to undertake risk stratification and individualized decisions, which is particularly challenging in the setting of ad hoc PCI and urgent procedures. This review analyzes the current evidence on pretreatment with oral and intravenous $P2Y_{12}$ inhibitors in patients undergoing coronary angiography with intent to undergo PCI.

Dual antiplatelet therapy (DAPT) is an essential component of treatment in patients with coronary artery disease treated with percutaneous coronary intervention (PCI). Recommendations for duration of DAPT after PCI should consider patient-specific risk, clinical presentation, stent characteristics, and procedural factors. Prolonged DAPT results in a reduction of stent thrombosis (ST) and myocardial infarction (MI) at the cost of increased bleeding. Studies of shorter-duration DAPT demonstrate similar mortality, MI, ST, and less bleeding when compared with longer DAPT duration in low risk populations. We review current evidence for strategies of prolonged DAPT and abbreviated DAPT following PCI.

> Cangrelor is an intravenous, non-thienopyridine, adenosine-triphosphate (ATP) analog that provides rapid and intensive inhibition of the platelet $P2Y_{12}$ receptor. Cangrelor is currently indicated as an adjunct to PCI to reduce the risk of myocardial infarction, repeat coronary revascularization, and stent thrombosis in patients who have not been treated with a $P2Y_{12}$. The pharmacology, clinical data, and rationale for the use of cangrelor is presented in detail. Platelet inhibitor and are not being given a glycoprotein IIb/IIIa inhibitor. Repeat coronary revascularization, and stent thrombosis in patients who have not been treated with a $P2Y_{12}$ platelet inhibitor and are not being given a glycoprotein IIb/IIIa inhibitor.

> Ticagrelor is a reversibly-binding, potent oral $P2Y_{12}$ inhibitor and a weak inhibitor of the ENT1 pathway for cellular adenosine uptake. In the PLATO trial, up to one year treatment with ticagrelor was superior to clopidogrel in ACS patients in reducing cardiovascular mortality. Consistent benefit was seen in the PEGASUS-TIMI 54 trial when ticagrelor was administered long-term. In addition to reduction in thrombotic events, these trials have shown disproportionate reduction of sudden death and, in PLATO, infection-related deaths with ticagrelor. It is therefore hypothesised that ticagrelor has significant "off-target" effects, independent of its antithrombotic effect. This review considers those effects.

> Thrombin is a potent platelet agonist, and protease-activated receptor-1 (PAR-1) is the main thrombin receptor in human platelets and thrombin. PAR-1 antagonism has attracted interest as a potential therapeutic target to reduce atherothrombotic events in patients with atherosclerotic disease, especially coronary artery disease. In this review, the author describes the rationale of PAR-1 antagonism for the reduction of atherothrombotic events and reviews the key phase 3 trial results, with special attention to analyses in percutaneous coronary intervention patients.

> Antiplatelet therapy with aspirin and a $P2Y_{12}$ receptor inhibitor is the cornerstone of treatment of patients with atherothrombotic disease manifestations. Switching between $P2Y_{12}$ inhibitors occurs commonly in clinical practice for a variety of reasons, including safety, efficacy, adherence, and economic considerations. There are concerns about the optimal approach for switching because of potential drug interactions, which may lead to ineffective platelet inhibition and thrombotic complications, or potential overdosing due to overlap in drug therapy, which might cause excessive platelet inhibition and increased bleeding. This review provides practical considerations of switching based on pharmacodynamic and clinical data available from the literature.

Stroke prevention is the main priority in the management cascade of atrial fibrillation. Most patients require long-term oral anticoagulation (OAC) and may require percutaneous coronary intervention. Prevention of recurrent cardiac ischemia and stent thrombosis necessitate dual antiplatelet therapy (DAPT) for up to 12 months. Triple antithrombotic therapy with OAC plus DAPT of shortest feasible duration is warranted, followed by dual antithrombotic therapy of OAC and antiplatelet agent, and OAC alone after 12 months. Because of elevated risk of hemorrhagic complications, new-generation drug-eluting stents, lower-intensity OAC, radial access, and routine use of gastric protection with proton pump inhibitors are recommended.

Patients with prior myocardial infarction (MI) are at long-term heightened risk for recurrent ischemic events. Several large randomized controlled trials have demonstrated the benefit of more intensive antiplatelet strategies for long-term secondary prevention of cardiovascular death, recurrent MI, and stroke in patients with a history of MI at a cost of increased bleeding. The bleeding risk associated with long-term intensive antiplatelet strategies requires careful patient selection and involvement of patients in shared decision making regarding risks and benefits of therapy. Clinical characteristics, adherence to therapy, and integrated risk scores may aid clinicians in translating clinical trials into individualized therapy.

Antithrombotic therapy is essential in the prevention of periprocedural death and myocardial infarction during and after percutaneous coronary intervention. In the pathogenesis of acute coronary syndromes (ACS), both platelets and the coagulation cascade play an important role. Therefore, periprocedural antithrombotic therapy is even more important in ACS than in elective PCI. The most used agents are aspirin, platelet P2Y12 blockers, platelet glycoprotein IIb/IIIa blockers, and parenteral anticoagulants. The P2Y12 blockers must be continued at least 12 months. High-risk patients should be treated with glycoprotein IIb/IIIa receptor antagonists, especially those undergoing primary angioplasty for ST-elevation acute coronary syndrome.

There is significant interpatient variability in clopidogrel effectiveness, which is due in part to cytochrome P450 (CYP) 2C19 genotype. Approximately 30% of individuals carry a *CYP2C19* loss-of-function allele, which has been consistently shown to reduce clopidogrel effectiveness after an acute coronary syndrome and percutaneous coronary intervention. Guidelines recommend consideration of prasugrel or ticagrelor in these patients. A clinical trial examining outcomes with *CYP2C19* genotype–guided antiplatelet therapy is ongoing. In the meantime, based on the evidence available to date, several institutions have started clinically implementing *CYP2C19* genotyping to assist with antiplatelet selection after percutaneous coronary intervention.

There is interindividual variability in the pharmacodynamic response to anti-platelet medications. High on-treatment platelet reactivity, reflecting a failure to achieve adequate platelet inhibition, is associated with a higher risk for thrombotic events. Low on-treatment platelet reactivity, or an enhanced response to antiplatelet medications, has been linked to a higher risk for bleeding. There is evidence for the prognostic value of platelet function testing for risk prediction. This review presents the current evidence regarding platelet function testing in patients undergoing percutaneous coronary intervention and coronary artery bypass grafting. The possible role of platelet function testing for individualized antiplatelet treatment is highlighted.

ANTIPLATELET AND ANTICOAGULATION THERAPY IN PCI

ISSUE OF RELATED INTEREST

Heart Failure Clinics, July 2016 (Vol. 12, No. 3)
Advanced Heart Failure
James C. Fang and Michael M. Givertz, *Editors*
Available at: http://www.heartfailure.theclinics.com/

THE CLINICS ARE NOW AVAILABLE ONLINE!

Access your subscription at:
www.theclinics.com

PREFACE

Antiplatelet and Anticoagulation Therapy in Percutaneous Coronary Intervention

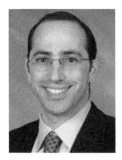 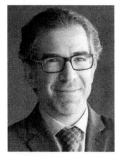

Dominick J. Angiolillo, MD, PhD   **Matthew J. Price, MD**

Editors

Ever-evolving devices and transcatheter techniques define the field of interventional cardiology and its core procedure, percutaneous coronary intervention (PCI). Yet, the success of PCI has been intertwined with advancements in and the optimal use of medical therapies, as adjunctive pharmacology critically influences post-PCI acute and long-term outcomes. The introduction of newer, more effective, and/or safer antiplatelet and anticoagulant agents over the past decade is a boon for patients but has also increased the complexity of the interventionalist's decision making. There is almost a dizzying array of antiplatelet agents that are now commercially available, studied in different populations and carrying different indications, contraindications, side effects, and drug-drug interactions. The clinician must also integrate new data that address the optimal timing to administer these agents and their treatment duration. The global burden of atrial fibrillation is increasing as the population ages, and a growing proportion of patients undergoing PCI are treated with vitamin K–dependent or non–vitamin K–dependent oral anticoagulants, further complicating short- and long-term treatment decisions.

This issue of *Interventional Cardiology Clinics* serves to put forth the current "state-of-the-art" for antiplatelet and anticoagulant therapy in patients undergoing PCI, written by leaders in the field. Dr Stalker and colleagues present the more nuanced picture of thrombosis that has recently emerged, incorporating the coordination of multiple signaling pathways across time and space, which may influence the efficacy and safety of different antithrombotic agents. Drs Angiolillo and Capodanno summarize the clinical data that address the role of pretreatment with oral $P2Y_{12}$ antagonists prior to angiography and in turn question the traditional status quo. Drs Price, Storey, and Tricoci discuss novel antiplatelet agents that are administered intravenously, have off-target effects, and provide inhibition through targets other than the platelet $P2Y_{12}$ receptor. Drs Rollini and Angiolillo lay forth a framework based on clinical and pharmacodynamic studies that can be followed when the clinician feels it is necessary to switch $P2Y_{12}$ antagonists. Dr Lip and Dr Verheught address the conundrum of "triple therapy" with anticoagulants and dual antiplatelet therapy after PCI and for the treatment of ACS, respectively. A large body of randomized clinical trial data that addresses the rationale for antiplatelet therapy beyond stent-related outcomes has recently been published, and Dr Bonaca synthesizes these results and how they should influence the practice of interventional cardiologists. Finally, Drs Cavallari and Sibbing provide an update of the role of precision medicine in the management of antiplatelet therapy in patients with coronary artery disease.

The goal of *Interventional Cardiology Clinics* is to provide the practicing and academic interventional cardiologist a resource that is more in-depth than a review journal but more fluid and

Intervent Cardiol Clin 6 (2017) xi–xii
http://dx.doi.org/10.1016/j.iccl.2016.10.001
2211-7458/17/© 2016 Published by Elsevier Inc

cutting edge than a textbook. We believe that this
issue meets—indeed, exceeds—that goal.

Dominick J. Angiolillo, MD, PhD
University of Florida College of
Medicine-Jacksonville
Division of Cardiology-ACC Building 5th Floor
655 West 8th Street
Jacksonville, FL 32209, USA

Matthew J. Price, MD
Scripps Clinic
9898 Genesee Avenue
Suite AMP-200
La Jolla, CA 92037, USA
E-mail addresses:
dominick.angiolillo@jax.ufl.edu (D.J. Angiolillo)
Price.Matthew@scrippshealth.org (M.J. Price)

Regulation of Platelet Activation and Coagulation and Its Role in Vascular Injury and Arterial Thrombosis

Maurizio Tomaiuolo, PhD, Lawrence F. Brass, MD, PhD, Timothy J. Stalker, PhD*

KEYWORDS

- Platelet activation • Coagulation • Vascular injury • Arterial thrombosis • Antithrombotic agents
- Hemostasis

KEY POINTS

- The platelet response to vascular injury involves multiple cell signaling pathways that are coordinated in both time and space.
- Local conditions within the evolving platelet plug microenvironment result in the development of platelet agonist gradients.
- Antiplatelet therapeutics targeting specific platelet activation pathways have disparate effects on platelet mass architecture depending on the spatiotemporal regulation of the target pathway.

INTRODUCTION

The hemostatic response to vascular injury is a complex process requiring regulated activation of coagulation proteins, platelets, and components of the vascular wall to form a localized hemostatic plug that prevents bleeding. Many aspects of this process have been well-characterized at the molecular and cellular levels in vitro, and the major biochemical pathways responsible for coagulation and platelet activation have been reviewed extensively elsewhere.[1–5]

This review focuses primarily on how the multiple components of the hemostatic system are integrated in time and space to generate an optimal response, including how fluid dynamics and the physical architecture of platelet plugs contribute to the formation of complex biochemical gradients at a site of vascular injury. Although presented in the context of hemostasis, all of the players and processes discussed have an important role in pathologic thrombosis as well, as indicated by the clinical usefulness of multiple therapeutics directed against platelet and coagulation targets as antithrombotics. As we continue to gain a better understanding of how coagulation and various cellular signaling pathways are coordinated in time and space during hemostasis, we are more likely to uncover differences that may exist between hemostasis and thrombosis that could be targeted for safer antithrombotic treatments.

THE HEMOSTATIC RESPONSE TO VASCULAR INJURY

In a fairly simplified view, the hemostatic response can be considered as a sequence of cellular and molecular events delineated into the overlapping phases of initiation, extension and stabilization. Each of these phases involves prohemostatic molecular processes that result

Department of Medicine, Perelman School of Medicine, University of Pennsylvania, 421 Curie Boulevard, Philadelphia, PA, 19104, USA
* Corresponding author.
E-mail address: tstalker@mail.med.upenn.edu

Intervent Cardiol Clin 6 (2017) 1–12
http://dx.doi.org/10.1016/j.iccl.2016.08.001
2211-7458/17/© 2016 Elsevier Inc. All rights reserved.

in the rapid plugging of a hole in the vessel wall to stem bleeding, balanced with antihemostatic processes that limit the response to the site of injury and prevent unwarranted vascular occlusion. The molecular players involved include adhesion molecules and their ligands, platelet surface receptors that initiate intracellular signaling pathways, and the coagulation cascade to generate thrombin and fibrin, among others.

Initiation

Hemostasis is triggered by the exposure of blood to a breach in the vessel wall. During the initiation phase, circulating platelets are recruited to the injury site via adhesive interactions between von Willebrand factor (vWf) bound to collagen fibers in the vessel wall and the platelet glycoprotein Ib (GPIb)–IX-V receptor complex. VWf is normally found circulating in the plasma in an inactive form, is secreted constitutively from endothelial cells as part of the extracellular matrix, and is also secreted from Weibel-Palade bodies of activated endothelial cells.[6,7] After a breach in the vessel wall, circulating vWf is deposited on collagen fibers exposed at the injury site.[8] Unfolding of the protein as a result of shear forces exposes binding sites for platelet surface GPIb to rapidly recruit platelets from the circulation.[6,7,9] Because the vWf–GPIb complex interaction is relatively weak, additional adhesive interactions mediated by integrin family adhesion molecules on the platelet surface are also required for firm platelet attachment at the site of injury. These include $\alpha_2\beta_1$ integrin binding to collagen and $\alpha_{IIb}\beta_3$ binding to vWf and other ligands. For platelet integrins to bind their ligands, they must undergo a conformational change from a resting to active state that requires platelet activation. Platelet activation during the initiation phase is likely mediated via multiple platelet signaling pathways, including activation of the GPVI collagen receptor, activation of platelet ATP and ADP receptors via release of these molecules from damaged cells and by signaling downstream of the GPIb–IX-V complex. In addition, escaping blood at the site of injury encounters tissue factor expressed by cells in the vessel wall and extravascular tissue initiating the generation of thrombin, which is a potent platelet activator.

Extension

After initial platelet adhesion and activation, additional platelets are recruited from the circulation to form a platelet aggregate via platelet–platelet cohesion during the extension phase. This cohesion is mediated primarily by binding of the plasma protein fibrinogen to $\alpha_{IIb}\beta_3$ integrin (aka GPIIbIIIa). Each fibrinogen molecule has 2 $\alpha_{IIb}\beta_3$ binding sites and can therefore mediate platelet–platelet interactions by binding to receptors on 2 adjacent platelets. Platelet recruitment and $\alpha_{IIb}\beta_3$–mediated cohesion require platelet activation by ADP released from platelet dense granules and thromboxane A_2 (TxA_2) generated by platelets already adherent at the site of injury. Thrombin activity also continues to contribute to platelet activation. The importance of $\alpha_{IIb}\beta_3$ in mediating platelet aggregation is demonstrated by the lack of aggregation of platelets from Glanzmann's thrombasthenia patients, which results in a bleeding diathesis. Inhibition of platelet aggregation using $\alpha_{IIb}\beta_3$ antagonists is effective to prevent thrombosis in the setting of percutaneous coronary intervention.[10,11]

Stabilization

Once formed, the nascent hemostatic plug must condense and become firmly anchored at the injury site to resist the force of flowing blood and prevent rebleeding. In addition to activating platelets, thrombin converts fibrinogen to fibrin, forming a network of fibrin fibers that helps to stabilize the platelet plug. Stabilization is also facilitated by consolidation of the platelet mass via actin-myosin–mediated platelet retraction. Platelet activation is reinforced by positive feedback from soluble agonists (thrombin, ADP, TxA_2), as well as contact-dependent signaling pathways that are initiated once platelets come in close proximity to one another such that receptor/ligand pairs on adjacent platelets become engaged. Again, $\alpha_{IIb}\beta_3$ integrin has an important role in this stage, now acting as a signaling molecule regulating platelet retractile processes.[12]

An Updated Model of Hierarchical Hemostatic Plug Architecture

This description of the hemostatic response provides a general sequence of events. It is consistent with, and in large part derived from, clinical experience regarding the importance of the various molecular players involved as defined by bleeding diatheses that result from either genetic or acquired deficiencies of specific molecular components. However, recent studies examining hemostasis and thrombosis in vivo show that this model is overly simplistic. Rather than a mass of uniformly activated platelets contained in a fibrin meshwork, hemostatic plugs formed in vivo develop a regional architecture where not all platelets are activated in the same way, and fibrin is distinctly localized (Fig. 1). Platelets in different regions are morphologically as well as molecularly distinct, reflecting differences in activation state. The architecture of a hemostatic plug has been described as consisting of a core of highly activated, densely packed, degranulated platelets overlaid by a shell of less activated, loosely associated platelets (Fig. 2A). This description is derived primarily from intravital imaging studies in the microcirculation,[13] but evidence suggests a similar hierarchical organization of platelet activation in large vessels as well. The mechanisms responsible for heterogeneity of platelet

activation include a complex interplay of platelet agonists and the physical microenvironment present within a platelet mass, resulting in the development of gradients of soluble platelet agonists such as thrombin, ADP, and TxA_2 (Fig. 2B). Critical concentrations of these agonists are reached in different regions within the hemostatic plug, which means that individual platelets are exposed to different combinations of agonists that can vary over time as well as space. Importantly, as a direct consequence of the variable contribution of platelet agonists in time and space, therapeutic approaches targeting specific platelet signaling pathways, such as $P2Y_{12}$ ADP receptor antagonists, aspirin, and thrombin inhibitors have distinct effects on hemostatic plug architecture.

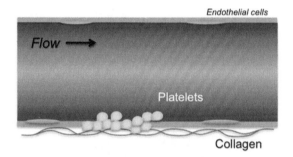

1. Initiation
Initial platelet adhesion at the site of injury is mediated by GPIb-vWF interactions and reinforced by adhesion to collagen.

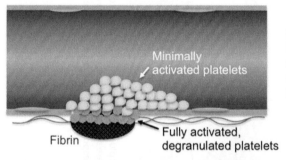

2. Extension
Platelet activation by collagen and thrombin occurs at the base of evolving plug. Additional platelet recruitment in outer shell requires ADP and/or TxA_2.

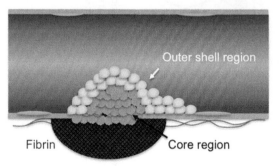

3. Stabilization
Formation of the core requires thrombin mediated platelet activation. Fibrin formation is localized to the core region and extends into the extravascular space.

Fig. 1. An updated model of the hemostatic response to vascular injury. This updated model takes into account the gradient of platelet activation observed emanating from the site of injury. GPIb, glycoprotein Ib; TxA_2, thromboxane A_2; vWF, von Willebrand factor.

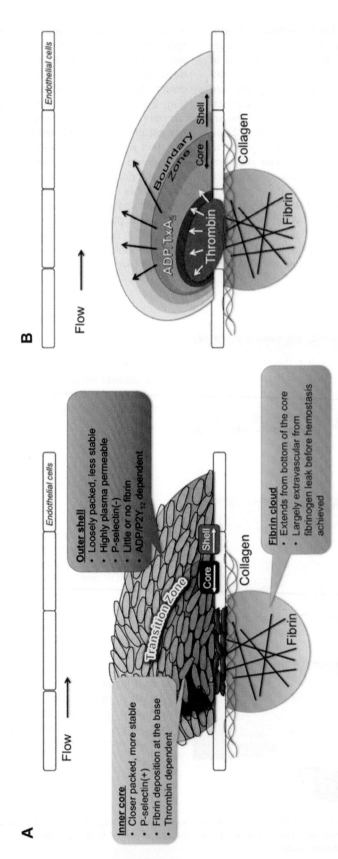

Fig. 2. Regional architecture of a hemostatic plug. (A) The properties of the core and shell regions of a hemostatic plug are described. (B) The core and shell architecture develops as a result of local platelet agonist gradients that are shaped by physical forces within the platelet mass microenvironment. TxA$_2$, thromboxane A$_2$. (From Stalker TJ, Traxler EA, Wu J, et al. Hierarchical organization in the hemostatic response and its relationship to the platelet-signaling network. Blood 2013;121(10):1875–85; with permission.)

REGULATION OF PLATELET ACTIVATION IN VIVO

Once platelets are captured at the damaged vessel wall, the primary drivers for platelet activation are collagen, thrombin, ADP, TxA$_2$ and, to a more limited extent, epinephrine (Fig. 3). With the exception of collagen, each of these agonists signal through 1 or more members of the G-protein–coupled receptor superfamily. In general terms, activation of receptors results in an increase in the cytosolic Ca^{2+} concentration, followed by a series of downstream cell signaling events leading to multiple cellular responses that in aggregate are referred to as platelet activation (see Fig. 3). Although often depicted as such, platelet activation is not a binary process, but rather a graded sequence of events, some of which are reversible and some that are not. Early, reversible components of platelet activation include shape change from a discoid morphology to a variety of other shapes, α$_{IIb}$β$_3$ integrin activation leading to platelet aggregation, and TxA$_2$ formation. Later, irreversible activation events include dense and alpha granule secretion, phosphtidylserine exposure supporting coagulation factor complex assembly, and finally membrane blebbing and microparticle formation. The degree to which platelets are activated at a site of injury depends on the integration of the activating inputs each platelet experiences.

As described and illustrated in Fig. 2, platelet activation within an evolving hemostatic plug or thrombus is heterogeneous, resulting in the development of a platelet mass with a gradient of platelet activation extending from the injury site.[13] The recognition that platelet activation is not uniform during the hemostatic response leads to the question of how such a platelet activation gradient develops and whether there are implications for both the use of existing antiplatelet therapies and the development of new ones. One possible explanation is that platelets with different degrees of activation represent subpopulations of circulating platelets with distinct properties. Although intriguing, there is at present little experimental evidence to support this hypothesis. Instead, the available evidence suggests that heterogeneity of platelet activation reflects nonuniformity in agonist distribution (see Fig. 2B). Herein, we discuss what is known about each of the major platelet agonist signaling pathways with regard to their contribution to the spatiotemporal regulation of platelet activation.

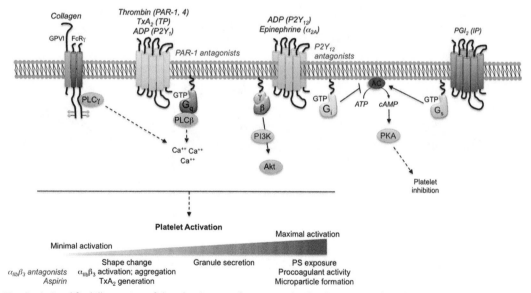

Fig. 3. A simplified illustration of the platelet signaling network. Platelets respond to chemical inputs in their local microenvironment via cell surface receptors that initiate multiple intracellular signaling cascades, ultimately leading to a graded series of platelet activation events, including shape change, integrin activation, aggregation, granule secretion, and procoagulant activity. The degree of activation achieved by individual platelets within a hemostatic plug or thrombus is the net result of the integration of multiple inputs. For the G-protein–coupled receptors (GPCRs) shown, the text in parentheses indicates the receptor(s) name for each agonist indicated. Red text indicates antiplatelet therapeutic targets. TxA$_2$, thromboxane A$_2$.

Thrombin

Thrombin is a key regulator of robust platelet activation in response to vascular injury. It activates platelets via 2 G-protein–coupled receptors on human platelets, PAR-1 and PAR-4. These receptors are coupled to Gq signaling pathways that lead to an increase in platelet cytosolic Ca^{2+} concentration, among other effects. Downstream signaling pathways culminate in activation of $\alpha_{IIb}\beta_3$ integrin and platelet aggregation, platelet granule secretion, generation of TxA_2 and platelet retraction (see Fig. 3).

In mouse models, inhibition of thrombin generation/activity or genetic deletion of the platelet thrombin receptor (PAR-4 on mouse platelets) results in significantly impaired platelet accumulation and a near complete lack of intracellular calcium mobilization[14,15] and P-selectin expression[13,16] as markers of platelet activation (Fig. 4A, B). Thus, thrombin activity is critical for development of a stable core composed of fully activated platelets. However, the localization of thrombin activity in time and space is limited. The prothrombinase complex (factors Va and Xa) that generates thrombin is localized to procoagulant membranes of platelets and endothelial cells at or immediately adjacent to the site of injury, thus limiting the distribution of thrombin within a platelet mass.[17–19] Once generated, thrombin distribution is limited by its ability to diffuse away from the site of generation (discussed in more detail elsewhere in this article) and by plasma-borne inhibitors that either directly inhibit its activity (eg, antithrombin) or generation (eg, tissue factor pathway inhibitor and activated protein C). This combination of factors limits thrombin activity to the core region of the hemostatic plug as demonstrated by studies using a fluorogenic thrombin sensor bound to the surface of platelets[20] and studies showing the localization of fibrin formation restricted to the core and extravascular space.[13,16,21]

Adenosine Diphosphate

ADP is released from damaged cells at the site of injury as well as from dense granules of activated platelets. It acts on 2 platelet receptors, $P2Y_1$ and $P2Y_{12}$, to reinforce platelet activation in a paracrine or autocrine fashion (see

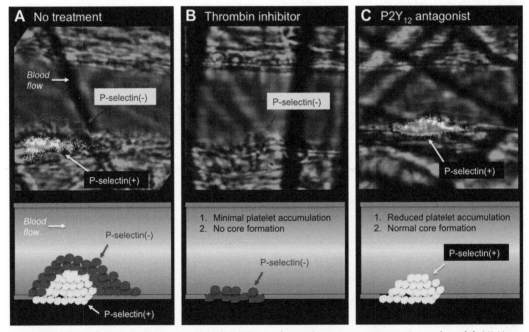

Fig. 4. The effect of antithrombotic agents on hemostatic plug architecture in an experimental model. (A) Hemostatic plug formation in the mouse cremaster microcirculation is characterized by formation of a core of P-selectin–positive platelets overlaid by a shell of P-selectin–negative platelets. (B) In the presence of the thrombin inhibitor hirudin, platelet accumulation is significantly attenuated and none of the adherent platelets become P-selectin positive. (C) In contrast, a $P2Y_{12}$ antagonist results in a decrease in platelet accumulation in the outer shell region with no effect on full platelet activation in the core region. (Data from Stalker TJ, Traxler EA, Wu J, et al. Hierarchical organization in the hemostatic response and its relationship to the platelet-signaling network. Blood 2013;121(10):1875–85.)

Fig. 2).[22–27] P2Y$_1$ is coupled to a Gq signaling pathway, although activation of Gq signaling by ADP is relatively weak compared with Gq signaling downstream of thrombin receptors, for example, P2Y$_{12}$ is coupled to a Gi signaling pathway.[28,29] Gi signaling results in inhibition of adenylyl cyclase and a decrease in cyclic AMP levels in platelets. Cyclic AMP is an important inhibitor of platelet activation, normally acting to keep platelets in a quiescent state in the circulation via stimulation of adenylyl cyclase as a result of prostacyclin receptor activation. One effect of P2Y$_{12}$ signaling, therefore, is to turn off this inhibitory pathway to facilitate platelet activation. P2Y$_{12}$ signaling also contributes to $\alpha_{IIb}\beta_3$ activation and granule secretion. P2Y$_{12}$/Gi signaling is required for platelet activation in response to weak agonist stimulation, such as ADP activation of P2Y$_1$, and it potentiates platelet activation in response to submaximal concentrations of thrombin or TxA$_2$. It is also required for maximal platelet activation downstream of the collagen receptor GPVI.

The importance of P2Y$_{12}$ in platelet activation in vivo is highlighted by the efficacy of P2Y$_{12}$ antagonists in inhibiting platelet activation and protecting against thrombotic events in humans.[30] This role for P2Y$_{12}$ signaling is recapitulated in animal models, where deletion of P2Y$_{12}$[23,31] and the introduction of P2Y$_{12}$ receptor antagonists have been shown to attenuate thrombus formation.[32] In general, these studies have ascribed a role for P2Y$_{12}$ in regulating thrombus stability.[31,33,34] Viewed from the perspective of the spatiotemporal regulation of platelet activation, the effect of P2Y$_{12}$ signaling on thrombus stability is owing to the importance of this signaling pathway in platelet recruitment and retention in the outer layers of a developing platelet plug, a region where thrombin activity rapidly declines. Inhibition of P2Y$_{12}$ activation greatly reduces platelet accumulation in the outer platelet shell (Fig. 4C), whereas a gain-of-function mutation in G$_{i2\alpha}$, the principal G protein coupled to P2Y$_{12}$ receptors, leads to an expansion of the shell.[13] In contrast, a P2Y$_{12}$ antagonist had no effect on robust platelet activation in the thrombus core, where thrombin activity is high (see Fig. 4C).[13] This latter finding may help to explain the relative safety of P2Y$_{12}$ antagonists used clinically.

Thromboxane A$_2$

Like ADP, TxA$_2$ generated and released by activated platelets acts to reinforce platelet activation in an autocrine and paracrine fashion. TxA$_2$ is generated via the aspirin sensitive cyclooxygenase-1 pathway in platelets. Upon release, it binds its receptors (TPα and β) on the platelet surface to activate a Gq signaling pathway (see Fig. 3). Like other Gq-coupled receptors, downstream signaling includes an increase in the cytosolic calcium concentration, activation of $\alpha_{IIb}\beta_3$, and granule release.[29]

The importance TxA$_2$ in platelet activation in vivo is shown by a number of large clinical studies demonstrating the efficacy of aspirin treatment in the prevention of platelet-mediated cardiovascular events (ie, myocardial infarction and stroke).[35] Thrombus formation is also attenuated in TP-deficient mice.[36] The spatiotemporal distribution of TxA$_2$ within a growing hemostatic plug is not yet well-defined. As a highly diffusible molecule, its localization will primarily be determined by its source (activated platelets) and its rapid metabolism in plasma to inactive metabolites. Initial studies indicate that, like ADP, TxA$_2$ contributes primarily to platelet recruitment and retention in the outer shell region of the hemostatic plug (Stalker et al, unpublished observation, 2016).

Collagen/von Willebrand factor

Collagen is a potent platelet agonist. Unlike most soluble platelet agonists, the collagen receptor GPVI is not a G-protein–coupled receptor, but instead belongs to the family of immune-type signaling receptors. GPVI is coupled to the Fc receptor gamma chain, which acts as the signaling component of the collagen receptor complex. Collagen binding to GPVI initiates a signaling cascade similar to Gq signaling in that it results in an increase in cytosolic Ca^{2+} concentration and subsequent downstream platelet activation events (see Fig. 3). In vitro, collagen-mediated platelet activation is highly dependent on secondary signaling by ADP and TxA$_2$.

In contrast with soluble platelet agonists, collagen is an insoluble component of the vessel wall and extravascular tissue. As such, its direct contribution to platelet signaling via activation of the collagen receptor GPVI is restricted to platelets in contact with the damaged vessel wall and those that escape into the extravascular compartment. The contribution of GPVI signaling in experimental models is therefore highly dependent on the mechanism and extent of injury, as well as the amount of thrombin generated.[37] This likely explains varying reports of GPVI being a critical regulator of platelet accumulation and activation in some settings, yet completely dispensable in others.[37–40] Thus, although collagen is clearly a potent activator of platelets in vitro, its contribution to hemostasis and thrombosis in vivo is likely much more context dependent than other platelet agonists, such as thrombin, ADP, and TxA$_2$.

The contribution of signaling from the GPIb–V–IX complex (the platelet vWf receptor) to platelet activation in vivo remains unclear. In vitro studies have suggested that GPIb–V-IX may act as a mechanosensor, including the demonstration of platelet calcium transients after GPIb complex engagement under flow conditions in vitro.[41,42] However, these results have not been directly recapitulated in an in vivo system. In fact, vWf mediated signaling seems to be dispensable for platelet activation as measured by cytoplasmic calcium concentration in the mouse cremaster laser injury model.[14] In contrast, a mouse line in which the cytoplasmic tail of GPIb-alpha was truncated showed defective thrombus formation in a FeCl$_3$ injury model.[43]

INFLUENCE OF LOCAL HEMODYNAMICS

The importance of the local hemodynamic conditions on platelet accumulation has been documented using in vivo and in vitro methods. The presence of geometric features that disrupt the local flow pattern, such as stenosis or aneurysms, can exacerbate preexisting conditions for platelet recruitment and activation. For instance, stenotic regions or developing platelet masses restrict the volume of the vessel available to blood flow, and in so doing generate zones of fluid acceleration and deceleration.[44–47] In the deceleration zones, platelet aggregation occurs via vWF/GPIb and $\alpha_{IIb}\beta_3$ integrin-dependent interactions.[44–46] Antiplatelet agents blocking the TxA$_2$ and ADP signaling pathways prevent the shear-dependent aggregation occurring in the deceleration zones, indicating that platelet activation is a necessary component of the deposition process.[44,46,47]

Aneurysms also present flow disturbances and are frequently associated with intramural thrombi.[48] A combination of experimental and computational studies shows that the presence of these thrombi further deteriorate the local conditions of the aneurysm via distinct mechanisms, including local release of degenerative enzymes,[49] flow-induced hypoxia, and changes in wall shear stress distribution.[50,51] All these mechanisms contribute to vessel wall weakening and may explain why the presence of intramural thrombi are associated with aneurysm growth,[52] rupture,[53] and mortality.[54]

Taken together, these studies indicate that flow disturbances affect platelet deposition,

and that platelet deposition in turn causes flow disturbances. This positive feedback can lead to disastrous consequences when platelet accumulation occurs at sites of atherosclerotic plaque formation. Platelet accumulation, however, in all cases discussed is always activation dependent.[45] Some in vitro evidence suggests that under conditions of nonphysiologic shear rates (>20,000 s^{-1}) vWF fibers become tissue plasminogen activator and ADAMTS13 resistant,[55] and can support activation-independent platelet aggregation.[56] This mechanism of platelet aggregation may be particularly problematic when blood moves through left ventricular assist and other artificial devices.

The Intrathrombus Microenvironment Shapes Agonist Distribution

Even as a growing platelet mass disturbs the bulk flow around it causing accelerations and decelerations, the flow conditions inside of the platelet mass are exceedingly calm. Within this calm domain, many chemical reactions occur that result in complex gradients of soluble platelet agonists. Location, mode of release, stability, and ease of movement are all factors that contribute to an agonist specific gradient. The movement of a soluble agonist within the platelet mass can become restricted owing to both agonist-dependent and platelet mass-dependent effects. Agonist-dependent effects include its size, charge, and binding interactions. The platelet mass-dependent effects are determined by the pore space formed between platelets, the size of the pores, and the connectivity and plasma velocity between the pores.

Although each of these factors has a physical meaning the net effect on a solute movement is estimated by measuring 2 multifactorial parameters, namely, permeability and diffusivity. Permeability measures the ability of a porous material to allow the passage of fluids. Diffusivity measures how quickly a solute spreads as a function of temperature and concentration. Studies have used experimental and computational approaches to estimate the permeability and diffusivity values of a platelet mass. Clot permeability, as measured in vitro, is small, has a value close to that of the endothelium (2 x 10^{-18} m^2), and is determined by platelet retraction and fibrin.[57] The small and heterogeneous permeability of a clot translates to a model of hindered or absent flow within the platelet mass microenvironment.[58–61]

When the contribution of flow becomes negligible, diffusion becomes the controlling factor for molecular movement.[57,60,61] In the platelet mass microenvironment, a solute's diffusivity is determined by the ratio of the solute size to the size of the pores. Solutes much smaller than the size of the pores diffuse faster, whereas solutes close to the size of the pores become excluded. Owing to differences in the extent of platelet packing density, diffusivity within the platelet mass is higher in the shell and lower in the core,[60–62] where it may even be absent owing to size exclusion.[13] Thus, the net effect of permeability and diffusivity is reduced and heterogeneous solute transport properties in a platelet mass, with lower transport in the core.[60,63,64]

Understanding how solute transport is regulated is critical to understand the delivery, removal, and depletion of procoagulant and anticoagulant factors within the platelet mass.[65–67] Studies have shown that individual reactions within the coagulation cascade can switch from being reaction limited to transport limited, depending on the local conditions.[68] Limited transport increases the residence time of solutes in the platelet mass, which translates into reduced generation of new thrombin, and at the same time increased biological activity of locally trapped thrombin. Evidence from experimental and theoretic studies show that, as the platelet mass develops, platelets physically cover tissue factor sites, which also leads to reduced thrombin generation.[67,69–71]

Taken together, these observations describe a progression of coordinated events that depend on the tight interaction between the hemodynamic environment and the biological response of platelets: (1) platelets accumulate at an injury site, (2) as the platelet mass grows the transport of soluble agonists is restricted and shifts from being convection to being diffusion dominated, (3) diffusion increases the residence time of larger agonists (eg, thrombin) more so than smaller agonists (eg, ADP), (4) the platelet mass consolidates in response to longer exposure to agonists creating zones that are closed to solute exchange, and (5) hemostasis is achieved.[60,63,64] When this balance is perturbed using mice deficient in platelet retraction, solute transport is increased resulting in fewer platelets becoming maximally activated.[63]

SUMMARY

Extensive research by many investigators over the past several decades has provided a thorough understanding of the major molecular mechanisms responsible for thrombin generation and platelet activation. We are now beginning to understand how the multiple cell signaling and biochemical events involved in the hemostatic response are integrated in time and space to achieve an optimal response to injury, and how perturbations in the regulation of these events cause pathologic thrombosis. Recent findings highlight the importance of the local microenvironment, including hemodynamic and other physical factors, in shaping the biochemical gradients present at a site of injury to elicit specific cellular responses. Finally, the spatiotemporal distribution of thrombin, ADP, and other platelet agonists helps to explain effects of therapeutic approaches that target these specific pathways. By gaining a better understanding of how coagulation and platelet activation are regulated in time and space, we may be able to better delineate differences between hemostasis and pathologic thrombosis, and identify novel targets for safer, effective antithrombotic treatment.

ACKNOWLEDGMENTS

The authors acknowledge research funding from the National Heart, Lung, and Blood Institute (P01-HL40387 and P01-HL120846) and The Medicines Company (MDCO 9256).

REFERENCES

1. Brass LF, Stalker TJ, Zhu L, et al. Signal transduction during initiation, extension and perpetuation of platelet plug formation. In: Michelson AD, editor. Platelets. 2nd edition. New York: Academic Press; 2006. p. 367–98.
2. Stalker TJ, Newman DK, Ma P, et al. Platelet signaling. Handb Exp Pharmacol 2012;(210):59–85.
3. Versteeg HH, Heemskerk JW, Levi M, et al. New fundamentals in hemostasis. Physiol Rev 2013; 93(1):327–58.
4. Mintz KP, Mann KG. Detection of procollagen biosynthesis using peptide-specific antibodies. Matrix 1990;10(3):186–99.
5. Mann KG, Jenny RJ, Krishnaswamy S. Cofactor proteins in the assembly and expression of blood clotting enzyme complexes. Annu Rev Biochem 1988; 57:915–56.
6. Ruggeri ZM. The role of von Willebrand factor in thrombus formation. Thromb Res 2007;120(Suppl 1):S5–9.
7. Ruggeri ZM, Mendolicchio GL. Adhesion mechanisms in platelet function. Circ Res 2007;100(12): 1673–85.
8. Rand JH, Glanville RW, Wu XX, et al. The significance of subendothelial von Willebrand factor. Thromb Haemost 1997;78(1):445–50.

9. Savage B, Saldivar E, Ruggeri ZM. Initiation of platelet adhesion by arrest onto fibrinogen or translocation on von Willebrand factor. Cell 1996; 84(2):289–97.

10. Use of a monoclonal antibody directed against the platelet glycoprotein IIb/IIIa receptor in high-risk coronary angioplasty. The EPIC Investigation. N Engl J Med 1994;330(14):956–61.

11. EPILOG Investigators. Platelet glycoprotein IIb/IIIa receptor blockade and low-dose heparin during percutaneous coronary revascularization. N Engl J Med 1997;336(24):1689–96.

12. Law DA, DeGuzman FR, Heiser P, et al. Integrin cytoplasmic tyrosine motif is required for outside-in alphaIIbbeta3 signalling and platelet function. Nature 1999;401(6755):808–11.

13. Stalker TJ, Traxler EA, Wu J, et al. Hierarchical organization in the hemostatic response and its relationship to the platelet-signaling network. Blood 2013;121(10):1875–85.

14. Dubois C, Panicot-Dubois L, Gainor JF, et al. Thrombin-initiated platelet activation in vivo is vWF independent during thrombus formation in a laser injury model. J Clin Invest 2007;117(4):953–60.

15. van Gestel MA, Reitsma S, Slaaf DW, et al. Both ADP and thrombin regulate arteriolar thrombus stabilization and embolization, but are not involved in initial hemostasis as induced by micropuncture. Microcirculation 2007;14(3):193–205.

16. Vandendries ER, Hamilton JR, Coughlin SR, et al. Par4 is required for platelet thrombus propagation but not fibrin generation in a mouse model of thrombosis. Proc Natl Acad Sci U S A 2007;104(1):288–92.

17. Hayashi T, Mogami H, Murakami Y, et al. Real-time analysis of platelet aggregation and procoagulant activity during thrombus formation in vivo. Pflugers Arch 2008;456(6):1239–51.

18. Munnix IC, Kuijpers MJ, Auger J, et al. Segregation of platelet aggregatory and procoagulant microdomains in thrombus formation: regulation by transient integrin activation. Arterioscler Thromb Vasc Biol 2007;27(11):2484–90.

19. Ivanciu L, Krishnaswamy S, Camire RM. New insights into the spatiotemporal localization of prothrombinase in vivo. Blood 2014;124(11):1705–14.

20. Welsh JD, Colace TV, Muthard RW, et al. Platelet-targeting sensor reveals thrombin gradients within blood clots forming in microfluidic assays and in mouse. J Thromb Haemost 2012;10(11):2344–53.

21. Falati S, Gross P, Merrill-Skoloff G, et al. Real-time in vivo imaging of platelets, tissue factor and fibrin during arterial thrombus formation in the mouse. Nat Med 2002;8(10):1175–81.

22. Daniel JL, Dangelmaier C, Jin J, et al. Molecular basis for ADP-induced platelet activation. I. Evidence for three distinct ADP receptors on human platelets. J Biol Chem 1998;273(4):2024–9.

23. Foster CJ, Prosser DM, Agans JM, et al. Molecular identification and characterization of the platelet ADP receptor targeted by thienopyridine antithrombotic drugs. J Clin Invest 2001;107(12):1591–8.

24. Hollopeter G, Jantzen HM, Vincent D, et al. Identification of the platelet ADP receptor targeted by antithrombotic drugs. Nature 2001;409(6817): 202–7.

25. Jin J, Daniel JL, Kunapuli SP. Molecular basis for ADP-induced platelet activation. II. The P2Y1 receptor mediates ADP-induced intracellular calcium mobilization and shape change in platelets. J Biol Chem 1998;273(4):2030–4.

26. Jin J, Kunapuli SP. Coactivation of two different G protein-coupled receptors is essential for ADP-induced platelet aggregation. Proc Natl Acad Sci U S A 1998;95(14):8070–4.

27. Zhang FL, Luo L, Gustafson E, et al. ADP is the cognate ligand for the orphan G protein-coupled receptor SP1999. J Biol Chem 2001;276(11):8608–15.

28. Yang J, Wu J, Jiang H, et al. Signaling through Gi family members in platelets. Redundancy and specificity in the regulation of adenylyl cyclase and other effectors. J Biol Chem 2002;277(48):46035–42.

29. Brass LF, Newman DK, Wannemacher KM, et al. Signal transduction during platelet plug formation. In: Michelson AD, editor. Platelets. 3rd edition. Boston: Academic Press; 2013. p. 367–98.

30. Cattaneo M. Platelet P2 receptors: old and new targets for antithrombotic drugs. Expert Rev Cardiovasc Ther 2007;5(1):45–55.

31. Andre P, Delaney SM, LaRocca T, et al. P2Y12 regulates platelet adhesion/activation, thrombus growth, and thrombus stability in injured arteries. J Clin Invest 2003;112(3):398–406.

32. Gachet C. The platelet P2 receptors as molecular targets for old and new antiplatelet drugs. Pharmacol Ther 2005;108(2):180–92.

33. Nergiz-Unal R, Cosemans JM, Feijge MA, et al. Stabilizing role of platelet P2Y(12) receptors in shear-dependent thrombus formation on ruptured plaques. PLoS One 2010;5(4):e10130.

34. Stolla M, Stefanini L, Roden RC, et al. The kinetics of alphaIIbbeta3 activation determines the size and stability of thrombi in mice: implications for antiplatelet therapy. Blood 2011;117(3):1005–13.

35. Lauer MS. Clinical practice. Aspirin for primary prevention of coronary events. N Engl J Med 2002; 346(19):1468–74.

36. Thomas DW, Mannon RB, Mannon PJ, et al. Coagulation defects and altered hemodynamic responses in mice lacking receptors for thromboxane A2. J Clin Invest 1998;102(11):1994–2001.

37. Mangin P, Yap CL, Nonne C, et al. Thrombin overcomes the thrombosis defect associated with platelet GPVI/FcRgamma deficiency. Blood 2006; 107(11):4346–53.

38. Dubois C, Panicot-Dubois L, Merrill-Skoloff G, et al. Glycoprotein VI-dependent and -independent pathways of thrombus formation in vivo. Blood 2006;107(10):3902–6.

39. Massberg S, Gawaz M, Gruner S, et al. A crucial role of glycoprotein VI for platelet recruitment to the injured arterial wall in vivo. J Exp Med 2003; 197(1):41–9.

40. Bender M, Hagedorn I, Nieswandt B. Genetic and antibody-induced glycoprotein VI deficiency equally protects mice from mechanically and FeCl(3) -induced thrombosis. J Thromb Haemost 2011;9(7):1423–6.

41. Mazzucato M, Pradella P, Cozzi MR, et al. Sequential cytoplasmic calcium signals in a 2-stage platelet activation process induced by the glycoprotein Ibalpha mechanoreceptor. Blood 2002;100(8):2793–800.

42. Nesbitt WS, Kulkarni S, Giuliano S, et al. Distinct glycoprotein Ib/V/IX and integrin alpha IIbbeta 3-dependent calcium signals cooperatively regulate platelet adhesion under flow. J Biol Chem 2002; 277(4):2965–72.

43. Jain S, Zuka M, Liu J, et al. Platelet glycoprotein Ib alpha supports experimental lung metastasis. Proc Natl Acad Sci U S A 2007;104(21):9024–8.

44. Maxwell MJ, Westein E, Nesbitt WS, et al. Identification of a 2-stage platelet aggregation process mediating shear-dependent thrombus formation. Blood 2007;109(2):566–76.

45. Nesbitt WS, Westein E, Tovar-Lopez FJ, et al. A shear gradient-dependent platelet aggregation mechanism drives thrombus formation. Nat Med 2009;15(6):665–73.

46. Westein E, van der Meer AD, Kuijpers MJ, et al. Atherosclerotic geometries exacerbate pathological thrombus formation poststenosis in a von Willebrand factor-dependent manner. Proc Natl Acad Sci U S A 2013;110(4):1357–62.

47. Jain A, Graveline A, Waterhouse A, et al. A shear gradient-activated microfluidic device for automated monitoring of whole blood haemostasis and platelet function. Nat Commun 2016;7:10176.

48. Harter LP, Gross BH, Callen PW, et al. Ultrasonic evaluation of abdominal aortic thrombus. J Ultrasound Med 1982;1(8):315–8.

49. Fontaine V, Jacob MP, Houard X, et al. Involvement of the mural thrombus as a site of protease release and activation in human aortic aneurysms. Am J Pathol 2002;161(5):1701–10.

50. Vorp DA, Lee PC, Wang DH, et al. Association of intraluminal thrombus in abdominal aortic aneurysm with local hypoxia and wall weakening. J Vasc Surg 2001;34(2):291–9.

51. Wang DH, Makaroun MS, Webster MW, et al. Effect of intraluminal thrombus on wall stress in patient-specific models of abdominal aortic aneurysm. J Vasc Surg 2002;36(3):598–604.

52. Wolf YG, Thomas WS, Brennan FJ, et al. Computed tomography scanning findings associated with rapid expansion of abdominal aortic aneurysms. J Vasc Surg 1994;20(4):529–35 [discussion: 535–8].

53. Stenbaek J, Kalin B, Swedenborg J. Growth of thrombus may be a better predictor of rupture than diameter in patients with abdominal aortic aneurysms. Eur J Vasc Endovasc Surg 2000;20(5):466–9.

54. Tsai TT, Evangelista A, Nienaber CA, et al. Partial thrombosis of the false lumen in patients with acute type B aortic dissection. N Engl J Med 2007;357(4): 349–59.

55. Herbig BA, Diamond SL. Pathological von Willebrand factor fibers resist tissue plasminogen activator and ADAMTS13 while promoting the contact pathway and shear-induced platelet activation. J Thromb Haemost 2015;13(9):1699–708.

56. Ruggeri ZM, Orje JN, Habermann R, et al. Activation-independent platelet adhesion and aggregation under elevated shear stress. Blood 2006; 108(6):1903–10.

57. Muthard RW, Diamond SL. Blood clots are rapidly assembled hemodynamic sensors: flow arrest triggers intraluminal thrombus contraction. Arterioscler Thromb Vasc Biol 2012;32(12):2938–45.

58. Kim OV, Xu Z, Rosen ED, et al. Fibrin networks regulate protein transport during thrombus development. PLoS Comput Biol 2013;9(6):e1003095.

59. Leiderman K, Fogelson AL. Grow with the flow: a spatial-temporal model of platelet deposition and blood coagulation under flow. Math Med Biol 2011;28(1):47–84.

60. Tomaiuolo M, Stalker TJ, Welsh JD, et al. A systems approach to hemostasis: 2. Computational analysis of molecular transport in the thrombus microenvironment. Blood 2014;124(11):1816–23.

61. Voronov RS, Stalker TJ, Brass LF, et al. Simulation of intrathrombus fluid and solute transport using in vivo clot structures with single platelet resolution. Ann Biomed Eng 2013;41(6):1297–307.

62. Leiderman K, Fogelson AL. The influence of hindered transport on the development of platelet thrombi under flow. Bull Math Biol 2013;75(8): 1255–83.

63. Stalker TJ, Welsh JD, Tomaiuolo M, et al. A systems approach to hemostasis: 3. Thrombus consolidation regulates intrathrombus solute transport and local thrombin activity. Blood 2014;124(11):1824–31.

64. Welsh JD, Stalker TJ, Voronov R, et al. A systems approach to hemostasis: 1. The interdependence of thrombus architecture and agonist movements in the gaps between platelets. Blood 2014; 124(11):1808–15.

65. Fogelson AL, Tania N. Coagulation under flow: the influence of flow-mediated transport on the initiation and inhibition of coagulation. Pathophysiol Haemost Thromb 2005;34(2–3):91–108.

66. Hathcock JJ, Nemerson Y. Platelet deposition inhibits tissue factor activity: in vitro clots are impermeable to factor Xa. Blood 2004;104(1):123–7.

67. Neeves KB, Illing DA, Diamond SL. Thrombin flux and wall shear rate regulate fibrin fiber deposition state during polymerization under flow. Biophys J 2010;98(7):1344–52.

68. Rana K, Neeves KB. Blood flow and mass transfer regulation of coagulation. Blood Rev 2016;30(5): 357–68.

69. Colace TV, Muthard RW, Diamond SL. Thrombus growth and embolism on tissue factor-bearing collagen surfaces under flow: role of thrombin with and without fibrin. Arterioscler Thromb Vasc Biol 2012;32(6):1466–76.

70. Okorie UM, Denney WS, Chatterjee MS, et al. Determination of surface tissue factor thresholds that trigger coagulation at venous and arterial shear rates: amplification of 100 fM circulating tissue factor requires flow. Blood 2008;111(7):3507–13.

71. Kuharsky AL, Fogelson AL. Surface-mediated control of blood coagulation: the role of binding site densities and platelet deposition. Biophys J 2001; 80(3):1050–74.

Pretreatment with Antiplatelet Agents in the Setting of Percutaneous Coronary Intervention
When and Which Drugs?

Davide Capodanno, MD, PhD[a],*,
Dominick J. Angiolillo, MD, PhD[b]

KEYWORDS

- Pretreatment • Preloading • Clopidogrel • Prasugrel • Ticagrelor • Cangrelor

KEY POINTS

- The evidence supporting pretreatment with clopidogrel in patients with stable coronary artery disease intended for percutaneous coronary intervention is weak.
- Patients with non–ST-segment–elevation acute coronary syndromes should not receive prasugrel before the coronary anatomy has been defined.
- European Society of Cardiology guidelines recommend that patients with ST-segment–elevation myocardial infarction should receive a $P2Y_{12}$ inhibitor as early as possible after the initial diagnosis.
- American College of Cardiology/American Heart Association guidelines recommend that patients with ST-segment–elevation myocardial infarction receive a $P2Y_{12}$ as early as possible or at the time of primary percutaneous coronary intervention.
- Intravenous cangrelor is a new treatment option for patients who have not been orally pretreated with $P2Y_{12}$ inhibitors.

INTRODUCTION

In patients undergoing coronary angiography with intent to undergo percutaneous coronary intervention (PCI), the term *pretreatment* typically refers to a variety of modalities of antiplatelet inhibitor(s) intake, including common clinical scenarios in which the drug (ie, aspirin, a $P2Y_{12}$ inhibitor, or a glycoprotein IIb/IIIa inhibitor [GPI]) is given before definition of the coronary anatomy (ie, in the ambulance, in the emergency department, in a peripheral hospital without a catheter laboratory, or in a primary hospital with a catheter laboratory before coronary angiography and/or PCI).[1]

Disclosure: Dr D. Capodanno reports receiving payments as an individual for consulting fee or honorarium from Eli Lilly, Daiichi-Sankyo, The Medicines Company, AstraZeneca, Bayer, Abbott Vascular. Dr D.J. Angiolillo reports receiving payments as an individual for: (a) Consulting fee or honorarium from Sanofi, Eli Lilly, Daiichi-Sankyo, The Medicines Company, AstraZeneca, Merck, Abbott Vascular and PLx Pharma; (b) Participation in review activities from CeloNova, Johnson & Johnson, and St. Jude Medical. Institutional payments for grants from GlaxoSmithKline, Eli Lilly, Daiichi-Sankyo, The Medicines Company, AstraZeneca, Janssen Pharmaceuticals, Osprey Medical Inc, Novartis, CSL Behring and Gilead.
[a] Cardio-Thoracic-Vascular Department, Ferrarotto Hospital, University of Catania, Via Citelli, 6, Catania 95124, Italy; [b] Division of Cardiology, Department of Medicine, University of Florida College of Medicine-Jacksonville, 655 West 8th Street, Jacksonville, FL 32209, USA
* Corresponding author.
E-mail address: dcapodanno@gmail.com

Early administration of antiplatelet drugs has advantages and disadvantages (Fig. 1). Platelet inhibition may be crucial to prevent the occurrence of thrombotic complications during and after PCI. However, stacking antithrombotic drugs—as frequently occurs in the setting of acute coronary syndromes (ACS)—may increase the risk of bleeding, which may be potentially fatal. This risk proves unnecessary and possibly unacceptable when patients initially thought to have coronary artery disease finally receive an alternative diagnosis or when they require prompt coronary artery bypass grafting. As such, pretreatment with antiplatelet agents is a frequent and controversial dilemma in clinical practice.[2–4] This article summarizes the current evidence on pretreatment with P2Y$_{12}$ inhibitors in the setting of PCI. Pharmacologic characteristics of these drugs are summarized in Table 1. A description of issues related to pretreatment with other established antiplatelet drugs (ie, aspirin) or drugs whose routine use upstream is discouraged (GPIs[5]) goes beyond the scope of this article.

PRETREATMENT WITH P2Y$_{12}$ INHIBITORS IN PATIENTS WITH STABLE CORONARY INTERVENTION UNDERGOING PERCUTANEOUS CORONARY INTERVENTION

Should Clopidogrel Be Given Before Percutaneous Coronary Intervention?

The CREDO (Clopidogrel for the Reduction of Events During Observation) trial failed to show a significant 28-day benefit of preloading with a 300-mg dose of clopidogrel compared with no preloading. However, in the same trial, there was a borderline significant 39% relative benefit in patients who received clopidogrel loading at least 6 hours before PCI, with no interaction depending on the clinical presentation (ACS vs no ACS).[6] On the other hand, a post-hoc analysis of CREDO found that it takes more than 15 days for the benefit of clopidogrel 300-mg loading to become clinically superior to that of placebo.[6,7] Although these findings seem to support the practice of early clopidogrel use before PCI, CREDO cannot be considered a true pretreatment study because of inclusion of patients mostly selected after coronary angiography

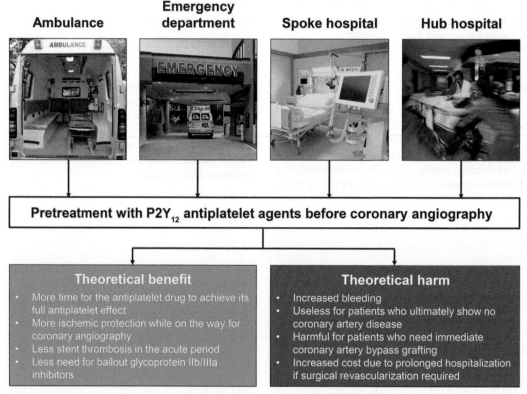

Ambulance   **Emergency department**   **Spoke hospital**   **Hub hospital**

Pretreatment with P2Y$_{12}$ antiplatelet agents before coronary angiography

Theoretical benefit	Theoretical harm
• More time for the antiplatelet drug to achieve its full antiplatelet effect • More ischemic protection while on the way for coronary angiography • Less stent thrombosis in the acute period • Less need for bailout glycoprotein IIb/IIIa inhibitors	• Increased bleeding • Useless for patients who ultimately show no coronary artery disease • Harmful for patients who need immediate coronary artery bypass grafting • Increased cost due to prolonged hospitalization if surgical revascularization required

Fig. 1. Potential advantages and disadvantages of pretreatment with P2Y$_{12}$ inhibitors.

Table 1
Pharmacologic characteristics of P2Y$_{12}$ inhibitors

	Clopidogrel	Prasugrel	Ticagrelor	Cangrelor
Structure				
Group	Thienopyridine	Thienopyridine	CPTP	ATP analog
Receptor blockade	Irreversible	Irreversible	Reversible	Reversible
Route of administration	Oral	Oral	Oral	Intravenous
Frequency of administration	Once a day	Once a day	Twice a day	Bolus + infusion
Prodrug	Yes	Yes	No[a]	No
% of active metabolite	15%	85%	90%–100%	100%
Onset of action	2–8 h	30 min–4 h[b]	30 min–4 h[b]	2 min
Offset of action	7–10 d	7–10 d	3–5 d	~60 min
CYP-targeted drugs interactions	CYP2C19	No	CYP3A4-5	No
Indications	ACS and PCI	ACS-PCI	ACS (any)	PCI

Abbreviations: ATP, Adenosine triphosphate; CPTP, cyclopentyl triazolo-pyrimidine.
[a] Although most ticagrelor-mediated antiplatelet effects are direct, approximately 30–40% are attributed to an active metabolite (AR-C124910XX).
[b] Depending on the clinical setting.

rather than before. In addition, CREDO did not compare preloading before PCI with loading at the time of PCI, the only design that can investigate meaningfully the effect of pretreatment.

Later pharmacodynamic studies supported the current practice shift into administering a 600-mg loading dose of clopidogrel instead of 300 mg, owing to evidence of faster platelet inhibition with the higher dose,[8,9] whereas administration of greater than 600 mg loading doses never proved to add significant additional benefits, possibly as the consequence of limited drug absorption.[10,11] A large-scale randomized clinical trial has consolidated on a clinical ground the benefit of doubling the loading dose of clopidogrel from 300 to 600 mg in patients with ACS,[12,13] renewing the interest in understanding the impact of pretreatment with a higher loading dose than that used in CREDO. The ISAR-REACT (Intracoronary Stenting and Antithrombotic Regimen-Rapid Early Action for Coronary Treatment) trial, which also was not a formal study of pretreatment versus no pretreatment, found no incremental benefit at 30 days for durations of pretreatment greater than 2 hours in patients undergoing PCI.[14] By contrast, the PRAGUE-8 trial—a true pretreatment study—did not find any difference in the combined ischemic endpoint between pretreatment with prehospital 600-mg clopidogrel compared with in-laboratory treatment and resulted in a higher risk of minor bleeding with pretreatment.[15] A meta-analysis of 1636 elective PCI patients from randomized, clinical trials and 5919 patients from observational analyses of randomized, clinical trials, conducted by the ACTION (Academic Research Organization) group, concluded that pretreatment with clopidogrel does not result in a significant mortality reduction compared with no pretreatment.[16] Although significant decreases in major coronary events were found with pretreatment when pooling observational studies, this was not confirmed when pooling randomized, clinical trials.

Overall, these findings suggest that pretreatment might have a role only if a 300-mg loading dose of clopidogrel is given, but this practice has been abandoned. Although using a 600-mg loading dose has become the standard of care, the need for pretreatment when using this dose is not supported by randomized data.

What About Prasugrel, Ticagrelor, and Cangrelor?

Prasugrel and ticagrelor are not approved for patients with stable coronary artery disease undergoing PCI; therefore, the impact of pretreatment with these drugs remains to be determined. Cangrelor is a novel adenosine triphosphate analogue administered intravenously and acting on the $P2Y_{12}$ receptor, which was recently approved for marketing in Europe and the United States. After 2 trials of cangrelor were terminated prematurely for futility,[17,18] the CHAMPION-PHOENIX (Cangrelor vs Standard Therapy to Achieve Optimal Management of Platelet Inhibition) trial found cangrelor to be superior to clopidogrel, 300 to 600 mg, in $P2Y_{12}$ inhibitor–naïve patients undergoing urgent or elective PCI.[19] The study was intended to be a large, generalizable trial across the spectrum of coronary artery disease and included patients who required PCI for stable angina, non–ST-segment–elevation acute coronary syndromes (NSTE-ACS), or ST-segment–elevation myocardial infarction (STEMI) and who did not receive pretreatment with platelet inhibitors. The primary efficacy endpoint was decreased significantly by 22%, and there was no increase in severe bleeding. There was a significant reduction in stent thrombosis within 48 hours from PCI with cangrelor. The benefit from cangrelor with respect to the primary endpoint was consistent across multiple prespecified subgroups. The US Food and Drug Administration approved cangrelor for patients who have not been treated with a $P2Y_{12}$ platelet inhibitor and are not being given a GPI. The European Medical Agency recommends cangrelor for patients undergoing PCI "who have not received an oral $P2Y_{12}$ inhibitor prior to the PCI procedure and in whom oral therapy with $P2Y_{12}$ inhibitors is not feasible or desirable." Because CHAMPION-PHOENIX was not a trial of pretreatment, the comparative effectiveness and safety of in-laboratory cangrelor versus pretreatment with clopidogrel remains undefined.[20]

What Do the Guidelines Say?

Although both the American College of Cardiology/American Heart Association (ACC/AHA) and European Society of Cardiology (ESC) guidelines are historically aligned in recommending aspirin before elective stenting,[21,22] there are differences over time regarding the timing of $P2Y_{12}$ inhibition with clopidogrel. In fact, the 2011 ACC/AHA guidelines for PCI regarded pretreatment as a practice of uncertain utility,[21] whereas the 2013 ESC guidelines for stable coronary artery disease issued a formal recommendation against pretreatment when coronary anatomy is not known (class III).[23] In 2014, the ESC guidelines recommended pretreatment with 600 mg clopidogrel "only after the coronary anatomy is known" and preferably ≥ 2 hours before PCI, whereas pretreatment with clopidogrel may be considered (class IIb) in patients with high probability for significant coronary artery disease and reloading (class IIb) in patients on a maintenance clopidogrel dose.[22] None of these mentioned documents include specific recommendations with respect to prasugrel, ticagrelor, or cangrelor use for patients with stable coronary artery disease undergoing elective PCI.

PRETREATMENT IN PATIENTS WITH NON-ST ELEVATION ACUTE CORONARY SYNDROMES UNDERGOING INVASIVE MANAGEMENT

Should Clopidogrel Be Given Before Coronary Angiography?

The CURE (Clopidogrel in Unstable Angina to Prevent Recurrent Events) trial is frequently conceived by advocates of pretreatment as a reasonable proof of the benefit of early clopidogrel initiation in patients with NSTE-ACS.[24,25] The trial randomly assigned patients who presented within 24 hours from symptoms onset to receive 300 mg of clopidogrel immediately (followed by a daily 75 mg dose) or placebo in addition to aspirin. The primary endpoint, a composite of death from cardiovascular causes, myocardial infarction, or stroke, was significantly reduced at 1 year by clopidogrel at the price of an increase in major but not life-threatening bleeding. The rate of the primary outcome was lower in the clopidogrel group both within 30 days after randomization and between 30 days and the end of the study. Further analyses found that the benefit of clopidogrel was apparent within a few hours from randomization, with the rate of death from cardiovascular causes, nonfatal myocardial infarction, stroke, or refractory or severe ischemia significantly reduced by 24 hours after randomization. In the PCI-CURE substudy, the benefit of combining clopidogrel with aspirin was noted not only after PCI but also before.[25] However, the median time from randomization to PCI was 10 days, which contrasts with the current practice of referring patients with NSTE-ACS to early invasive management. Although another post-hoc analysis of CURE suggested that the benefit of clopidogrel therapy in addition to aspirin was significant irrespective of the timing of PCI,[26] PCI-CURE remains to date the only evidence to support pretreatment with clopidogrel in NSTE-ACS. By contrast, another small clinical trial,[27] 2 observational analyses from randomized clinical trials,[28,29] and a meta-analysis[16] did not find any benefit of clopidogrel pretreatment in these patients. In CREDO, 67% of patients

had unstable angina or recent myocardial infarction and—as mentioned before—there was no interaction between the null effect of clopidogrel preloading and clinical presentation.[6] Finally, in a nonrandomized study of 1041 patients with NSTE-ACS, pretreatment with clopidogrel (chronic 75-mg clopidogrel therapy, a 300-mg loading dose $\geq$12 hours, or a 600-mg loading dose $\geq$2 hours before angiography) was associated with similar adjusted short-term ischemic and bleeding outcomes compared with in-laboratory 600-mg clopidogrel loading (ie, <2 hours before or after PCI).[30] Collectively, the evidence supporting pretreatment with clopidogrel non-ST elevation ACS is scarce.

What About Prasugrel, Ticagrelor, and Cangrelor?

Pretreatment was not allowed in non-ST elevation ACS patients enrolled in the TRITON-TIMI 38 (Trial to Assess Improvement in Therapeutic Outcomes by Optimizing Platelet Inhibition With Prasugrel—Thrombolysis in Myocardial Infarction 38) trial, the landmark trial of prasugrel in invasively managed ACS.[31] This trial set the rationale for designing ACCOAST (A Comparison of Prasugrel at the Time of Percutaneous Coronary Intervention or as Pretreatment at the Time of Diagnosis in Patients With Non–ST Segment– Elevation Myocardial Infarction), a trial of pretreatment with a halved dose of prasugrel (30 mg) followed by a second 30-mg dose at the time of PCI, which was compared with standard of care (ie, 60-mg loading dose at the time of PCI once the coronary anatomy has been defined).[32] In ACCOAST, pretreatment did not reduce significantly the primary ischemic endpoint and increased by 90% the risk of major bleeding, including non–coronary artery bypass grafting–related major bleeding and life-threatening bleeding. There was no evidence of heterogeneity in these results across study subgroups, including patients undergoing PCI.[33] Notably, in ACCOAST, the median time to coronary angiography was only 4 hours, but when patients were stratified into quartiles of time from the first loading dose to coronary angiography, there was again no evidence of a significant interaction effect with the primary endpoint, even when patients with longer (>14 hours) duration of pretreatment were considered (Eli Lilly/Daiichi Sankyo, unpublished data, 2013). A new meta-analysis from the AC-TION group, incorporating data from ACCOAST, failed to show a significant reduction in mortality with pretreatment in NSTE-ACS, and concluded that patients who are pretreated experience significantly more major bleeding.[34] There was a reduction in major adverse cardiovascular events in the analysis of all patients, driven by the data from CURE and CREDO, but the difference was not significant for the cohort of patients undergoing PCI.[34]

Pretreatment with ticagrelor has never been formally tested in NSTE-ACS. In contrast to TRITON, the protocol of PLATO (Study of Platelet Inhibition and Patient Outcomes)—the landmark study of ticagrelor in patients with ACS—allowed patients to be given the study drug before coronary angiography, and patients pretreated with clopidogrel before randomization were not excluded.[35] There was no interaction between pretreatment and the primary outcomes of the trial, which led to the common opinion that pretreatment with ticagrelor is feasible and safe in patients with NSTE-ACS. In reality, because PLATO was not a trial of pretreatment, the evidence supporting this strategy remains insufficient. Given the lack of data on ticagrelor use in $P2Y_{12}$ receptor inhibitor–naïve patients with unstable angina (troponin-negative NSTE-ACS) undergoing ad-hoc PCI, a recent study was conducted in this setting that proved in-laboratory ticagrelor to be associated with more prompt and potent platelet inhibition compared with clopidogrel.[36]

The availability of a fast-acting intravenous $P2Y_{12}$ inhibitor like cangrelor is intuitively attractive for patients undergoing ad-hoc PCI in the setting of NSTE-ACS (about 25% of those randomized in CHAMPION-PHOENIX) and in other potential candidates.[37,38] However, as observed earlier in this article, CHAMPION-PHOENIX was not a trial of pretreatment, and the comparative effectiveness and safety of in-laboratory cangrelor versus pretreatment with oral $P2Y_{12}$ inhibitors (particularly prasugrel or ticagrelor), or pretreatment with cangrelor itself, remains to be elucidated.[20]

What Do the Guidelines Say?

For many years, the ESC guidelines for NSTE-ACS recommended early initiation of $P2Y_{12}$ inhibitors. This position was revised in the 2015 update, with the ESC writing committee deciding to avoid any recommendation favoring or disfavoring the practice of pretreatment with clopidogrel or ticagrelor because of lack of dedicated studies with these drugs.[39] In contrast, the recommendation for pretreatment with prasugrel is class III (ie, harm). Based on the same guidelines, intravenous cangrelor may now be considered in patients undergoing PCI who are $P2Y_{12}$ inhibitor naïve (class IIb). The ACC/AHA guidelines currently do not discuss in detail the issue of pretreatment in NSTE-ACS, and the only relevant (and neutral) recommendation is to administer a loading dose of a $P2Y_{12}$ inhibitor before PCI with stenting.[40]

PRETREATMENT IN PATIENTS WITH ST ELEVATION MYOCARDIAL INFARCTION UNDERGOING PRIMARY PERCUTANEOUS CORONARY INTERVENTION

Should $P2Y_{12}$ Inhibitors Be Given as Soon as Possible?

Few randomized studies, with small sample sizes and surrogate primary endpoints, have explored the issue of pretreatment with antiplatelet agents in the setting of STEMI.[41–43] The largest of these studies was ATLANTIC (Administration of Ticagrelor in the Cath Lab or in the Ambulance for New ST Elevation Myocardial Infarction to Open the Coronary Artery), which randomly assigned 1862 patients with ongoing STEMI and symptom onset within 6 hours to prehospital versus in-hospital treatment with ticagrelor. ATLANTIC did not show a benefit of ticagrelor pretreatment with respect to 2 coprimary surrogate endpoints (ie, proportion of patients who did not have a 70% or greater resolution of ST-segment elevation before PCI and proportion of patients who did not have a thrombolysis in myocardial infarction flow grade 3 in the infarct-related artery at initial angiography).[43] When interpreting the negative results of ATLANTIC, one should consider the short median time between the 2 loading doses in the pretreatment and no pretreatment groups (about 30 minutes), which was likely insufficient to allow for a significant separation in platelet inhibition between the 2 groups at the time of PCI. Indeed, some benefits of ticagrelor pretreatment emerged at later time points.[43,44] Moreover, although ATLANTIC did not formally show a benefit of ticagrelor pretreatment with respect to its ischemic coprimary endpoints, a positive finding was the lack of significant bleeding hazard with early initiation of the drug (a concern previously noted with prasugrel in NSTE-ACS patients from ACCOAST). No studies have explored the impact of prasugrel pretreatment in STEMI in the context of a randomized trial. Yet, administration of prasugrel is acceptable in this setting for patients undergoing primary PCI within 12 hours from symptoms, in line with the TRITON-TIMI 38 design, which allowed only for STEMI patients with planned primary PCI to be pretreated.[31,45] With respect to cangrelor, STEMI patients were only about 18% of those randomly assigned in CHAMPION-PHOENIX.[46,47] In the trial, the effect of cangrelor was consistent irrespective of the clinical presentation (for interaction, $P= .98$). As previously noted for NSTE-ACS, how cangrelor compares with the more potent and faster-acting P2Y$_{12}$ receptor inhibitors prasugrel and ticagrelor and the impact of cangrelor pretreatment compared with in-laboratory initiation are unknown.[20]

What Do the Guidelines Say?
The ESC STEMI guidelines, published in 2012, indirectly support antiplatelet pretreatment, stating that "patients undergoing primary PCI should receive a combination of DAPT with aspirin and an adenosine diphosphate receptor blocker, as early as possible before angiography."[48] The 2014 ESC guidelines for myocardial revascularization more recently made this

statement even more explicit, with a class I recommendation for pretreatment with a P2Y$_{12}$ inhibitor "at the time of first medical contact."[22] Similarly, in the ACC/AHA guidelines, pretreatment "as early as possible or at time of primary PCI" is clearly endorsed (class I).[49]

Pretreatment with Antiplatelet Agents in the Setting of Percutaneous Coronary Intervention: When and Which Drugs?
Pretreatment with P2Y$_{12}$ inhibitors is currently an uncertain strategy in all clinical presentations across the spectrum of coronary artery disease (Figs. 2 and 3). In patients undergoing elective PCI, the only randomized trial of pretreatment with active control (PRAGUE-8) was negative. Similarly, the largest randomized

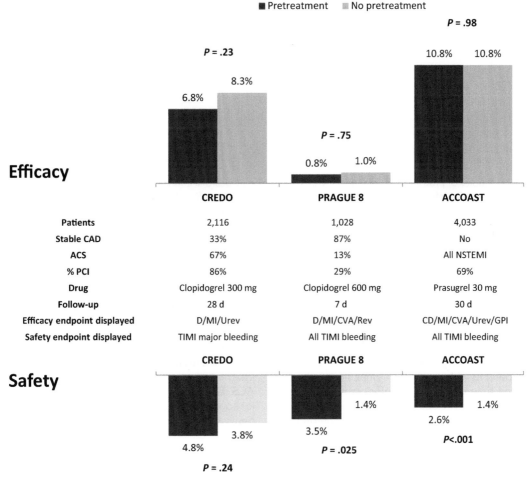

Fig. 2. Studies of pretreatment in patients with stable coronary artery disease and NSTE-ACS. CAD, coronary artery disease; CD, cardiovascular death; CVA, cerebrovascular accidents; D, death; MI, myocardial infarction; NSTEMI, non–ST-segment–elevation myocardial infarction; Rev, revascularization; TIMI, thrombolysis in myocardial infarction; Urev, urgent revascularization. (From Capodanno D, Angiolillo DJ. Pretreatment with antiplatelet drugs in invasively managed patients with coronary artery disease in the contemporary era: review of the evidence and practice guidelines. Circ Cardiovasc Interv 2015;8(3):e002301; with permission.)

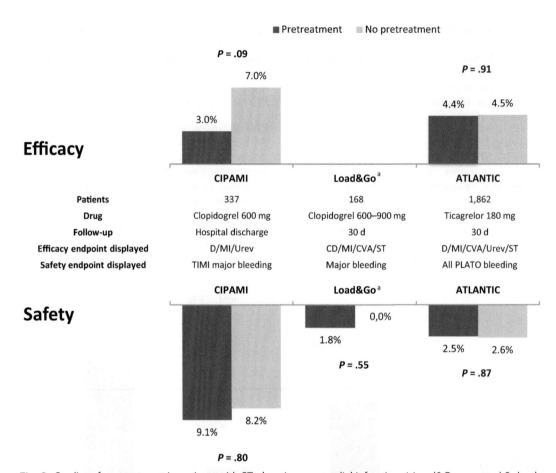

Fig. 3. Studies of pretreatment in patients with ST-elevation myocardial infarction. * Load&Go reported 2 deaths and 1 myocardial infarction in the overall population (P, nonsignificant [NS] for comparison between groups). CD, cardiovascular death; CVA, cerebrovascular accidents; D, death; MI, myocardial infarction; PLATO, study of platelet inhibition and patient outcomes; ST, stent thrombosis; TIMI, thrombolysis in myocardial infarction; Urev, urgent revascularization. (*From* Capodanno D, Angiolillo DJ. Pretreatment with antiplatelet drugs in invasively managed patients with coronary artery disease in the contemporary era: review of the evidence and practice guidelines. Circ Cardiovasc Interv 2015;8(3):e002301; with permission.)

studies conducted in NSTE-ACS (ACCOAST) and STEMI (ATLANTIC) did not support the practice of pretreatment with prasugrel and ticagrelor, respectively. Finally, CHAMPION-PHOENIX introduced cangrelor, a new treatment option for patients with no oral $P2Y_{12}$ inhibitors on board at the time of coronary angiography, but it was compared with clopidogrel initiated at the time or after PCI; hence, no recommendation on pretreatment can be given with this drug.

Pretreatment with Antiplatelet Agents in Current Practice: What Are the Challenges?

A significant proportion of patients with ischemia-producing stable coronary artery disease undergoes ad-hoc PCI after coronary angiography. Delaying PCI to allow for pretreatment with antiplatelet agents is considered unpractical in many

centers (ie, if a simple lesion needs to be treated with 1 stent), and pretreatment is undertaken only for complex angiographic presentations or scheduled PCI in patients whose coronary anatomy is already known. The evolution in thrombotic pharmacotherapy and management strategies for ACS has culminated in more fast-acting antiplatelet agents available than in the past and more patients undergoing early invasive management and ad-hoc PCI. As such, more and more patients undergo coronary angiography when the oral antiplatelet agents have not reached their full inhibitory effect (ie, as the result of delayed absorption in STEMI). Time to coronary angiography is critical to decide whether a benefit can be expected from pretreatment in NSTE-ACS. If the median time to coronary angiography is short (ie, <6–12 hours), there is probably not much to gain from antiplatelet pretreatment, particularly when fast-acting oral agents are used. In such circumstances, defining the coronary anatomy before administering antiplatelet agents allows for personalizing treatment decisions and avoids delays in case urgent cardiac surgery is needed or unnecessary antiplatelet management if no coronary artery disease is found. Conversely, if the median time to coronary angiography is long (ie, >24 hours), considerations on providing early antiplatelet protection may prevail. In STEMI, trials of pretreatment are limited by the low power in detecting differences in clinical endpoints. In aggregate, the data are reassuring in that pretreatment is not associated with significant bleeding risk, which indirectly supports the current guidelines recommendation of administering P2Y$_{12}$ inhibitors at the time of the first medical contact. However, a limitation of pretreatment in STEMI remains the theoretic probability of administering antiplatelet drugs to patients who finally prove to have an alternative diagnosis (ie, aortic dissection).

What Next?

Trials such as ACCOAST and ATLANTIC cannot be considered conclusive on the topic of pretreatment in NSTE-ACS and STEMI, respectively. In fact, they reflect an ideal practice in which the difference in time between coronary angiography and PCI is much shorter than in many real-world settings.[50] Therefore, these results apply only to clinical scenarios in which rapid invasive management is undertaken. In addition, both ACCOAST and ATLANTIC investigated one of the newer oral P2Y$_{12}$ inhibitors, and their results do not apply automatically to other agents in this category. Finally, these studies were underpowered for hard clinical endpoints. Among new trials of pretreatment that will try to add more clarity in the field, DUBIUS (Downstream vs Upstream Strategy for the Administration of P2Y$_{12}$ Receptor Blockers)—a randomized study of ticagrelor upstream versus prasugrel or ticagrelor downstream—is under way in patients with NSTE-ACS (NCT02618837). Another unsolved issue is how cangrelor will fit into local protocol schemes in which oral P2Y$_{12}$ inhibitors are currently used. Based on pharmacodynamic studies, prasugrel and ticagrelor require 4 to 6 hours to achieve an adequate level of platelet inhibition in STEMI, even with the use of high-loading dose regimens.[51–53] Therefore, inadequate platelet inhibition at the time of primary PCI might be one of the contributing factors for the lack of observed effect on pre-PCI reperfusion noted in ATLANTIC. Crushing oral P2Y$_{12}$

receptor inhibitors has represented a strategy to accelerate drug absorption and their platelet inhibitory effects.[54,55] However, this cannot overcome the speed of an intravenous agent.[56] With its fast onset of action and weaning of platelet inhibitory effects at drug discontinuation, cangrelor has many theoretic advantages over oral P2Y$_{12}$ inhibitors, particularly in ACS.[57] In keeping with the design of CHAMPION-PHOENIX, cangrelor is indicated only in patients who have not been pretreated with a P2Y$_{12}$ platelet inhibitor and are not being given a GPI. Therefore, studies that compare different antiplatelet strategies with and without cangrelor are now warranted.

REFERENCES

1. Capodanno D, Angiolillo DJ. Pretreatment with antiplatelet drugs in invasively managed patients with coronary artery disease in the contemporary era: review of the evidence and practice guidelines. Circ Cardiovasc interv 2015;8(3):e002301.
2. Valgimigli M. Pretreatment with P2Y12 inhibitors in non-ST-segment-elevation acute coronary syndrome is clinically justified. Circulation 2014;130(21):1891–903 [discussion: 1903].
3. Collet JP, Silvain J, Bellemain-Appaix A, et al. Pretreatment with P2Y12 inhibitors in non-ST-Segment-elevation acute coronary syndrome: an outdated and harmful strategy. Circulation 2014;130(21):1904–14 [discussion: 14].
4. Capodanno D, Angiolillo DJ. Reviewing the controversy surrounding pre-treatment with P2Y inhibitors in acute coronary syndrome patients. Expert Rev Cardiovasc Ther 2016;14(7):811–20.
5. Muniz-Lozano A, Rollini F, Franchi F, et al. Update on platelet glycoprotein IIb/IIIa inhibitors: recommendations for clinical practice. Ther Adv Cardiovasc Dis 2013;7(4):197–213.
6. Steinhubl SR, Berger PB, Mann JT 3rd, et al. Early and sustained dual oral antiplatelet therapy following percutaneous coronary intervention: a randomized controlled trial. JAMA 2002;288(19): 2411–20.
7. Steinhubl SR, Berger PB, Brennan DM, et al. Optimal timing for the initiation of pre-treatment with 300 mg clopidogrel before percutaneous coronary intervention. J Am Coll Cardiol 2006;47(5): 939–43.
8. Angiolillo DJ, Fernandez-Ortiz A, Bernardo E, et al. High clopidogrel loading dose during coronary stenting: effects on drug response and inter-individual variability. Eur Heart J 2004;25(21): 1903–10.
9. Lotrionte M, Biondi-Zoccai GG, Agostoni P, et al. Meta-analysis appraising high clopidogrel loading

in patients undergoing percutaneous coronary intervention. Am J Cardiol 2007;100(8):1199–206.

10. von Beckerath N, Taubert D, Pogatsa-Murray G, et al. Absorption, metabolization, and antiplatelet effects of 300-, 600-, and 900-mg loading doses of clopidogrel: results of the ISAR-CHOICE (Intracoronary Stenting and Antithrombotic Regimen: choose between 3 high oral doses for immediate clopidogrel Effect) Trial. Circulation 2005;112(19):2946–50.

11. Montalescot G, Sideris G, Meuleman C, et al. A randomized comparison of high clopidogrel loading doses in patients with non-ST-segment elevation acute coronary syndromes: the ALBION (Assessment of the Best Loading Dose of Clopidogrel to Blunt Platelet Activation, Inflammation and Ongoing Necrosis) trial. J Am Coll Cardiol 2006;48(5):931–8.

12. Mehta SR, Bassand JP, Chrolavicius S, et al. Dose comparisons of clopidogrel and aspirin in acute coronary syndromes. N Engl J Med 2010;363(10):930–42.

13. Mehta SR, Tanguay JF, Eikelboom JW, et al. Double-dose versus standard-dose clopidogrel and high-dose versus low-dose aspirin in individuals undergoing percutaneous coronary intervention for acute coronary syndromes (CURRENT-OASIS 7): a randomised factorial trial. Lancet 2010;376(9748):1233–43.

14. Kandzari DE, Berger PB, Kastrati A, et al. Influence of treatment duration with a 600-mg dose of clopidogrel before percutaneous coronary revascularization. J Am Coll Cardiol 2004;44(11):2133–6.

15. Widimsky P, Motovska Z, Simek S, et al. Clopidogrel pre-treatment in stable angina: for all patients > 6 h before elective coronary angiography or only for angiographically selected patients a few minutes before PCI? A randomized multicentre trial PRAGUE-8. Eur Heart J 2008;29(12):1495–503.

16. Bellemain-Appaix A, O'Connor SA, Silvain J, et al. Association of clopidogrel pretreatment with mortality, cardiovascular events, and major bleeding among patients undergoing percutaneous coronary intervention: a systematic review and meta-analysis. JAMA 2012;308(23):2507–16.

17. Bhatt DL, Lincoff AM, Gibson CM, et al. Intravenous platelet blockade with cangrelor during PCI. N Engl J Med 2009;361(24):2330–41.

18. Harrington RA, Stone GW, McNulty S, et al. Platelet inhibition with cangrelor in patients undergoing PCI. N Engl J Med 2009;361(24):2318–29.

19. Bhatt DL, Stone GW, Mahaffey KW, et al. Effect of platelet inhibition with cangrelor during PCI on ischemic events. N Engl J Med 2013;368(14):1303–13.

20. Franchi F, Angiolillo DJ. Novel antiplatelet agents in acute coronary syndrome. Nat Rev Cardiol 2015;12(1):30–47.

21. Levine GN, Bates ER, Blankenship JC, et al. 2011 ACCF/AHA/SCAI guideline for percutaneous coronary intervention. A report of the American college of cardiology foundation/American heart association task force on practice guidelines and the society for cardiovascular angiography and interventions. J Am Coll Cardiol 2011;58(24):e44–122.

22. Windecker S, Kolh P, Alfonso F, et al. 2014 ESC/EACTS guidelines on myocardial revascularization: the task force on myocardial revascularization of the European society of cardiology (esc) and the European association for cardio-thoracic surgery (EACTS) developed with the special contribution of the European association of percutaneous cardiovascular interventions (EAPCI). Eur Heart J 2014;35(37):2541–619.

23. Montalescot G, Sechtem U, Achenbach S, et al. 2013 ESC guidelines on the management of stable coronary artery disease: the task force on the management of stable coronary artery disease of the European society of cardiology. Eur Heart J 2013;34(38):2949–3003.

24. Yusuf S, Zhao F, Mehta SR, et al. Effects of clopidogrel in addition to aspirin in patients with acute coronary syndromes without ST-segment elevation. N Engl J Med 2001;345(7):494–502.

25. Mehta SR, Yusuf S, Peters RJ, et al. Effects of pretreatment with clopidogrel and aspirin followed by long-term therapy in patients undergoing percutaneous coronary intervention: the PCI-CURE study. Lancet 2001;358(9281):527–33.

26. Lewis BS, Mehta SR, Fox KA, et al. Benefit of clopidogrel according to timing of percutaneous coronary intervention in patients with acute coronary syndromes: further results from the clopidogrel in unstable angina to prevent recurrent events (CURE) study. Am Heart J 2005;150(6):1177–84.

27. Di Sciascio G, Patti G, Pasceri V, et al. Effectiveness of in-laboratory high-dose clopidogrel loading versus routine pre-load in patients undergoing percutaneous coronary intervention: results of the ARMYDA-5 PRELOAD (Antiplatelet therapy for reduction of MYocardial damage during angioplasty) randomized trial. J Am Coll Cardiol 2010;56(7):550–7.

28. Stone GW, White HD, Ohman EM, et al. Bivalirudin in patients with acute coronary syndromes undergoing percutaneous coronary intervention: a subgroup analysis from the acute catheterization and urgent intervention triage strategy (ACUITY) trial. Lancet 2007;369(9565):907–19.

29. Wang TY, White JA, Tricoci P, et al. Upstream clopidogrel use and the efficacy and safety of early eptifibatide treatment in patients with acute coronary syndrome: an analysis from the early glycoprotein IIb/IIIa inhibition in patients with Non-ST-segment elevation acute coronary syndrome (EARLY ACS) trial. Circulation 2011;123(7):722–30.

30. Feldman DN, Fakorede F, Minutello RM, et al. Efficacy of high-dose clopidogrel treatment (600 mg) less than two hours before percutaneous coronary intervention in patients with non-ST-segment elevation acute coronary syndromes. Am J Cardiol 2010;105(3):323–32.

31. Wiviott SD, Braunwald E, McCabe CH, et al. Prasugrel versus clopidogrel in patients with acute coronary syndromes. N Engl J Med 2007;357(20):2001–15.

32. Montalescot G, Bolognese L, Dudek D, et al. Pretreatment with prasugrel in non-ST-segment elevation acute coronary syndromes. N Engl J Med 2013;369(11):999–1010.

33. Montalescot G, Collet JP, Ecollan P, et al. Effect of prasugrel pre-treatment strategy in patients undergoing percutaneous coronary intervention for NSTEMI: the ACCOAST-PCI study. J Am Coll Cardiol 2014;64(24):2563–71.

34. Bellemain-Appaix A, Kerneis M, O'Connor SA, et al. Reappraisal of thienopyridine pretreatment in patients with non-ST elevation acute coronary syndrome: a systematic review and meta-analysis. BMJ 2014;349:g6269.

35. Wallentin L, Becker RC, Budaj A, et al. Ticagrelor versus clopidogrel in patients with acute coronary syndromes. N Engl J Med 2009;361(11):1045–57.

36. Angiolillo DJ, Franchi F, Waksman R, et al. Effects of ticagrelor versus clopidogrel in troponin-negative patients with low-risk ACS undergoing Ad Hoc PCI. J Am Coll Cardiol 2016;67(6):603–13.

37. Angiolillo DJ, Firstenberg MS, Price MJ, et al. Bridging antiplatelet therapy with cangrelor in patients undergoing cardiac surgery: a randomized controlled trial. JAMA 2012;307(3):265–74.

38. Capodanno D, Angiolillo DJ. Management of antiplatelet therapy in patients with coronary artery disease requiring cardiac and noncardiac surgery. Circulation 2013;128(25):2785–98.

39. Roffi M, Patrono C, Collet JP, et al. 2015 ESC guidelines for the management of acute coronary syndromes in patients presenting without persistent ST-segment elevation: task force for the management of acute coronary syndromes in patients presenting without persistent ST-segment elevation of the european society of cardiology (ESC). Eur Heart J 2016;37(3):267–315.

40. Amsterdam EA, Wenger NK, Brindis RG, et al. 2014 AHA/ACC guideline for the management of patients with Non-ST-elevation acute coronary syndromes: a report of the American college of cardiology/American heart association task force on practice guidelines. Circulation 2014;130(25):2354–94.

41. Zeymer U, Arntz HR, Mark B, et al. Efficacy and safety of a high loading dose of clopidogrel administered prehospitally to improve primary percutaneous coronary intervention in acute myocardial infarction: the randomized CIPAMI trial. Clin Res Cardiol 2012;101(4):305–12.

42. Ducci K, Grotti S, Falsini G, et al. Comparison of pre-hospital 600 mg or 900 mg vs. peri-interventional 300 mg clopidogrel in patients with ST-elevation myocardial infarction undergoing primary coronary angioplasty. The Load&Go randomized trial. Int J Cardiol 2013;168(5):4814–6.

43. Montalescot G, Hof AW, Lapostolle F, et al. Prehospital ticagrelor in ST-segment elevation myocardial infarction. N Engl J Med 2014;371(24):2338–9.

44. Montalescot G, van 't Hof AW, Bolognese L, et al. Effect of pre-hospital ticagrelor during the first 24 h after primary percutaneous coronary intervention in patients with ST-segment elevation myocardial infarction: the ATLANTIC-H(24) analysis. JACC Cardiovasc Interv 2016;9(7):646–56.

45. Wiviott SD, Antman EM, Gibson CM, et al. Evaluation of prasugrel compared with clopidogrel in patients with acute coronary syndromes: design and rationale for the trial to assess improvement in therapeutic outcomes by optimizing platelet inhibition with prasugrel thrombolysis in myocardial infarction 38 (TRITON-TIMI 38). Am Heart J 2006;152(4):627–35.

46. Angiolillo DJ, Bhatt DL, Steg PG, et al. Impact of cangrelor overdosing on bleeding complications in patients undergoing percutaneous coronary intervention: insights from the CHAMPION trials. J Thromb Thrombolysis 2015;40(3):317–22.

47. Franchi F, Rollini F, Park Y, et al. A Safety evaluation of cangrelor in patients undergoing PCI. Expert Opin Drug Saf 2016;15(2):275–85.

48. Steg PG, James SK, Atar D, et al. ESC guidelines for the management of acute myocardial infarction in patients presenting with ST-segment elevation. Eur Heart J 2012;33(20):2569–619.

49. O'Gara PT, Kushner FG, Ascheim DD, et al. 2013 ACCF/AHA guideline for the management of ST-elevation myocardial infarction: a report of the American college of cardiology foundation/American heart association task force on practice guidelines. J Am Coll Cardiol 2013;61(4):e78–140.

50. De Luca L, Leonardi S, Cavallini C, et al. Contemporary antithrombotic strategies in patients with acute coronary syndrome admitted to cardiac care units in Italy: the EYESHOT Study. Eur Heart J Acute Cardiovasc Care 2015;4(5):441–52.

51. Parodi G, Valenti R, Bellandi B, et al. Comparison of prasugrel and ticagrelor loading doses in ST-segment elevation myocardial infarction patients: RAPID (Rapid Activity of Platelet Inhibitor Drugs) primary PCI study. J Am Coll Cardiol 2013;61(15):1601–6.

52. Parodi G, Bellandi B, Valenti R, et al. Comparison of double (360 mg) ticagrelor loading dose with

standard (60 mg) prasugrel loading dose in ST-elevation myocardial infarction patients: the rapid activity of platelet inhibitor drugs (RAPID) primary PCI 2 study. Am Heart J 2014;167(6):909–14.

53. Franchi F, Rollini F, Cho JR, et al. Impact of escalating loading dose regimens of ticagrelor in patients With ST-segment elevation myocardial infarction undergoing primary percutaneous coronary intervention: results of a prospective randomized pharmacokinetic and pharmacodynamic investigation. JACC Cardiovasc Interv 2015;8(11): 1457–67.

54. Parodi G, Xanthopoulou I, Bellandi B, et al. Ticagrelor crushed tablets administration in STEMI patients: the MOJITO study. J Am Coll Cardiol 2015;65(5):511–2.

55. Rollini F, Franchi F, Hu J, et al. Crushed prasugrel tablets in patients with STEMI undergoing primary

percutaneous coronary intervention: the CRUSH study. J Am Coll Cardiol 2016;67(17):1994–2004.

56. Valgimigli M, Tebaldi M, Campo G, et al. Prasugrel versus tirofiban bolus with or without short post-bolus infusion with or without concomitant prasugrel administration in patients with myocardial infarction undergoing coronary stenting: the FABOLUS PRO (Facilitation through Aggrastat By drOpping or shortening Infusion Line in patients with ST-segment elevation myocardial infarction compared to or on top of PRasugrel given at loading dOse) trial. JACC Cardiovasc Interv 2012;5(3):268–77.

57. Angiolillo DJ, Schneider DJ, Bhatt DL, et al. Pharmacodynamic effects of cangrelor and clopidogrel: the platelet function substudy from the cangrelor versus standard therapy to achieve optimal management of platelet inhibition (CHAMPION) trials. J Thromb Thrombolysis 2012;34(1):44–55.

Optimal Duration of Dual Antiplatelet Therapy After Percutaneous Coronary Intervention

Arjun Majithia, MD[a], Deepak L. Bhatt, MD, MPH[b],*

KEYWORDS

• Dual antiplatelet therapy • Percutaneous coronary intervention • Coronary artery disease

KEY POINTS

- Dual antiplatelet therapy (DAPT) remains an essential component of treatment in patients with coronary artery disease, treated with and without percutaneous coronary intervention (PCI).
- Recommendations for duration of DAPT after PCI should consider patient-specific risk, clinical presentation, stent characteristics, and technical and procedural factors.
- Overall, primary studies and meta-analyses of prolonged DAPT longer than 12 months after PCI demonstrate reduction in rates of stent thrombosis (ST) and myocardial infarction (MI), at the cost of increased bleeding.
- Studies of shorter-duration DAPT after PCI in non–acute coronary syndrome populations treated with a second-generation drug-eluting stent, suggest similar mortality, MI, ST, and lower bleeding when compared with longer DAPT duration.

INTRODUCTION

Antiplatelet therapy is a cornerstone in the management of patients with coronary artery disease (CAD) after percutaneous coronary intervention (PCI).[1] Historically, dual antiplatelet therapy (DAPT) with aspirin and a P2Y12 inhibitor is administered for a period of at least 1 month to 1 year after implantation of a bare-metal stent (BMS) or drug-eluting stent (DES), respectively, to mitigate stent thrombosis (ST) and future myocardial infarctions (MIs). This standard was supported by studies of patients presenting with acute coronary syndromes (ACS), and electively, treated with PCI.[2,3] However, the optimal duration of antiplatelet therapy after PCI remains uncertain. Longer DAPT exposure decreases ischemic events, but leads to an increase in clinically meaningful bleeding. Strategies for both prolonged DAPT of longer than 1 year, and abbreviated DAPT for 3 to 6 months have been proposed.

Here, we review current evidence for strategies of prolonged DAPT and abbreviated DAPT following PCI.

PROLONGED DUAL ANTIPLATELET THERAPY OF LONGER THAN 12 MONTHS FOLLOWING PERCUTANEOUS CORONARY INTERVENTION

Rationale for Studies of Prolonged Dual Antiplatelet Therapy (Longer than 12 Months)

First-generation DESs were developed to address the high restenosis rates associated

Disclosures: See last page of article.
[a] Landsman Heart and Vascular Center, Lahey Hospital and Medical Center, 41 Burlington Mall Road, Burlington, MA 01805, USA; [b] Heart & Vascular Center, Brigham and Women's Hospital, Harvard Medical School, 75 Francis Street, Boston, MA 02115, USA
* Corresponding author.
E-mail address: dlbhattmd@post.harvard.edu

Intervent Cardiol Clin 6 (2017) 25–37
http://dx.doi.org/10.1016/j.iccl.2016.08.003
2211-7458/17/© 2016 Elsevier Inc. All rights reserved.

with BMS, but were limited by higher rates of late ST. The BASKET-LATE (Basel Stent Kosten Effektivitäts Trial-Late Thrombotic Events) trial followed 746 patients treated with DES or BMS for 1 year after discontinuation of clopidogrel, and demonstrated no difference in overall 18-month cardiovascular death or MI.[4] However, the study demonstrated higher rates of death and MI in the DES group after discontinuation of clopidogrel (between months 7–18), with twice as frequent late ST (2.6% vs 1.3%). These results suggested that despite an initial benefit of reducing target vessel revascularization (TVR) compared with BMS, the benefit of first-generation DES may be attenuated by late ST, leading to increased cardiac death and MI.

Several factors affect the likelihood of ST. First-generation, polymer-based, drug-coated stents elute sirolimus or paclitaxel to attenuate aggressive neointimal hyperplasia and subsequent restenosis within the stent lumen. However, autopsy studies of patients treated with first-generation DES who have died from late ST demonstrate delayed arterial healing, characterized by persistent fibrin deposition, and poor stent endothelialization.[5,6] Clinical presentation at the time of index PCI also affects the likelihood of ST. The use of DES in patients with acute MI (AMI) is associated with greater incidence of late ST when compared with those with stable plaques.[6] Procedural factors, such as stent underexpansion, malapposition, and stent edge dissection also influence the likelihood of ST, although these factors tend to promote early ST, and affect both BMS and DES similarly, as evidenced by the similar rate of early ST with BMS and DES.[5] A strategy of prolonged DAPT was proposed to mitigate ST and ischemic events involving and unrelated to the index lesion. However, the safety of long-term DAPT exposure is uncertain.

Recent studies have identified potential safety concerns with prolonged antiplatelet therapy. The CHARISMA (Clopidogrel for High Atherothrombotic Risk and Ischemic Stabilization, Management, and Avoidance) trial randomized 15,603 with cardiovascular disease or multiple risk factors to clopidogrel and aspirin versus aspirin alone.[7] At a median of 28 months, the primary efficacy endpoint of MI, stroke, or death from cardiovascular causes was not significantly different between groups. In the subgroup of patients with multiple risk factors (but without clinically evident atherosclerotic disease), the incidence of death was higher in the group treated with clopidogrel. In the subgroup of patients with clinically evident atherothrombotic disease, there was a suggestion of benefit in

the clopidogrel group. The subgroup with prior ischemic events such as MI seemed to derive particular benefit from prolonged dual antiplatelet therapy with aspirin plus clopidogrel.[8] Among the entire population of patients, those treated with clopidogrel plus aspirin demonstrated a significant increase in moderate bleeding, and a trend toward an increase in severe bleeding.

Studies Evaluating Prolonged Dual Antiplatelet Therapy (of Longer than 12 Months)

Studies of prolonged DAPT exposure and PCI have reported conflicting results with regard to the efficacy of extending therapy beyond 1 year. The DES-LATE (Optimal Duration of Dual Antiplatelet Therapy After Drug-Eluting Stent Implantation) trial, randomized 5045 patients who received DES and were event free at 12 months to aspirin or aspirin and clopidogrel.[9] The study demonstrated no difference in a composite endpoint of death, MI, or stroke at 24 months, and similar bleeding rates between groups. Similarly, the ARCTIC-Interruption (Assessment by a double Randomisation of a Conventional antiplatelet strategy vs a monitoring-guided strategy for DES implantation and, of Treatment Interruption vs Continuation 1 year after stenting-Interruption) trial, an extension of the ARCTIC-Monitoring trial, demonstrated no clinical benefit with prolonged DAPT, but a significant increase in major or minor bleeding with prolonged therapy.[10]

Other studies have demonstrated results in favor of prolonged DAPT. The DAPT (Dual Antiplatelet Therapy) study, a large, multicenter, blinded, placebo-controlled trial addressed several limitations of previous studies.[11] A total of 9961 patients who had undergone DES were randomly assigned to continued thienopyridine (clopidogrel or prasugrel) plus aspirin versus aspirin plus placebo for a period of 18 months after completing 12 months of DAPT after PCI. Prolonged DAPT resulted in a reduced rate of ST and major adverse cardiovascular or cerebrovascular events (MACCE), a composite of death, MI, or stroke, driven by a reduction in the rate of MI (including nonstent thrombosis–related MI). The study also demonstrated an increase in moderate or severe bleeding, and a signal for increased noncardiovascular death with prolonged therapy. An analysis of ST and MI in the period surrounding discontinuation revealed elevated risk during the 3 months after discontinuation of thienopyridines in both groups. Most recently, the OPTIDUAL (OPTImal DUAL Antiplatelet Therapy Trial) study randomized 1966 patients treated with DES for stable CAD or ACS to 12 months or 48 months of DAPT, and demonstrated a net clinical benefit with prolonged therapy, with no difference in bleeding.[12] However, the trial was terminated early for low recruitment. A summary of trials evaluating prolonged DAPT can be seen in Table 1.

Although most studies of prolonged DAPT after PCI have focused on evaluating a combination of aspirin and clopidogrel (with the exception of the DAPT study, which also included prasugrel), the use of ticagrelor in addition to aspirin beyond 1 year has been evaluated in patients with a history of prior MI. The PEGASUS-TIMI 54 (Prevention of Cardiovascular Events in Patients with Prior Heart Attack Using Ticagrelor Compared to Placebo on a Background of Aspirin–Thrombolysis in Myocardial Infarction 54) study randomized 21,161 patients with a history of AMI, most with a history of PCI, to aspirin and ticagrelor (60 mg twice a day [BID] or 90 mg BID) versus aspirin and placebo. After a median follow-up of 33 months, the groups receiving ticagrelor had significantly lower rates of MACCE and higher rates of TIMI major bleeding (with a numerically higher rate of bleeding with ticagrelor 90 mg orally [PO] BID vs 60 mg PO BID), with similar rates of intracranial hemorrhage or fatal bleeding among the 3 groups.[13] The study is important in demonstrating the efficacy of prolonged DAPT in high-risk patients using more-potent P2Y12 inhibitors, and also supports the safety of this strategy in carefully selected patients, confirming the earlier CHARISMA subgroup analysis. A recently published PEGASUS-TIMI 54 substudy demonstrated a reduction in ischemic events, cardiovascular deaths, and coronary heart disease deaths in diabetic patients receiving ticagrelor in addition to aspirin, suggesting a clinically meaningful role for DAPT, and particularly ticagrelor, for secondary prevention in high-risk subgroups.[14] A separate substudy demonstrated a significant reduction in major adverse cardiac events (MACE) in the peripheral arterial disease subgroup and a reduction in major adverse limb outcomes in the entire PEGASUS-TIMI 54 population.[15] Other studies have also suggested a benefit of prolonged DAPT in high-risk patients. A post hoc DAPT substudy demonstrated a far greater benefit in reduction of MI and MACCE in patients presenting with MI versus those without MI.[16] These analyses confirm findings from a prior substudy of the CHARISMA trial analyzing 9478 patients with prior MI, stroke, or peripheral arterial disease, demonstrated significantly lower MACE

with prolonged DAPT.[8] Together, the results from CHARISMA, DAPT, and PEGASUS-TIMI 54, suggest that patients presenting with ACS, treated with or without PCI, derive substantial benefit from prolonged DAPT.

A number of meta-analyses have been performed to study the safety and efficacy of prolonged DAPT. A recently published meta-analysis using multiple analytical approaches examined mortality outcomes in 31,666 patients treated with extended DAPT after DES.[17] The study demonstrated lower all-cause mortality with shorter DAPT compared with longer DAPT, attributable to noncardiac mortality. Shorter DAPT duration was associated with lower rates of major bleeding and higher rates of MI and ST. In a separate meta-analysis of randomized trials comparing more than 1 year of DAPT with aspirin alone in 33,425 patients with a history of MI, extended DAPT decreased MACE, MI, stroke, ST, and cardiovascular death, with no increase in noncardiovascular death.[18] There was an increase of major, nonfatal bleeding, and no overall effect on all-cause mortality.[19]

The results of these meta-analyses corroborate several important findings. When considering all patients treated with DES (and largely elective DES in patients with low ischemic risk), longer duration of DAPT decreases the rates of future ischemic events, including ST and MI, at the cost of increased bleeding, and possibly noncardiovascular death. When specifically considering patients with prior MI, treated with or without PCI, prolonged DAPT of longer than 1 year decreases ischemic events, including ST, and MI, at the cost of increased bleeding, with no net effect on mortality. Thus, it is the patient with prior ACS that is most likely to benefit from longer durations of DAPT and more intense DAPT, assuming that they are at low bleeding risk at baseline and during follow-up.

SHORTER DURATION OF DUAL ANTIPLATELET THERAPY (3–6 MONTHS) AFTER PERCUTANEOUS CORONARY INTERVENTION
Rationale for Shorter Duration of Dual Antiplatelet Therapy After Percutaneous Coronary Intervention
Extending DAPT duration has the potential to reduce late ST and ischemic events remote from the target lesion. However, the benefits of longer DAPT exposure may be mitigated by the use of newer-generation stents, which have lower rates of late ST, and by the increase in at

Table 1
Studies evaluating prolonged DAPT duration after PCI

Trial	Study Design, Size	DAPT Duration	Patient Population	ACS, %	2nd Gen DES, %	Endpoints	ST	MI	Bleeding	Death
DES-LATE, Lee et al,[9] 2014	Open-label RCT, n = 5045	12 mo vs >12 mo	Inclusion: DES, event free at 12–18 mo; Exclusion: ACS, ischemia, bleeding before randomization	61	30	Primary: CV death, MI, stroke at 24 mo: 2.4% vs 2.6%, P = .75	0.5% vs 0.3%, P = .34	1.2% vs 0.8%, P = .23	1.1% vs 1.4%, P = .20	1.4% vs 2.0%, P = .12
ARCTIC-INTERRUPTION, Collet et al,[10] 2014	Open-label RCT, n = 1259	12 mo vs >12 mo	Inclusion: patients event free at 12 mo (extension of ARCTIC-MONITORING); Exclusion: PCI for STEMI, bleeding	26	63	Primary: death, MI, ST, CVA, or urgent TVR: 4% vs 4%, P = .58	1% vs 0%	1% vs 1%, P = .94	<0.5% vs 1%, P = .073	1% vs 1%, P = .58
DAPT Study, Mauri et al,[11] 2014	Placebo-controlled RCT, n = 9961	12 mo vs 30 mo	Inclusion: patients treated with BMS or DES; Exclusion: MI, stroke repeat revascularization, ST, bleeding	43	60	Primary: ST: 1.4% vs 0.4%, P = .001; MACCE (death, MI, CVA): 5.9% vs 4.3%, P<.001	1.4% vs 0.4%, P = .001	4.1% vs 2.1%, P<.001	1.6% vs 2.6%, P = .001	1.5% vs 2.0%, P = .05

Trial	Design	Duration	Inclusion/Exclusion			Primary outcome				
OPTIDUAL, Helft et al,[12] 2016	Open-label RCT, n = 1966	12 mo vs 48 mo	Inclusion: DES for stable CAD or ACS; Exclusion: unprotected LM, anticoagulation	36	59	Primary: death, MI, CVA, or bleeding: 7.5% vs 5.8%, P = .017	0% vs 0.4%	2.3% vs 1.6%, P = .31	2.0% vs 2.0%, P = .95	3.5% vs 2.3%, P = .18
ITALIC, Gilard et al,[23] 2015	Open-label RCT, noninferiority	6 mo vs 24 mo	Inclusion: Patients undergoing PCI; Exclusion: STEMI, LM PCI	23	100	Primary: death, MI, urgent TVR, CVA, major bleeding at 12 mo: 1.6% vs 1.5%, P = .85 (P<.00002 for noninferiority)	0% vs 0.3%	0.4% vs 0.7%, P = .53	0 vs 0.3%	0.8% vs 0.9%, P = .80
PRODIGY, Valgimigli et al,[24] 2012	RCT, n = 2013	6 mo vs 24 mo	Inclusion: stable CAD or ACS undergoing PCI	74.6	50	Primary: death, MI, or CVA at 24 mo: 10.1% vs 10.0%, P = .91	0.8% vs 0.7%, P = .80	4.0% vs 4.2%, P = .80	7.4% vs 3.5%, P = .0002	6.6% vs 6.6%, P = .98

Abbreviations: ACS, acute coronary syndrome; BMS, bare-metal stent; CV, cardiovascular; CVA, cerebrovascular accident; DAPT, dual antiplatelet therapy; DES, drug-eluting stent; Gen, generation; LM, left main; MACCE, major adverse cardiac and cardiovascular event; MACE, major adverse cardiac event; MI, myocardial infarction; PCI, percutaneous coronary intervention; RCT, randomized controlled trial; ST, stent thrombosis; STEMI, ST-elevation myocardial infarction; TVR, target vessel revascularization.

least moderate bleeding. In patients who are not at high risk for ischemic events, some studies suggest that prolonging DAPT may increase noncardiovascular mortality. In patients who have high bleeding risk, treated with second-generation DES, or who may require interruption of DAPT, it is reasonable to consider a strategy of abbreviated DAPT duration of less than 1 year after PCI. Several studies have been performed to evaluate this strategy.

Studies Evaluating Shorter Duration of Dual Antiplatelet Therapy

Most studies of shorter DAPT duration have evaluated a strategy of 3 to 6 months of DAPT after PCI versus 1 year of DAPT after DES. The first such study, the EXCELLENT study, evaluated 6 versus 12 months of DAPT in 1443 patients undergoing DES implantation (most treated with everolimus-eluting stents [EES]).[20] In this randomized study, the rate of target vessel failure (cardiac death, MI, ischemia driven TVR at 12 months) was similar using either strategy. There was a trend toward increased ST in the shorter DAPT group, with no difference in risk of death or MI. However, target vessel failure occurred more frequently with shorter DAPT in diabetic patients, a predefined subgroup. Notably, the study excluded several high-risk patients, including those who presented with MI within 72 hours, patients with left-main disease, or with severe left ventricular dysfunction. Nonetheless, the results suggested noninferiority of shorter DAPT duration in lower-risk populations, although the results cannot be extrapolated to higher-risk subgroups, including patients with diabetes, who suffered higher event rates with shorter therapy. Three other studies comparing 6 versus 12 months of DAPT after DES in low-risk populations, treated predominantly with second-generation DES, demonstrated noninferiority in net clinical outcome (composite of ischemic and bleeding outcomes) with abbreviated DAPT following PCI.[21–23]

The PRODIGY (Prolonging Dual-Antiplatelet Treatment after Grading Stent-induced Intimal Hyperplasia) study evaluated a strategy of 6 months versus 24 months of DAPT in a high-risk patient cohort, most who presented with MI, receiving a mixture of BMS, zotarolimus-eluting stents (ZES), paclitaxel-eluting stents, or EESs.[24] The primary outcome of all-cause death, MI, or cerebrovascular event was similar between the 2 groups at the 2-year follow-up, with consistently higher bleeding in the group randomized to 24 months of DAPT.

The RESET (REal Safety and Efficacy of 3-month dual antiplatelet therapy following

Endeavor zotarolimus-eluting stent implantation) study evaluated a strategy of even shorter DAPT, randomizing 2117 patients with CAD to 3 months of DAPT after ZES implantation versus 12 months of DAPT following ZES, EES, or sirolimus-eluting stent implantation.[25] The primary endpoint, a composite of cerebrovascular (CV) death, MI, ST, TVR, or bleeding at 1 year was similar between groups, with no difference in rates of ST. Furthermore, there was no increase in ST after discontinuation of DAPT, unlike that observed in the DAPT trial. The results were consistent across all clinical subgroups, including patients with diabetes, although there was a nonsignificant trend favoring longer DAPT in patients with ACS, and in patients with long lesion length. The OPTIMIZE study also evaluated a strategy of 3 months of DAPT after ZES implantation versus 12 months of therapy, and demonstrated noninferiority of shorter DAPT in a population of patients with stable CAD or low-risk ACS.[26]

A summary of trials evaluating a strategy of shorter DAPT duration can be seen in Table 2.

It is difficult to draw definitive, generalizable conclusions from any of the 7 trials of short versus standard or prolonged DAPT. Each of the studies is underpowered to detect differences in individual endpoints. Multiple trials were terminated early because of slow enrollment. Most studies had follow-up periods of only 1 year, limiting the ability to assess for late clinical events. All of the studies, except for the PRODIGY study, primarily recruited patients with stable CAD or low-risk ACS. It also should be noted that every study primarily used second-generation stents, and 3 studies used second-generation stents exclusively.

A recent meta-analysis of short versus long duration of DAPT after DES compared clinical outcomes between less than 6 months of DAPT and 1 year of DAPT, as well as among patients exposed for 3 months, 6 months, and 1 year of DAPT.[27] This study included 4 trials, and 8180 patients, and found that at 1 year, short-term DAPT after DES (mostly second-generation DES) was associated with similar MACE and lower bleeding compared with prolonged DAPT in an overall low-risk patient population. No increase in MACE was seen after discontinuing short-term DAPT, and no differences were captured among those treated with 3 months, 6 months, or 12 months of therapy.

Most studies of PCI and DAPT duration have excluded patients with high bleeding risk or clinically evident bleeding. Patients at high risk for bleeding requiring PCI are usually treated with BMS followed by 1 month of DAPT. However,

Table 2
Studies evaluating abbreviated DAPT duration after PCI

Trial	Study Design, Size	DAPT Duration	Patient Population	ACS, %	2nd Gen DES, %	Endpoints	ST	MI	Bleeding	Death
EXCELLENT, Gwon et al,[20] 2012	Open-label RCT, noninferiority, n = 1443	6 mo vs 12 mo	Inclusion: stenosis >50%, evidence of myocardial ischemia; Exclusion: MI within 72 hours, EF <25%, CV shock, LM disease, CTO, bifurcation lesion	51	75	Primary: TVR (CV death, MI, ischemia driven revascularization) at 1 year: 4.8% vs 4.3%, P = .001 for noninferiority	0.9% vs 0.1%, P = .10	1.8% vs 1.0%, P = .19	0.3% vs 0.6%, P = .42	0.6% vs 1.0%, P = .37
RESET, Kim et al,[25] 2012	Open-label RCT, noninferiority; n = 2117	3 mo vs 12 mo	Inclusion: angina or acute MI, with planned elective DES; Exclusion: STEMI, CV shock, LM disease	55	71.5	Primary: CV death, MI, ST, TVR, or bleeding at 1 year: 4.7% vs 4.7%, P<.001 for noninferiority	0.2% vs 0.3%, P = .65	0.2% vs 0.4%, P = .41	0.2% vs 0.6%, P = .16	0.5% vs 1.0%, P = .39
OPTIMIZE, Feres et al,[26] 2013	Open-label, RCT, noninferiority	3 mo vs 12 mo	Inclusion: stable angina, low-risk ACS (not acute MI, not biomarker positive on presentation); Exclusion: STEMI, previous DES, SVG lesions, DES stenoses	31	100	Primary: Death, MI, stroke, or major bleeding at 12 mo: 6.0% vs 5.8%, P = .002 for noninferiority	0.8% vs 0.8%, P = .86	3.2% vs 2.7%, P = .47	0.6% vs 0.9%, P = .41	2.8% vs 2.9%, P = .82
SECURITY, Colombo et al,[21] 2014	Open-label RCT, noninferiority; n = 1399	6 mo vs 12 mo	Inclusion: stable angina, unstable angina, silent ischemia; Exclusion: STEMI, non-STEMI, EF<30%, LM PCI, SVG PCI, CKD	38.4	100	Primary: CV death, MI, CVA, ST, BARC type 3 or 5 bleeding at 12 mo: 4.5% vs 3.7%, P = .469 (P<.05 for noninferiority)	0.3% vs 0.4%, P = .69	2.3% vs 2.1%, P = .75	0.6% vs 1.1%, P = .28	1.1% vs 1.2%, P = .41
ISAR-SAFE, Schulz-Schupke et al,[22] 2015	Double-blind, placebo-controlled RCT, noninferiority, n = 4005	6 mo vs 12 mo	Inclusion: patients on DAPT 6 mo after DES for CAD or ACS; Exclusion: LM PCI, MI within 6 mo after PCI, prior ST	40	72	Primary: Death, MI ST, CVA, or TIMI major bleeding 15 mo after stent: 1.5% vs 1.6%, P<.001 for noninferiority	0.3% vs 0.2%, P = .49	0.7% vs 0.7%, P = .85	0.2% vs 0.3%, P = .74	0.4% vs 0.6%, P = .37

Abbreviations: ACS, acute coronary syndrome; CKD, chronic kidney disease; CTO, chronic total occlusion; CV, cardiovascular; CVA, cerebrovascular accident; DAPT, dual antiplatelet therapy; DES, drug-eluting stent; EF, ejection fraction; Gen, generation; LM, left main; MI, myocardial infarction; PCI, percutaneous coronary intervention; RCT, randomized controlled trial; ST, stent thrombosis; STEMI, ST-elevation myocardial infarction; SVG, saphenous vein graft; TVR, target vessel revascularization.

more recent studies have evaluated the efficacy of DES in this high-risk cohort. The ZEUS (Zotarolimus-eluting Endeavor Sprint Stent in Uncertain DES Candidates) Study randomly assigned patients with uncertain DES candidacy to ZES or BMS, followed by a tailored regimen for DAPT based on patient characteristics.[28] After a median DAPT duration of 32 days, patients treated with ZES demonstrated a significant reduction in 1-year MACE. In a substudy of participants with high bleeding risk, treatment with ZES and 30 days of DAPT led to significant reductions in MACE and TVR versus treatment with BMS.[29] It should be noted that outcomes with the Endeavor ZES, which was exclusively used in the ZEUS study, may not reflect those of currently used DES, given differences in drug elution kinetics and endothelialization. The LEADERS-FREE (Prospective Randomized Comparison of the BioFreedom Biolimus A9 Drug-Coated Stent vs the Gazelle Bare-Metal Stent in Patients at High Bleeding Risk) trial evaluated a strategy of 1 month of DAPT following PCI with a polymer-free stent versus BMS in patients with high bleeding risk.[30] At 390 days, treatment with the drug-coated stent was associated with a significant reduction in composite cardiac death, MI, or ST, and significant reduction in clinically driven TVR. In a substudy of patients who presented with ACS, treatment with the drug-coated stent demonstrated superior safety, driven by significant reductions in cardiac death and MI, and superior efficacy evidenced by a significant reduction in TVR.[31] Notably, there are no clinical trial data assessing other commonly used stents in patients with high bleeding risk or compared with BMS. However, these studies suggest that in patients with high bleeding risk, treatment with current-generation DES may provide superior safety and efficacy compared with BMS, and that a minimum duration of 1 month of DAPT after DES in high-risk patients may be reasonable.

Overall, when considering the several primary studies and meta-analyses of short-duration DAPT after PCI, the results suggest that 3 to 6 months of DAPT after PCI may be reasonable in patients with stable CAD or low-risk ACS after treatment with a second-generation DES. In patients with high bleeding risk, treatment with DES and a minimum DAPT duration of 1 month is reasonable.

Guideline-Based Management of Dual Antiplatelet Therapy After Percutaneous Coronary Intervention

The 2011 American College of Cardiology/American Heart Association (ACC/AHA) guideline for PCI recommended a minimum of 12 months of DAPT after PCI (BMS or DES) for ACS (Class I, level of evidence [LOE] B), and after DES for a non-ACS indication (Class I, LOE B).[32] On account of several recent studies assessing shorter or longer duration of DAPT, a focused update addressing DAPT duration in patients with CAD was published by the ACC/AHA.[33]

For patients with stable ischemic heart disease (SIHD), and no history of PCI or coronary artery bypass graft, DAPT is not recommended (Class III). Patients with SIHD treated with BMS should be treated with DAPT for at least 1 month (Class I), and DAPT may be continued in patients without high bleeding risk (Class IIb). Current guidelines recommend that patients with SIHD treated with DES should be treated with DAPT for at least 6 months (Class I), and DAPT may be continued for longer in patients without high bleeding risk (Class IIb). In patients with SIHD who develop a high risk of bleeding or have a bleeding complication, the current guideline suggests that discontinuation of the P2Y12 agent after 3 months is reasonable (Class IIb).

Patients with acute or recent ACS are considered separately. Patients presenting with ACS treated with BMS or DES, should be treated with DAPT for at least 12 months (Class I), and prolonging DAPT for longer than 12 months may be reasonable (Class IIb). In patients with ACS treated with DAPT after DES who develop a high risk of bleeding or have a bleeding complication, the current guideline suggests that discontinuation of the P2Y12 agent after 6 months is reasonable (Class IIb). In all cases, aspirin should be continued indefinitely, with a recommended daily dose of 81 mg (Class I).

The updated guideline also addresses the use of other P2Y12 inhibitors in place of clopidogrel. The guideline recommends that for patients with ACS, treated with or without PCI, it is reasonable to use ticagrelor in place of clopidogrel for maintenance of a P2Y12 inhibitor (Class IIa).[34] The guideline also recommends that for patients with ACS treated with PCI who are not at high risk for bleeding and who do not have a history of stroke or transient ischemic attack, it is reasonable to choose prasugrel over clopidogrel for maintenance P2Y12 inhibitor therapy (Class IIa).[35]

The current recommendations more closely mirror the 2014 European Society of Cardiology guidelines, which suggest that patients with ACS, treated with BMS or DES, continue DAPT for 12 months, and that patients without ACS treated with DES continue DAPT for 6 months.[36] Recommendations for antiplatelet management of bioabsorbable stents and stents with bioabsorbable polymers are not specifically addressed in current guidelines. However, a recent meta-analysis suggests that first-generation bioabsorbable stents appear to have a higher rate of ST, and therefore longer durations of DAPT should be considered if these stents are going to be used.[37]

Assessing Ischemic and Bleeding Risk

Exposure to DAPT protects the target vessel treated with PCI by decreasing early and late ST. However, exposure to DAPT also decreases the frequency of MI involving sites remote from the target vessel, and in certain high-risk populations treated without PCI. Longer exposure to DAPT unequivocally increases clinically significant bleeding. It is therefore imperative to understand which factors increase the propensity for future ischemic events or ST vs bleeding events when determining the appropriate duration of antiplatelet therapy.

Several factors influence the likelihood of future ischemic events, and can be broadly thought of in 4 categories: (1) patient-specific risk factors, (2) clinical presentation, (3) procedural and technical consideration, and (4) stent characteristics. Patient-specific risk factors that have been associated with high ischemic risk include advanced age, history of prior MI, extensive CAD, diabetes mellitus, and chronic kidney disease (CKD). Patient-specific risk factors that increase the likelihood of ST include prior stent thrombosis, diabetes mellitus, and left ventricular ejection fraction less than 40%.[33] Clinical presentation at the time of the index event or procedure can broadly be categorized as ACS and non-ACS presentations. ACS presentation increases ischemic risk and the risk of ST. Procedural considerations that increase the likelihood of ST include stent undersizing, smaller stent diameter, greater stent length, and bifurcation lesion stenting. The presence of in-stent restenosis also increases the likelihood of ST.[33,38]

Factors that increase the likelihood of bleeding include a history of bleeding, concurrent anticoagulant therapy, female sex, advanced age, low body weight, CKD, diabetes mellitus (in some analyses), anemia, and chronic steroid or nonsteroidal anti-inflammatory drug use.[33]

Recently, multiple risk prediction tools have been created to stratify patients into those who would benefit from prolonged DAPT after PCI.[39–41] The "DAPT score," derived from DAPT study data, incorporates several weighted factors to predict whether a patient's ischemic potential outweighs the risk of bleeding. A score

of ≥2 predicts a favorable risk-to-benefit ratio for prolonged DAPT. Separately, using data from 4190 patients with DES enrolled in the PARIS (Patterns of Non-Adherence to Anti-Platelet Regimen in Stented Patients) registry, risk scores were developed to predict coronary thrombotic events and major bleeding.[41] Before being used as a tool to help guide actual clinical decision making, the clinical risk score needs to be validated in multiple prospective patient cohorts.

Proton Pump Inhibitors to Reduce Gastrointestinal Bleeding in Patients on Dual Antiplatelet Therapy

Therapies that diminish the risk of bleeding of DAPT may further influence the risk-to-benefit ratio of prolonged DAPT. There is emerging evidence surrounding the potential role of proton pump inhibitors (PPI) in reducing gastrointestinal (GI) bleeding in patients on DAPT.[42] Initial pharmacodynamic studies of clopidogrel and the PPI omeprazole, a moderate CYP2C19 inhibitor, demonstrated a metabolic drug-drug interaction between the drugs, prompting a Food and Drug Administration box warning to alert physicians about this interaction.[43,44] However, large randomized clinical studies suggest that coadministration of clopidogrel and omeprazole does not lead to an increase in cardiovascular events.[42] The Clopidogrel with or without Omeprazole in Coronary Artery Disease (COGENT) study randomly assigned 3873 patients with an indication for DAPT to receive clopidogrel in combination with either omeprazole or placebo, in addition to aspirin.[45] The primary GI endpoint of overt or occult bleeding, symptomatic gastroduodenal ulcers or erosions, obstruction, or perforation occurred in 1.1% with omeprazole versus 2.9% with placebo at 180 days ($P<.001$). Importantly, there was a significant reduction in overt upper GI bleeding with omeprazole. The COGENT study did not show any significant interaction between omeprazole use and cardiovascular outcomes. A post hoc analysis dividing COGENT patients into those who received low-dose versus high-dose aspirin demonstrated a similar rate of composite GI endpoints, as well as a similar reduction of adverse GI endpoints with PPI administration.[46] These results suggest that even patients on low-dose aspirin may benefit from prophylactic, concurrent PPI administration. A separate analysis demonstrated improvement of dyspepsia with addition of PPIs to DAPT, a finding that may have implications in improving patient compliance with DAPT.[47]

SUMMARY

DAPT remains an essential component of treatment in patients with CAD, treated with and without PCI. Recommendations for duration of DAPT after PCI should consider patient-specific risk (ischemic potential vs bleeding risk), clinical presentation (ACS vs non-ACS, diabetes vs no diabetes), stent characteristics (first-generation vs second-generation DES), as well as technical and procedural factors (procedural complexity, lesion length, bifurcation stenting) (Table 3). Overall, primary studies and meta-analyses of prolonged DAPT of longer than 12 months after PCI demonstrate reduction in rates of ST and MI, at the cost of increased bleeding. Prolonged DAPT after ACS, in both PCI and non-PCI patients, reduces cardiovascular events without an increase in mortality. In patients with ACS treated with PCI, DAPT should be continued for at least 1 year. In those patients with high bleeding risk, a duration of less than 1 year with a minimum of 1 month is acceptable if using BMS or current-generation DES.[1] Duration of DAPT shorter than 1 year also may be considered in low-risk patients treated with second-generation DES. Overall, studies of shorter-duration DAPT after PCI in non-ACS populations treated with second-generation DES suggest similar mortality, MI, ST, and lower bleeding when compared with longer DAPT duration. This approach also may be reasonable in patients at high risk of bleeding or who require interruption, with a minimum duration of 1 month of DAPT.

DISCLOSURE

Dr D.L. Bhatt discloses the following relationships: *Advisory Board*: Cardax, Elsevier Practice Update Cardiology, Medscape Cardiology, Regado Biosciences; *Board of Directors*: Boston VA Research Institute, Society of Cardiovascular Patient Care; *Chair*: American Heart Association Quality Oversight Committee; *Data Monitoring Committees*: Duke Clinical Research Institute, Harvard Clinical Research Institute, Mayo Clinic, Population Health Research Institute; *Honoraria*: American College of Cardiology (Senior Associate Editor, Clinical Trials and News, ACC.org), Belvoir Publications (Editor in Chief, Harvard Heart Letter), Duke Clinical Research Institute (clinical trial steering committees), Harvard Clinical Research Institute (clinical trial steering committee), HMP Communications (Editor in Chief, Journal of Invasive Cardiology), Journal of the American College of Cardiology (Guest Editor; Associate Editor), Population Health Research Institute (clinical trial steering committee), Slack Publications (Chief Medical Editor, Cardiology

Table 3 Factors to consider when determining the optimal duration of DAPT after PCI		
	≤12 mo DAPT	**≥12 mo DAPT**
Patient-related factors	Patients with stable CAD	Patients with ACS
	Patients with a history of bleeding Patients with high risk of bleeding	Patients with diabetes mellitus Patients with renal dysfunction Patients with CHF Patients with previous ST Patients with PAD
Anatomy-related factors	Short lesion Single-vessel disease	Long lesion Small vessel Bifurcation lesion Complex anatomy Left-main coronary artery
Stent-related factors	Second-generation DES	First-generation DES Long stent Multiple stents

Abbreviations: ACS, acute coronary syndromes; CAD, coronary artery disease; CHF, congestive heart failure; DAPT, dual antiplatelet therapy; DES, drug-eluting stent; PAD, peripheral artery disease; PCI, percutaneous coronary intervention; ST, stent thrombosis.
From Eisen A, Bhatt DL. Antiplatelet therapy: defining the optimal duration of DAPT after PCI with DES. Nat Rev Cardiol 2015;12(8):456; with permission.

REFERENCES

1. Bagai A, Bhatt DL, Eikelboom JW, et al. Individualizing duration of dual antiplatelet therapy after
acute coronary syndrome or percutaneous coronary intervention. Circulation 2016;133(21):2094–8.
2. Mehta SR, Yusuf S, Peters RJG, et al. Effects of pretreatment with clopidogrel and aspirin followed by
long-term therapy in patients undergoing percutaneous coronary intervention: the PCI-CURE study.
Lancet 2001;358(9281):527–33.
3. Steinhubl SR, Berger PB, Mann JT 3rd, et al. Early
and sustained dual oral antiplatelet therapy
following percutaneous coronary intervention: a
randomized controlled trial. JAMA 2002;288(19):
2411–20.
4. Pfisterer M, Brunner-La Rocca HP, Buser PT, et al.
Late clinical events after clopidogrel discontinuation may limit the benefit of drug-eluting stents:
an observational study of drug-eluting versus
bare-metal stents. J Am Coll Cardiol 2006;48(12):
2584–91.
5. Nakazawa G. Stent thrombosis of drug eluting
stent: pathological perspective. J Cardiol 2011;
58(2):84–91.
6. Nakazawa G, Finn AV, Joner M, et al. Delayed arterial healing and increased late stent thrombosis at
culprit sites after drug-eluting stent placement for
acute myocardial infarction patients: an autopsy
study. Circulation 2008;118(11):1138–45.
7. Bhatt DL, Fox KA, Hacke W, et al. Clopidogrel and
aspirin versus aspirin alone for the prevention of
atherothrombotic events. N Engl J Med 2006;
354(16):1706–17.
8. Bhatt DL, Flather MD, Hacke W, et al. Patients with
prior myocardial infarction, stroke, or symptomatic
peripheral arterial disease in the CHARISMA trial.
J Am Coll Cardiol 2007;49(19):1982–8.
9. Lee CW, Ahn JM, Park DW, et al. Optimal duration
of dual antiplatelet therapy after drug-eluting stent

implantation: a randomized, controlled trial. Circulation 2014;129(3):304–12.
10. Collet J-P, Silvain J, Barthélémy O, et al. Dual-antiplatelet treatment beyond 1 year after drug-eluting
stent implantation (ARCTIC-Interruption): a randomised trial. Lancet 2014;384(9954):1577–85.
11. Mauri L, Kereiakes DJ, Yeh RW, et al. Twelve or 30
months of dual antiplatelet therapy after drug-
eluting stents. N Engl J Med 2014;371(23):2155–66.
12. Helft G, Steg PG, Le Feuvre C, et al. Stopping or
continuing clopidogrel 12 months after drug-
eluting stent placement: the OPTIDUAL randomized trial. Eur Heart J 2016;37(4):365–74.
13. Bonaca MP, Bhatt DL, Cohen M, et al. Long-term
use of ticagrelor in patients with prior myocardial
infarction. N Engl J Med 2015;372(19):1791–800.
14. Bhatt DL, Bonaca MP, Bansilal S, et al. Reduction in
ischemic events with ticagrelor in diabetic patients:
from the PEGASUS-TIMI 54 trial. J Am Coll Cardiol
2016;67(23):2732–40.
15. Bonaca MP, Bhatt DL, Storey RF, et al. Efficacy and
safety of ticagrelor as long-term secondary prevention in patients with peripheral artery disease and
prior myocardial infarction. J Am Coll Cardiol
2016;67(23):2719–2.
16. Yeh RW, Kereiakes DJ, Steg PG, et al. Benefits and
risks of extended duration dual antiplatelet therapy
after PCI in patients with and without acute
myocardial infarction. J Am Coll Cardiol 2015;
65(20):2211–21.
17. Palmerini T, Benedetto U, Bacchi-Reggiani L, et al.
Mortality in patients treated with extended duration dual antiplatelet therapy after drug-eluting
stent implantation: a pairwise and Bayesian
network meta-analysis of randomised trials. Lancet
2015;385(9985):2371–82.
18. Udell JA, Bonaca MP, Collet JP, et al. Long-term
dual antiplatelet therapy for secondary prevention
of cardiovascular events in the subgroup of
patients with previous myocardial infarction: a
collaborative meta-analysis of randomized trials.
Eur Heart J 2016;37(4):390–9.
19. FDA. FDA Drug safety communication: FDA review
finds long-term treatment with bloodthinning
medicine Plavix (clopidogrel) does not change risk
of death. Available at: http://www.fda.gov/Drugs/
DrugSafety/ucm471286.htm. Accessed September
1, 2016.
20. Gwon HC, Hahn JY, Park KW, et al. Six-month
versus 12-month dual antiplatelet therapy after
implantation of drug-eluting stents: the Efficacy of
Xience/Promus Versus Cypher to Reduce Late
Loss After Stenting (EXCELLENT) randomized,
multicenter study. Circulation 2012;125(3):505–13.
21. Colombo A, Chieffo A, Frasheri A, et al. Second-
generation drug-eluting stent implantation
followed by 6- versus 12-month dual antiplatelet

therapy: the SECURITY randomized clinical trial. J Am Coll Cardiol 2014;64(20):2086–97.

22. Schulz-Schupke S, Byrne RA, Ten Berg JM, et al. ISAR-SAFE: a randomized, double-blind, placebo-controlled trial of 6 vs. 12 months of clopidogrel therapy after drug-eluting stenting. Eur Heart J 2015;36(20):1252–63.

23. Gilard M, Barragan P, Noryani AA, et al. 6- versus 24-month dual antiplatelet therapy after implantation of drug-eluting stents in patients nonresistant to aspirin: the randomized, multicenter ITALIC trial. J Am Coll Cardiol 2015;65(8):777–86.

24. Valgimigli M, Campo G, Monti M, et al. Short-versus long-term duration of dual-antiplatelet therapy after coronary stenting: a randomized multicenter trial. Circulation 2012;125(16):2015–26.

25. Kim BK, Hong MK, Shin DH, et al. A new strategy for discontinuation of dual antiplatelet therapy: the RESET Trial (REal Safety and Efficacy of 3-month dual antiplatelet therapy following Endeavor zotarolimus-eluting stent implantation). J Am Coll Cardiol 2012;60(15):1340–8.

26. Feres F, Costa RA, Abizaid A, et al. Three vs twelve months of dual antiplatelet therapy after zotarolimus-eluting stents: the OPTIMIZE randomized trial. JAMA 2013;310(23):2510–22.

27. Palmerini T, Sangiorgi D, Valgimigli M, et al. Short-versus long-term dual antiplatelet therapy after drug-eluting stent implantation: an individual patient data pairwise and network meta-analysis. J Am Coll Cardiol 2015;65(11):1092–102.

28. Valgimigli M, Patialiakas A, Thury A, et al. Zotarolimus-eluting versus bare-metal stents in uncertain drug-eluting stent candidates. J Am Coll Cardiol 2015;65(8):805–15.

29. Ariotti S, Adamo M, Costa F, et al. Is bare-metal stent implantation still justifiable in high bleeding risk patients undergoing percutaneous coronary intervention? A pre-specified analysis from the ZEUS trial. JACC Cardiovasc Interv 2016;9(5):426–36.

30. Urban P, Meredith IT, Abizaid A, et al. Polymer-free drug-coated coronary stents in patients at high bleeding risk. N Engl J Med 2015;373(21): 2038–47.

31. Naber CK, Urban P, Ong PJ, et al. Biolimus-A9 polymer-free coated stent in high bleeding risk patients with acute coronary syndrome: a Leaders Free ACS sub-study. Eur Heart J 2016. [Epub ahead of print].

32. Levine GN, Bates ER, Blankenship JC, et al. 2011 ACCF/AHA/SCAI guideline for percutaneous coronary intervention. A report of the American College of Cardiology Foundation/American Heart Association task force on practice guidelines and the Society for Cardiovascular Angiography and interventions. J Am Coll Cardiol 2011;58(24): e44–122.

33. Levine GN, Bates ER, Bittl JA, et al. 2016 ACC/AHA guideline focused update on duration of dual antiplatelet therapy in patients with coronary artery disease: a report of the American College of Cardiology/American Heart Association task force on clinical practice guidelines: an update of the 2011 ACCF/AHA/SCAI guideline for percutaneous coronary intervention, 2011 ACCF/AHA guideline for coronary artery bypass graft surgery, 2012 ACC/AHA/ACP/AATS/PCNA/SCAI/STS guideline for the diagnosis and management of patients with stable ischemic heart disease, 2013 ACCF/AHA guideline for the management of ST-elevation myocardial infarction, 2014 AHA/ACC guideline for the management of patients with non-ST-elevation acute coronary syndromes, and 2014 ACC/AHA guideline on perioperative cardiovascular evaluation and management of patients undergoing noncardiac surgery. Circulation 2016; 134(10):e123–55.

34. Wallentin L, Becker RC, Budaj A, et al. Ticagrelor versus clopidogrel in patients with acute coronary syndromes. N Engl J Med 2009;361(11):1045–57.

35. Wiviott SD, Braunwald E, McCabe CH, et al. Prasugrel versus clopidogrel in patients with acute coronary syndromes. N Engl J Med 2007; 357(20):2001–15.

36. Authors/Task Force Members, Windecker S, Kolh P, Alfonso F, et al. 2014 ESC/EACTS guidelines on myocardial revascularization: the task force on myocardial revascularization of the European Society of Cardiology (ESC) and the European Association for Cardio-Thoracic Surgery (EACTS) developed with the special contribution of the European Association of Percutaneous Cardiovascular Interventions (EAPCI). Eur Heart J 2014;35(37): 2541–619.

37. Bangalore S, Toklu B, Bhatt DL. Outcomes with bioabsorbable vascular scaffolds versus everolimus eluting stents: insights from randomized trials. Int J Cardiol 2016;212:214–22.

38. Eisen A, Bhatt DL. Antiplatelet therapy: defining the optimal duration of DAPT after PCI with DES. Nat Rev Cardiol 2015;12(8):445–6.

39. Yeh RW, Secemsky EA, Kereiakes DJ, et al. Development and validation of a prediction rule for benefit and harm of dual antiplatelet therapy beyond 1 year after percutaneous coronary intervention. JAMA 2016;315(16):1735–49.

40. Kereiakes DJ, Yeh RW, Massaro JM, et al. DAPT score utility for risk prediction in patients with or without previous myocardial infarction. J Am Coll Cardiol 2016;67(21):2492–502.

41. Baber U, Mehran R, Giustino G, et al. Coronary thrombosis and major bleeding after PCI with drug-eluting stents: risk scores from PARIS. J Am Coll Cardiol 2016;67(19):2224–34.

42. Moukarbel GV, Bhatt DL. Antiplatelet therapy and proton pump inhibition: clinician update. Circulation 2012;125(2):375–80.

43. Angiolillo DJ, Gibson CM, Cheng S, et al. Differential effects of omeprazole and pantoprazole on the pharmacodynamics and pharmacokinetics of clopidogrel in healthy subjects: randomized, placebo-controlled, crossover comparison studies. Clin Pharmacol Ther 2011;89(1):65–74.

44. Frelinger AL 3rd, Lee RD, Mulford DJ, et al. A randomized, 2-period, crossover design study to assess the effects of dexlansoprazole, lansoprazole, esomeprazole, and omeprazole on the steady-state pharmacokinetics and pharmacodynamics of clopidogrel in healthy volunteers. J Am Coll Cardiol 2012;59(14):1304–11.

45. Bhatt DL, Cryer BL, Contant CF, et al. Clopidogrel with or without omeprazole in coronary artery disease. N Engl J Med 2010;363(20):1909–17.

46. Vaduganathan M, Bhatt DL, Cryer BL, et al. Proton-pump inhibitors reduce gastrointestinal events regardless of aspirin dose in patients requiring dual antiplatelet therapy. J Am Coll Cardiol 2016;67(14):1661–71.

47. Vardi M, Cryer BL, Cohen M, et al. The effects of proton pump inhibition on patient-reported severity of dyspepsia when receiving dual antiplatelet therapy with clopidogrel and low-dose aspirin: analysis from the clopidogrel and the optimization of gastrointestinal events trial. Aliment Pharmacol Ther 2015;42(3):365–74.

Cangrelor

Pharmacology, Clinical Data, and Role in Percutaneous Coronary Intervention

Matthew J. Price, MD

KEYWORDS

- Cangrelor • P2Y$_{12}$ receptor • Stent thrombosis • Myocardial infarction
- Percutaneous coronary intervention • Thienopyridine

KEY POINTS

- Cangrelor is an intravenous, non-thienopyridine, adenosine-triphosphate (ATP) analog that provides rapid and intensive inhibition of the platelet P2Y$_{12}$ receptor.
- In the CHAMPION PHOENIX trial, cangrelor reduced ischemic events at 48 hours compared with conventional clopidogrel therapy in thienopyridine-naive patients undergoing PCI, driven by reductions in myocardial infarction (MI) according to the universal definition and in stent thrombosis, with similar rates of major bleeding.
- Cangrelor reduces intraprocedural stent thrombosis, an uncommon event but one that is strongly associated with adverse cardiovascular outcomes.
- There is a pharmacodynamic interaction between the thienopyridines (clopidogrel and prasugrel) and cangrelor; the loading dose of clopidogrel should be given at the time of discontinuation of the cangrelor infusion, and the loading dose of prasugrel should be given at the end of the infusion or up to 30 minutes before it is stopped.
- Cangrelor is currently indicated as an adjunct to PCI to reduce the risk of MI, repeat coronary revascularization, and stent thrombosis in patients who have not been treated with a P2Y$_{12}$ platelet inhibitor and are not being given a glycoprotein IIb/IIIa inhibitor.

INTRODUCTION

The platelet P2Y$_{12}$ receptor plays a central role in the initiation and amplification of platelet activation that occurs due to endothelial disruption from spontaneous plaque rupture and iatrogenically during percutaneous coronary intervention (PCI). The oral P2Y$_{12}$ receptor antagonists, clopidogrel, prasugrel, and ticagrelor, reduce thrombotic events after acute coronary syndrome (ACS) and PCI.[1–5] However, these agents share several characteristics that may limit their ability to provide optimal protection from thrombotic events in the acute setting. Their onsets of action are fairly slow, with peak effects after a loading dose ranging from 4 to 6 hours with clopidogrel[6,7] to approximately 2 hours with prasugrel[7] and ticagrelor,[8] although the latter agents can provide more prompt antiplatelet effects when they are administered as crushed tablets.[9,10] This slow onset of action may be problematic in the acute setting of PCI, particularly in ACS, when the time from presentation to treatment may be short and where the onset of action of prasugrel and ticagrelor is further delayed.[11,12] In addition, the oral agents have a prolonged offset of action: as long as 5 to 7 days for clopidogrel,[6,13,14] 7 to 9 days for prasugrel,[13] and 3 to 5 days for ticagrelor.[8] This delay in the recovery of platelet function can result in increased bleeding, length of hospital

Division of Cardiovascular Diseases, Scripps Clinic, 9898 Genesee Avenue, Suite AMP-200, La Jolla, CA 92037, USA
E-mail address: price.matthew@scrippshealth.org

Intervent Cardiol Clin 6 (2017) 39–47
http://dx.doi.org/10.1016/j.iccl.2016.08.012
2211-7458/17/© 2016 Elsevier Inc. All rights reserved.

stay, and resource use in patients who require coronary artery bypass grafting (CABG) after pretreatment with the oral agents.[15] In the case of clopidogrel, a substantial interindividual variability in antiplatelet effect results in high levels of on-treatment platelet reactivity in a significant proportion of patients, which has been strongly associated with thrombotic and ischemic events during and after PCI.[16–18]

Therefore, there is an unmet clinical need for a $P2Y_{12}$ antagonist with a rapid onset of action and a consistent and potent antiplatelet effect while allowing for a prompt return of platelet function after discontinuation. Cangrelor is an intravenous, nucleotide-mimetic, directly acting $P2Y_{12}$ receptor antagonist indicated as an adjunct to PCI in patients who have not been treated with a $P2Y_{12}$ inhibitor. Herein, the pharmacology, clinical data, and rationale for the use of cangrelor is presented in detail.

PHARMACOLOGY AND METABOLISM

Cangrelor is a non-thienopyridine adenosine triphosphate analogue (ie, a nucleotide-mimetic) with the chemical structure shown in Fig. 1. Cangrelor is administered intravenously and exerts its antiplatelet effects by directly and reversibly interacting with the $P2Y_{12}$ receptor. The mechanism of action has not been well defined, although competitive binding at the adenosine diphosphate (ADP)-binding site has

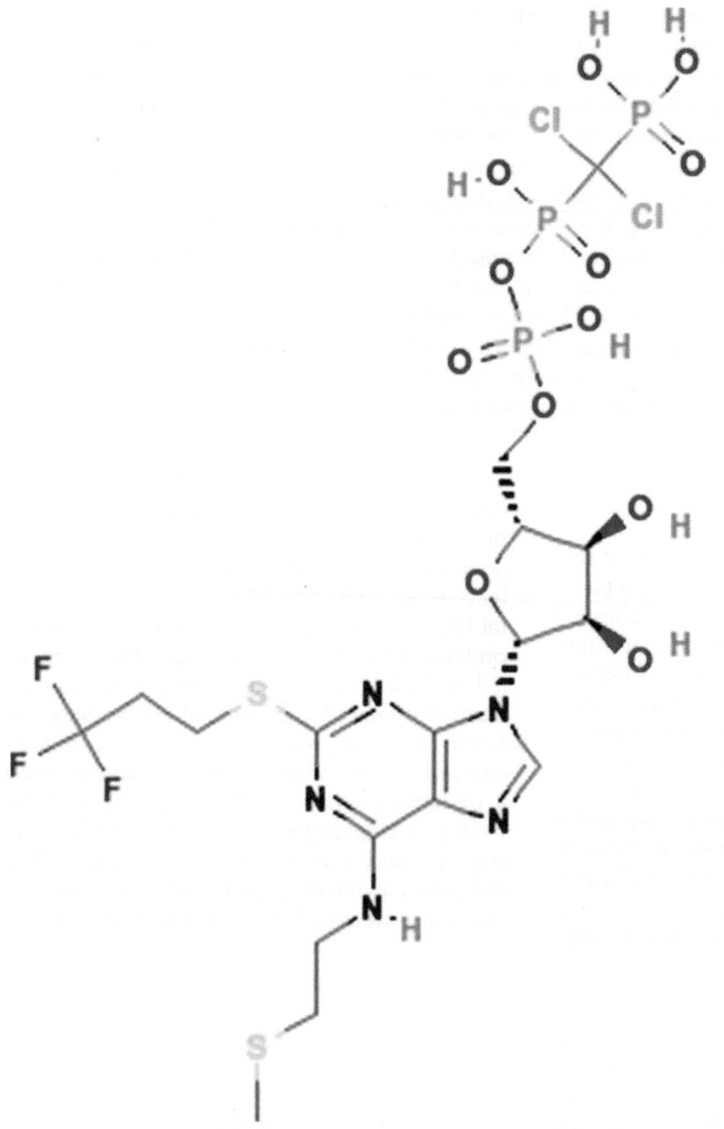

Fig. 1. Chemical structure of cangrelor. Cangrelor is an ATP analogue that directly and reversibly interacts with the platelet $P2Y_{12}$ receptor to inhibit ADP-induced platelet activation. ATP, adenosine triphosphate.

been proposed,[19] which would explain the observed interaction when thienopyridines are administered during a cangrelor infusion.[20] The average half-life is 3.5 to 6 minutes in healthy volunteers. Cangrelor is metabolized through dephosphorylation by ectonucleotidase (CD39) to form a nucleoside (AR-C69712XX). AR-C69412XX is further metabolized into several products and is primarily eliminated in the urine and to a lesser degree in the feces. The plasma concentration-time profiles for cangrelor and its primary metabolite are comparable between patients with renal insufficiency and healthy volunteers, and therefore, dose adjustment based on renal function is not required or recommended.

PHARMACODYNAMICS

A cangrelor bolus followed by infusion provides near complete $P2Y_{12}$ receptor occupancy and inhibition of ADP-induced $P2Y_{12}$ platelet aggregation within minutes of administration. In healthy volunteers, a 30-μg/kg bolus followed by a 4-μg/kg/min infusion provided extensive inhibition of platelet aggregation by 2 minutes after the bolus dose, and 80% of subjects returned to near-baseline platelet activity within 60 minutes (Fig. 2).[21] In the BRIDGE (Maintenance of Platelet Inhibition With Cangrelor After Discontinuation of Thienopyridines in Patients Undergoing Surgery) trial,[22] which randomly assigned patients who had received a thienopyridine and were awaiting cardiac surgery to either placebo or 0.75-μg/kg infusion of cangrelor until surgery was performed, patients treated with cangrelor had low levels of platelet reactivity throughout the treatment period (a median infusion duration of 2.8 days), and platelet reactivity

was not significantly different between cangrelor-treated patients before surgical incision at a median of 3.2 hours after discontinuation of the infusion and patients treated with placebo (Fig. 3).[22]

THIENOPYRIDINE-CLOPIDOGREL INTERACTION

Pharmacodynamic studies demonstrate a substantial interaction when a thienopyridine loading dose is administered during cangrelor infusion. Specifically, the antiplatelet effect of a clopidogrel or prasugrel loading dose is substantially attenuated when given in the midst of the infusion (and therefore will not provide the anticipated $P2Y_{12}$ inhibition once the infusion is discontinued), likely because the labile, short-lived active metabolite of clopidogrel and prasugrel cannot bind to the $P2Y_{12}$ receptor when it is occupied by cangrelor.[23–26] Therefore, a clopidogrel loading dose should be administered at the end of the cangrelor infusion, and a prasugrel loading dose should be administered at the end of the infusion or up to 30 minutes before it is stopped.[27] Ticagrelor, which appears to have a $P2Y_{12}$ binding site separate from cangelor,[19] can be administered at any time during cangrelor administration.[27]

CLINICAL SAFETY AND EFFICACY

CHAMPION (Cangrelor vs Standard Therapy to Achieve Optimal Management of Platelet Inhibition) PHOENIX was a double-blind, double-dummy, placebo-controlled trial that randomly assigned 11,145 patients who were undergoing PCI to either intravenous cangrelor or clopidogrel.[28] Patients were eligible to be enrolled if they

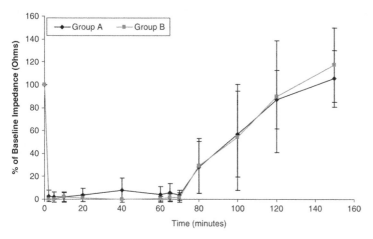

Fig. 2. Effect of cangrelor on ADP-induced (20 μM) platelet aggregation by whole-blood electrical impedance in healthy volunteers. Group A, cangrelor 15-μg/kg bolus + 2-μg/kg/min infusion for 1 hour; group B, cangrelor 30-μg/kg bolus + 4-μg/kg/min infusion for 1 hour. Data are presented as mean ± SD. (*Adapted from* Akers WS, Oh JJ, Oestreich JH, et al. Pharmacokinetics and pharmacodynamics of a bolus and infusion of cangrelor: a direct, parenteral P2Y12 receptor antagonist. J Clin Pharmacol 2010;50:27–35; with permission.)

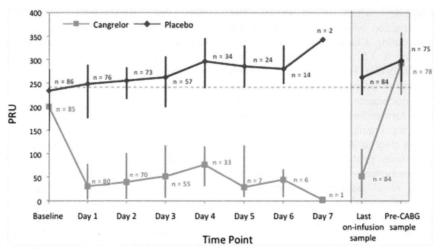

Fig. 3. Platelet reactivity as assessed by PRU using the VerifyNow P2Y12 assay during the study time course of the BRIDGE trial (at baseline and up to 7 days of study drug infusion and at last sample taken before CABG). The infusion dose was 0.75 µg/kg/min (lower than the PCI infusion dose of 4 µg/kg/min) and was discontinued a median of 3.2 hours (interquartile range, 2–5 hours) before surgical incision. At the time of surgical incision, platelet reactivity was not significantly different to placebo (P = .21), and there were no significant differences in CABG-related major bleeding. PRU, P2Y12 reaction units. (Adapted from Angiolillo DJ, Firstenberg MS, Price MJ, et al. Bridging antiplatelet therapy with cangrelor in patients undergoing cardiac surgery. JAMA 2012;307:265–74; with permission.)

had not been treated previously with platelet inhibitors and were undergoing PCI for ST-elevation myocardial infarction (STEMI), non-ST-segment elevation acute coronary syndrome (NSTE-ACS), or stable angina. Patients randomly assigned to cangrelor received a cangrelor bolus and infusion (30-µg/kg bolus followed by a 4 µg/kg/min) and placebo capsules; cangrelor was continued for at least 2 hours or for the duration of the procedure, whichever was longer. At the end of the infusion, patients received a clopidogrel 600-mg loading dose. Patients randomly assigned to clopidogrel received either 600 mg or 300 mg of clopidogrel based on clinician preference as well as a placebo bolus and infusion followed by placebo capsules. The primary endpoint was a composite of death, myocardial infarction (MI), ischemia-driven revascularization, or stent thrombosis at 48 hours. The definition of periprocedural MI was based on the universal definition of MI and involved an assessment of patients' baseline biomarker status. In patients with normal biomarkers at baseline, an MI was considered to have occurred if there was post-PCI elevation in creatine kinase-MB (CK-MB) 3 times or more than the upper limit of normal (ULN). If baseline biomarkers were abnormal, additional clinical evidence of ischemia was required.[29] Stent thrombosis included definite stent thrombosis according to the Academic Research Consortium definition,[30] or intraprocedural stent thrombosis, which was assessed by a blinded angiographic core laboratory. The primary safety end point was severe bleeding not related to CABG at 48 hours, according to the Global Use of Strategies to Open Occluded Coronary Arteries (GUSTO) criteria.[31]

Cangrelor significantly reduced the primary efficacy endpoint at 48 hours (4.7 vs 5.9%, odds ratio [OR] 0.78, 95% confidence interval [CI] 0.66–0.93, P = .005), driven by reductions in MI and stent thrombosis. The treatment effect of cangrelor was consistent across subgroups, and whether the patient received a clopidogrel 300 mg or 600 mg loading dose. The reduction in periprocedural MI with cangrelor was consistent regardless of definition used: cangrelor decreased the rate of MI according to the per-protocol definition (3.8% vs 4.7%; OR 0.80; 95% CI, 0.67–0.97; P = .02), the Society for Cardiovascular Angiography and Intervention definition (OR 0.65; 95% CI, 0.46–0.92; P = .01), and the rate of MI with peak CK-MB $\geq$ 10 $\times$ ULN (OR 0.64; 95% CI, 0.45–0.91).[29] There was a significant association between the occurrence of MI by any of these definitions and mortality at 30 days (Fig. 4). Cangrelor reduced the primary endpoint consistently in patients presenting with stable angina or ACS (OR 0.83; 95% CI, 0.67–1.01; OR 0.71; 95% CI, 0.52–0.96, respectively, interaction P = .41). The reduction in stent thrombosis was also consistent across patients presenting with stable angina and ACS (interaction P = .62).

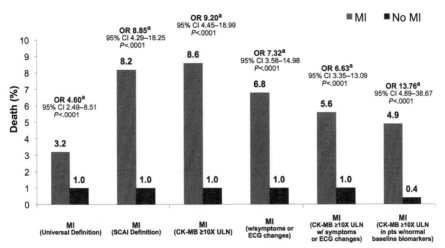

Fig. 4. Association between the type of MI using various definitions and the risk of death at 30 days in the CHAMPION PHOENIX randomized clinical trial. [a] Adjusted for treatment, patient status, age (≥65 years), history of congestive heart failure (CHF), diabetes, prior MI, country (United States vs non-United States), PCI duration. ECG, electrocardiogram; SCAI, Society for Cardiovascular Angiography and Intervention. (*Adapted from* Cavender MA, Bhatt DL, Stone GW, et al, CHAMPION PHOENIX Investigators. Consistent reduction in peri-procedural myocardial infarction with cangrelor as assessed by multiple definitions: findings from CHAMPION PHOENIX (Cangrelor versus standard therapy to achieve optimal management of platelet inhibition). Circulation 2016;134(10):723–33; with permission.)

Patients treated with cangrelor were less likely to need bailout glycoprotein IIb/IIIa inhibitors (2.3% vs 3.5%, OR 0.65; 95% CI, 0.52–0.82; P<.001) and had less procedural complications (3.4% vs 4.5%, OR 0.74; 95% CI, 0.61–0.90; P = .002).

A unique aspect of the CHAMPION PHOENIX trial was the assessment of all procedural angiograms by a blinded core laboratory for the occurrence of intraprocedural stent thrombosis. Thrombus was defined as any discrete, mobile, intraluminal filling defect with defined borders, with or without associated contrast staining or a total occlusion with convex edges and staining. Intraprocedural stent thrombosis occurred in 89 of the 10,939 patients (0.8%) in whom angiograms were available for review. According to adjusted analyses, intraprocedural stent thrombosis was strongly associated with subsequent ischemic events, including out-of-laboratory stent thrombosis, MI, and death. Cangrelor significantly reduced the rate of intraprocedural stent thrombosis compared with clopidogrel (0.6% vs 1.0%, OR 0.65; 95% CI: 0.42–0.99; P = .04), contributing to its efficacy in reducing the individual endpoints of MI and stent thrombosis compared with clopidogrel.[32]

The primary safety endpoint, GUSTO severe bleeding, occurred uncommonly and the rates were not significantly different between groups (0.16% vs 0.11%, OR 1.50; 95% CI 0.53–4.22; P = .44), although ACUITY major bleeding, which is a more sensitive definition, was more frequent with cangrelor (4.3% vs 2.5%, OR 1.72; 95% CI 1.39–2.13; P<.001). There was no interaction between the effect of cangrelor on bleeding and whether femoral or radial access was used (interaction P = .54), although the absolute rates of bleeding were much lower with the radial approach (ACUITY major bleeding: femoral cohort, 5.2% with cangrelor vs 3.1% with clopidogrel [OR 1.69, 95% CI 1.35–2.12, P<.0001]; radial cohort, 1.5% with cangrelor vs 0.7% with clopidogrel [OR 2.17, 95% CI 1.02–4.62], P = .04).[33] In a post hoc, adjusted analysis of the pooled cangrelor trial experience, cangrelor alone was associated with similar ischemic risk and a trend toward lower risk-adjusted severe bleeding risk compared with clopidogrel plus routine glycoprotein IIb/IIIa inhibitor use.

Based on the results of the CHAMPION PHOENIX trial, the US Food and Drug Administration (FDA) has approved the use of cangrelor as an adjunct to PCI to reduce the risk of MI, repeat coronary revascularization, and stent thrombosis in patients who have not been treated with a $P2Y_{12}$ platelet inhibitor and are not being given a glycoprotein IIb/IIIa inhibitor.

CHAMPION PCI and PLATFORM

CHAMPION PCI and CHAMPION PLATFORM were 2 other randomized clinical trials that preceded CHAMPION PHOENIX and also

Table 1
The phase III clinical trials of cangrelor

Trial	Trial Size (N)	Prior Exposure to Thienopyridine	Comparator	Endpoint	Duration (h)	Outcome
CHAMPION PCI	8877	Prior exposure allowed	Clopidogrel 600 mg within 30 min before PCI	Death, MI,[a] or IDR	48	7.5% vs 7.1%, P = .59
CHAMPION PLATFORM	5362	Naive patients only	Clopidogrel 600 mg at end of PCI	Death, MI,[a] or IDR	48	7.0% vs 8.0%, P = .17
CHAMPION PHOENIX	11,145	Naive patients only	Clopidogrel 300 or 600 mg, dose and timing per operator	Death, MI (universal definition), IDR, or ST	48	4.7% vs 5.9%, P = .005

Abbreviations: IDR, ischemia-driven revascularization; ST, stent thrombosis.
[a] CHAMPION PCI and PLATFORM did not use the universal definition of MI.

evaluated the safety and efficacy of cangrelor in patients undergoing PCI (Table 1). The CHAMPION PCI trial randomly assigned 8716 patients to receive a bolus and infusion of cangrelor followed by transition to clopidogrel or to receive a clopidogrel 600 mg loading dose within 30 minutes of the start of PCI.[34] The CHAMPION PLATFORM trial randomly assigned 5362 patients who had not been treated with a thienopyridine to receive a bolus and infusion of cangrelor followed by transition to clopidogrel or to receive a clopidogrel 600 mg loading dose immediately after the procedure.[35] In CHAMPION PCI, patients with stable angina, NSTE-ACS, and STEMI were eligible to be enrolled, whereas in CHAMPION PLATFORM, most enrolled patients had NSTE-ACS. Therefore, the 2 trials differed according to the types of patients included and the timing of clopidogrel administration in the control group. Cangrelor was not superior to clopidogrel in either trial with respect to the primary endpoint of death from any cause, MI, or ischemia-driven revascularization at 48 hours. However, a post hoc analysis of the pooled CHAMPION PCI and CHAMPION PLATFORM trials demonstrated a significant reduction in the primary endpoint of death, MI, and ischemia-driven revascularization with cangrelor when the universal definition of MI (similar to the definition in CHAMPION PHOENIX) was used (OR 0.82, 95% CI 0.68–0.99, $P = .037$), rather than the per-protocol definition.[36] The short times from randomization to PCI in CHAMPION PCI and PLATFORM may represent a diagnostic challenge to identify a PCI-related MI in patients with elevated biomarkers at presentation, because in these cases, increased biomarker levels after the procedure may reflect the initial thrombotic event rather than a result of the procedure. Therefore, the universal definition of MI, similar to that used in the subsequent CHAMPION PHOENIX trial, may enhance discrimination in detecting PCI-related MI and may allow a more rigorous assessment of the therapeutic benefit of adjunctive pharmacologic interventions.[37]

Pooled Analyses

A patient-level, pooled meta-analysis of all 3 phase III trials, involving in total 24,910 patients, demonstrated that cangrelor significantly reduced the rate of the composite outcome of death, MI according to the universal definition, ischemia-driven revascularization, or stent thrombosis at 48 hours compared with clopidogrel (3.8% vs 4.7%, OR 0.81; 95% CI, 0.71–0.91, $P = .0007$).[38] Cangrelor also reduced the rate of the individual endpoint of stent thrombosis (0.5% vs 0.8%; OR 0.59, 95% CI 0.43–0.80, $P = .0008$). Cangrelor did not increase the risk of GUSTO severe bleeding, GUSTO moderate bleeding, or the need for blood transfusion, but did increase bleeding according to more sensitive indices such as ACUITY major bleeding (4.2 vs 2.8%, $P<.0001$). However, when excluding hematomas greater than 5 cm in diameter, the absolute difference in ACUITY major bleeds was small, although still statistically significant (1.3 vs 1.0%, $P = .007$).

CANGRELOR FOR SURGICAL BRIDGING

At least 5 and 7 days are required for platelet functional recovery after discontinuation of clopidogrel and prasugrel, respectively.[13,14] This slow offset results in surgical delays in patients with ACSs and also represents a clinical dilemma in patients with drug-eluting stents who require surgery. BRIDGE was a phase II trial that evaluated the use of cangrelor for bridging thienopyridine-treated patients to CABG. A total of 210 patients with ACS or treated with a coronary stent, who had received a thienopyridine and were awaiting CABG surgery, were randomly assigned to receive either cangrelor infusion or placebo. The primary efficacy endpoint was platelet reactivity measured by the VerifyNow P2Y12 test (Accriva, San Diego, CA, USA), and the main safety endpoint was excessive CABG-related bleeding. A greater proportion of patients treated with cangrelor had low levels of platelet reactivity throughout the treatment period (98.8% vs 19%, $P<.001$) (see Fig. 3); there were no significant differences in major bleeding before CABG or excessive CABG-related bleeding.[22] This study was not powered to address ischemic outcomes. At present, cangrelor does not have an FDA indication for use in the setting of bridging to surgery.

SUMMARY

Cangrelor is an intravenous antiplatelet agent that provides intensive P2Y$_{12}$ inhibition with rapid onset and offset. Cangrelor reduces ischemic events compared with conventional clopidogrel therapy in thienopyridine-naive patients undergoing PCI, driven by reductions in MI according to the universal definition and in stent thrombosis, with similar rates of major bleeding and blood transfusions but at the cost of more minor bleeding events. Keen attention should be paid to the timing of thienopyridine loading in patients receiving cangrelor: given the well-documented pharmacodynamic interaction that may negate the antiplatelet effect of the oral drug if given during infusion, a thienopyridine loading dose should be given at the time of discontinuation of the cangrelor infusion. Cangrelor represents an important addition to the pharmacologic armamentarium of the interventional cardiologist for the acute care of patients undergoing PCI, because it does not require oral administration and reduces periprocedural MI and early stent thrombosis without increasing major bleeding or the need for transfusion.

REFERENCES

1. Yusuf S, Zhao F, Mehta SR, et al. Effects of clopidogrel in addition to aspirin in patients with acute coronary syndromes without ST-segment elevation. N Engl J Med 2001;345:494–502.
2. Mehta SR, Yusuf S, Peters RJ, et al. Effects of pretreatment with clopidogrel and aspirin followed by long-term therapy in patients undergoing percutaneous coronary intervention: the PCI-CURE study. Lancet 2001;358:527–33.
3. Wiviott SD, Braunwald E, McCabe CH, et al. Prasugrel versus clopidogrel in patients with acute coronary syndromes. N Engl J Med 2007;357:2001–15.
4. Wallentin L, Becker RC, Budaj A, et al. Ticagrelor versus clopidogrel in patients with acute coronary syndromes. N Engl J Med 2009;361:1045–57.
5. Lindholm D, Varenhorst C, Cannon CP, et al. Ticagrelor vs. clopidogrel in patients with non-ST-elevation acute coronary syndrome with or without revascularization: results from the PLATO trial. Eur Heart J 2014;35:2083–93.
6. Price MJ, Coleman JL, Steinhubl SR, et al. Onset and offset of platelet inhibition after high-dose clopidogrel loading and standard daily therapy measured by a point-of-care assay in healthy volunteers. Am J Cardiol 2006;98:681–4.
7. Wallentin L, Varenhorst C, James S, et al. Prasugrel achieves greater and faster P2Y12 receptor-mediated platelet inhibition than clopidogrel due to more efficient generation of its active metabolite in aspirin-treated patients with coronary artery disease. Eur Heart J 2008;29:21–30.
8. Gurbel PA, Bliden KP, Butler K, et al. Randomized double-blind assessment of the ONSET and OFFSET of the antiplatelet effects of ticagrelor versus clopidogrel in patients with stable coronary artery disease: the ONSET/OFFSET study. Circulation 2009;120:2577–85.
9. Parodi G, Xanthopoulou I, Bellandi B, et al. Ticagrelor crushed tablets administration in STEMI patients: the MOJITO study. J Am Coll Cardiol 2015;65:511–2.
10. Rollini F, Franchi F, Hu J, et al. Crushed prasugrel tablets in patients with STEMI undergoing primary percutaneous coronary intervention: the CRUSH study. J Am Coll Cardiol 2016;67:1994–2004.
11. Alexopoulos D, Xanthopoulou I, Gkizas V, et al. Randomized assessment of ticagrelor versus prasugrel antiplatelet effects in patients with ST-segment-elevation myocardial infarction. Circ Cardiovasc Interv 2012;5:797–804.
12. Parodi G, Valenti R, Bellandi B, et al. Comparison of prasugrel and ticagrelor loading doses in ST-segment elevation myocardial infarction patients: RAPID (Rapid Activity of Platelet Inhibitor Drugs) primary PCI study. J Am Coll Cardiol 2013;61:1601–6.
13. Price MJ, Walder JS, Baker BA, et al. Recovery of platelet function after discontinuation of prasugrel or clopidogrel maintenance dosing in aspirin-treated patients with stable coronary disease: the recovery trial. J Am Coll Cardiol 2012;59:2338–43.
14. Price MJ, Teirstein PS. Dynamics of platelet functional recovery following a clopidogrel loading dose in healthy volunteers. Am J Cardiol 2008;102:790–5.
15. Fox KA, Mehta SR, Peters R, et al. Benefits and risks of the combination of clopidogrel and aspirin in patients undergoing surgical revascularization for non-ST-elevation acute coronary syndrome: the Clopidogrel in Unstable angina to prevent Recurrent ischemic Events (CURE) trial. Circulation 2004;110:1202–8.
16. Price MJ, Angiolillo DJ, Teirstein PS, et al. Platelet reactivity and cardiovascular outcomes after percutaneous coronary intervention: a time-dependent analysis of the gauging responsiveness with a VerifyNow P2Y12 assay: impact on thrombosis and safety (GRAVITAS) trial. Circulation 2011;124:1132–7.
17. Stone GW, Witzenbichler B, Weisz G, et al. Platelet reactivity and clinical outcomes after coronary artery implantation of drug-eluting stents (ADAPT-DES): a prospective multicentre registry study. Lancet 2013;382:614–23.
18. Tantry US, Bonello L, Aradi D, et al, Working Group on On-Treatment Platelet Reactivity. Consensus and update on the definition of on-treatment platelet reactivity to adenosine diphosphate associated with ischemia and bleeding. J Am Coll Cardiol 2013;62:2261–73.
19. Zhang J, Zhang K, Gao ZG, et al. Agonist-bound structure of the human P2Y12 receptor. Nature 2014;509:119–22.
20. Price MJ. The pharmacodynamics of switching between P2Y12 receptor antagonists. JACC Cardiovasc Interv 2016;9:1099–101.
21. Akers WS, Oh JJ, Oestreich JH, et al. Pharmacokinetics and pharmacodynamics of a bolus and infusion

of cangrelor: a direct, parenteral P2Y12 receptor antagonist. J Clin Pharmacol 2010;50:27–35.

22. Angiolillo DJ, Firstenberg MS, Price MJ, et al. Bridging antiplatelet therapy with cangrelor in patients undergoing cardiac surgery. JAMA 2012; 307:265–74.

23. Dovlatova NL, Jakubowski JA, Sugidachi A, et al. The reversible P2Y antagonist cangrelor influences the ability of the active metabolites of clopidogrel and prasugrel to produce irreversible inhibition of platelet function. J Thromb Haemost 2008;6:1153–9.

24. Schneider DJ, Agarwal Z, Seecheran N, et al. Pharmacodynamic effects when clopidogrel is given before cangrelor discontinuation. J Interv Cardiol 2015;28:415–9.

25. Schneider DJ, Seecheran N, Raza SS, et al. Pharmacodynamic effects during the transition between cangrelor and prasugrel. Coron Artery Dis 2015; 26:42–8.

26. Steinhubl SR, Oh JJ, Oestreich JH, et al. Transitioning patients from cangrelor to clopidogrel: pharmacodynamic evidence of a competitive effect. Thromb Res 2008;121:527–34.

27. Schneider DJ. Transition strategies from cangrelor to oral platelet P2Y12 receptor antagonists. Coron Artery Dis 2016;27:65–9.

28. Bhatt DL, Stone GW, Mahaffey KW, et al. Effect of platelet inhibition with cangrelor during PCI on ischemic events. N Engl J Med 2013;368:1303–13.

29. Cavender MA, Bhatt DL, Stone GW, et al, CHAMPION PHOENIX Investigators. Consistent reduction in peri-procedural myocardial infarction with cangrelor as assessed by multiple definitions: findings from CHAMPION PHOENIX (Cangrelor versus standard therapy to achieve optimal management of platelet inhibition). Circulation 2016;134(10): 723–33.

30. Cutlip DE, Windecker S, Mehran R, et al. Clinical end points in coronary stent trials: a case for standardized definitions. Circulation 2007;115:2344–51.

31. An international randomized trial comparing four thrombolytic strategies for acute myocardial infarction. The GUSTO investigators. N Engl J Med 1993; 329:673–82.

32. Genereux P, Stone GW, Harrington RA, et al. Impact of intraprocedural stent thrombosis during percutaneous coronary intervention: insights from the CHAMPION PHOENIX Trial (clinical trial comparing cangrelor to clopidogrel standard of care therapy in subjects who require percutaneous coronary intervention). J Am Coll Cardiol 2014;63:619–29.

33. Gutierrez JA, Harrington RA, Blankenship JC, et al. The effect of cangrelor and access site on ischaemic and bleeding events: insights from CHAMPION PHOENIX. Eur Heart J 2016;37:1122–30.

34. Harrington RA, Stone GW, McNulty S, et al. Platelet inhibition with cangrelor in patients undergoing PCI. N Engl J Med 2009;361:2318–29.

35. Bhatt DL, Lincoff AM, Gibson CM, et al. Intravenous platelet blockade with cangrelor during PCI. N Engl J Med 2009;361:2330–41.

36. White HD, Chew DP, Dauerman HL, et al. Reduced immediate ischemic events with cangrelor in PCI: a pooled analysis of the CHAMPION trials using the universal definition of myocardial infarction. Am Heart J 2012;163:182–90.e4.

37. Leonardi S, Truffa AA, Neely ML, et al. A novel approach to systematically implement the universal definition of myocardial infarction: insights from the CHAMPION PLATFORM trial. Heart 2013;99:1282–7.

38. Steg PG, Bhatt DL, Hamm CW, et al. Effect of cangrelor on periprocedural outcomes in percutaneous coronary interventions: a pooled analysis of patient-level data. Lancet 2013;382:1981–92.

Ticagrelor
Effects Beyond the P2Y$_{12}$ Receptor

Wael Sumaya, MD, MRCP*,
Robert F. Storey, BM, DM, MRCP, FESC

KEYWORDS

- Ticagrelor • Adenosine • P2Y$_{12}$ antagonist • Inflammation • Acute coronary syndrome

KEY POINTS

- Ticagrelor is a potent, reversibly binding inhibitor of platelet P2Y$_{12}$ receptors, inhibiting both platelet aggregation and release of platelets' stored inflammatory mediators.
- Ticagrelor also weakly inhibits cellular adenosine uptake via the equilibrative nucleoside transporter-1 transporter protein and this might explain some of the positive and adverse effects of ticagrelor.
- Ticagrelor positively modulates fibrin clot in a human model of sepsis-induced inflammation and this effect might contribute to the reduction in sepsis-related deaths in ticagrelor-treated patients observed in the PLATO trial.
- Some evidence suggests that ticagrelor positively impacts endothelial function.

INTRODUCTION

The development of platelet P2Y$_{12}$ inhibitors has been pivotal in the era of percutaneous coronary intervention (PCI) as a mainstay treatment of coronary artery disease (CAD). Platelets play a central role in arterial thrombosis. Following plaque rupture, platelets adhere to exposed collagen through the glycoprotein VI receptor, leading to platelet activation that is reinforced by thrombin generated as a consequence of tissue factor expression. This leads to the release of multiple agonists, including adenosine diphosphate (ADP), which amplifies and sustains platelet activation through the platelet P2Y$_{12}$ receptor. Activated platelets undergo shape change and express activated glycoprotein IIb/IIIa receptors that bind fibrinogen, which mediates platelet-platelet cross-linking and consequent platelet aggregation and thrombus formation.[1–3] Targeting the platelet P2Y$_{12}$ receptor has proved successful in reducing ischemic events and dual antiplatelet therapy with aspirin, and a P2Y$_{12}$ receptor antagonist is recommended following acute coronary syndrome (ACS) and PCI.[4,5]

The PLATelet inhibition and patient Outcomes (PLATO) trial[6] compared the novel P2Y$_{12}$ inhibitor ticagrelor with clopidogrel in moderate-risk to high-risk patients with ACS, and found it to be superior to clopidogrel in reducing major adverse cardiovascular events. Ticagrelor was also associated with improved all-cause mortality out of proportion to what was observed with other trials using different

Disclosure Statement: W. Sumaya is funded by a BHF clinical research training fellowship (grant number FS/15/82/31824) and reports no conflicts of interest; R.F. Storey has received Institutional Research Grants from AstraZeneca; consultancy fees from AstraZeneca, Aspen, Correvio, The Medicines Company, PlaqueTec, and Thermo-Fisher Scientific; as well as speaker fees from AstraZeneca and Medscape.
Department of Infection, Immunity and Cardiovascular Disease, University of Sheffield, Beech Hill Road, Sheffield S10 2RX, UK
* Corresponding author.
E-mail address: w.sumaya@sheffield.ac.uk

P2Y$_{12}$ inhibitors.[7,8] The rates of sudden death, lower respiratory tract infections, and sepsis-related deaths were lower in the ticagrelor-treated group as compared with the clopidogrel-treated group.[9–11] This has led to the hypothesis that ticagrelor might exhibit unintended ("off-target") effects beyond those related to prevention of thrombosis and that these might be relevant to its clinical efficacy. This has attracted a plethora of research into the pleiotropic effects of ticagrelor. In this article we aim to review those effects and elucidate some of the potential mechanisms of actions driving those effects.

TICAGRELOR AND INFLAMMATION

Platelets play a central role in hemostasis, but their role in inflammation and immune response is increasingly recognized.[12] Platelets are anucleate cells generated from bone marrow megakaryocytes. On activation, they release several agonists (ADP, adenosine triphosphate [ATP], serotonin) from their dense granules and many inflammatory cytokines, adhesion molecules, von Willebrand factor, and some coagulation factors from their α-granules.[2,13] Inflammatory mediators include P-selectin, platelet factor 4 (PF4), RANTES, interleukin (IL)-1, and CD40L among many others.[13] These mediators chemoattract and stimulate leukocytes. Activated platelets express P-selectin on their surface and interact with leukocytes and endothelial cells expressing P-selectin glycoprotein-1 (PSGL-1). This interaction leads to mutual stimulation of both cell types, promoting the inflammatory cascade.[14,15]

Blocking platelet P2Y$_{12}$ receptors not only inhibits platelet aggregation but also dampens release of inflammatory mediators from α-granules, thereby modulating platelet-leukocyte interaction and other proinflammatory responses.

Clopidogrel is a thienopyridine prodrug, irreversible inhibitor of the platelet P2Y$_{12}$ receptor. Most of clopidogrel is converted to inactive metabolites by plasma carboxylesterases and approximately 15% is converted to its active metabolite by the cytochrome P450 (CYP) enzymes.[16] Because of the variable efficiency of metabolism of clopidogrel, in part due to common *CYP2C19* loss-of-function alleles, there is wide interindividual variability in pharmacodynamic response.[17] Clopidogrel attenuates the levels of inflammatory mediators in patients with CAD, including P-selectin, CD40L, and RANTES, and also reduces the formation of platelet-leukocyte aggregates.[18,19] Clopidogrel

also reduced inflammatory marker level C-reactive protein (CRP) in patients with stable CAD, ACS, and those undergoing PCI.[18,20,21] Tumor necrosis factor α (TNF-α) levels are also reduced in patients with ACS treated with clopidogrel.[20]

Unlike clopidogrel, ticagrelor is a cyclopentyl-triazolopyrimidine, directly acting, and reversibly binding P2Y$_{12}$ inhibitor. Because it is not a prodrug, this reduces the chance of varying interindividual pharmacodynamic response such as that observed with clopidogrel, and allows it to offer rapid platelet inhibition within 30 to 60 minutes in stable patients.[22] In patients with ST-elevation myocardial infarction, onset of action may be delayed, at least partly due to effects of opiate analgesia on gastric transit time.[23] Platelet inhibition with ticagrelor is significantly more pronounced and consistent than with clopidogrel.[24]

Our group has recently demonstrated that both ticagrelor and clopidogrel were able to attenuate inflammatory responses in association with reduced platelet-monocyte aggregate formation in a human model of sepsis-related inflammation induced by endotoxin in healthy volunteers. Peak levels of IL-6, TNF-α, and other chemokines were significantly reduced in both the ticagrelor and the clopidogrel groups as compared with the control group, with greater effects in the ticagrelor group. These effects are likely to be mediated through P2Y$_{12}$ inhibition, as clopidogrel and ticagrelor share no other feature except for blocking the P2Y$_{12}$ receptor. In addition, ticagrelor reduced IL-8 levels and increased the level of the anti-inflammatory IL-10, potentially through the effect of ticagrelor on adenosine (discussed later in this article) (Fig. 1). Endotoxin also induced prothrombotic changes in fibrin clot dynamics and ticagrelor was able to attenuate these prothrombotic changes.[25]

Despite the evidence that ticagrelor more effectively inhibits the inflammatory response induced by endotoxin, associated with its more effective platelet P2Y$_{12}$ inhibition, paradoxic findings were observed in the PLATO trial: leukocyte counts, including neutrophils, and other inflammatory markers were significantly higher in the ticagrelor compared with the clopidogrel group during maintenance therapy.[11] After discontinuation of study medication, these small but significant differences disappeared, mainly due to an increase in leukocyte count after cessation of clopidogrel, although a very slight fall also was noted after discontinuation of ticagrelor.[11] These data suggest complex and differential effects of clopidogrel and

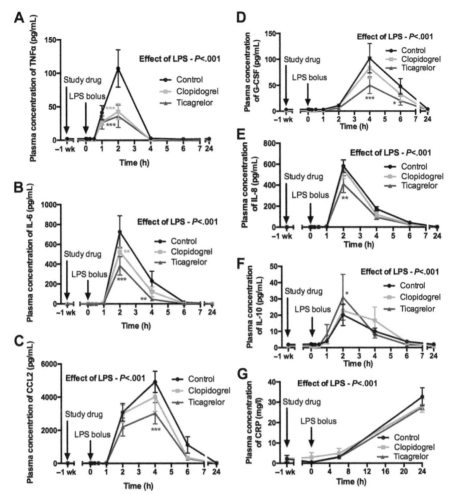

Fig. 1. Levels of proinflammatory cytokines TNF-α (A), IL-6 (B), CCL2 (C), granulocyte colony-stimulating factor (G-CSF) (D), IL-8 (E), IL-10 (F), and high-sensitivity (hs)CRP (G) before and after 1 week of antiplatelet treatment and following lipopolysaccharide administration (t = 0 hours). Compared with control, both P2Y$_{12}$ inhibitors had a marked effect on the proinflammatory cytokine response, reducing peak levels of TNF-α, IL-6, and CCL2. In addition, ticagrelor, but not clopidogrel, significantly reduced peak levels of G-CSF and IL-8, and significantly increased peak levels of the anti-inflammatory cytokine IL-10. Neither drug significantly modified the hsCRP response (G). (*Adapted from* Thomas MR, Outteridge SN, Ajjan RA, et al. Platelet P2Y12 inhibitors reduce systemic inflammation and its prothrombotic effects in an experimental human model. Arterioscler Thromb Vasc Biol 2015;35(12):2562–70; with permission.)

ticagrelor on inflammatory responses that may vary under different circumstances, partly related to differences in levels of platelet P2Y$_{12}$ inhibition but also related to different off-target effects of the 2 drugs.

TICAGRELOR AND ADENOSINE

Adenosine is a purine nucleoside primarily produced by endothelial cells in response to oxidative stress, ischemia, or inflammation.[26] ATP and ADP are metabolized by nucleotidases to produce adenosine. Adenosine is then rapidly taken up by cells via 4 transporter proteins: the sodium-independent equilibrative nucleoside transporters (ENT) 1 and 2 and the sodium-dependent concentrative nucleoside transporters (CNT) 1 and 2. This leads to the very short plasma half-life of adenosine.[27,28] Intracellular adenosine is then converted to either ATP or inosine through the action of adenosine kinase or adenosine deaminase, respectively.[29]

The biological actions of adenosine are mediated by 4 G-protein-coupled adenosine receptors; A$_1$R, A$_{2A}$R, A$_{2B}$R, and A$_3$R. A$_1$R and A$_3$R inhibit adenylate cyclase, thus reducing intracellular levels of cyclic adenosine monophosphate (cAMP), whereas $A_{2A}R$ and $A_{2B}R$ stimulate adenylate cyclase and therefore increase intracellular cAMP.[30] Adenosine has a multitude of effects, including coronary vasodilatation,[31] platelet inhibition,[32] modulation of inflammation,[33] reduced atrioventricular conduction,[34] sensory nerve stimulation,[35] and reduction in glomerular filtration rate.[36]

In a quest to unravel the mechanisms leading to the off-target effects of ticagrelor, adenosine uptake by human red blood cells was measured in the presence of ticagrelor; this demonstrated inhibition of uptake in a similar dose-dependent fashion to dipyridamole but with lower affinity for the ENT-1 transporter.[37] Moreover, ticagrelor augmented the increase in coronary blood flow in response to ischemia or adenosine infusion in a canine model.[37] In healthy volunteers, ticagrelor treatment also augmented coronary blood flow velocity in response to intravenous adenosine infusion.[38]

Adenosine plasma concentrations are higher in ticagrelor-treated patients with ACS as compared with clopidogrel-treated patients, with no change in adenosine deaminase activity, indicating that the mechanism of increased adenosine is the inhibition of adenosine cellular uptake rather than adenosine degradation (Fig. 2).[39] The specific mechanisms of ticagrelor-induced adenosine uptake inhibition have been further characterized in recombinant Madin-Darby canine kidney cells: adenosine inhibition in response to clinically relevant concentrations of ticagrelor was evident only in cells expressing ENT-1, confirming ticagrelor to be an ENT-1 inhibitor.[40]

POTENTIAL ADENOSINE-MEDIATED CLINICAL EFFECTS

There are numerous potential adenosine-mediated clinical effects of ticagrelor therapy (Fig. 3). Similar to that seen in healthy volunteers, ticagrelor potentiated adenosine-mediated increases in coronary blood flow as compared to prasugrel in a randomized study of 56 patients with non–ST-elevation myocardial infarction.[41] In vitro studies also suggest that ticagrelor may be able to achieve platelet inhibitory effects independent of $P2Y_{12}$ receptor inhibition as a consequence of increasing plasma adenosine levels that then reduce platelet reactivity by stimulation of platelet A_{2A} receptors.[42] This might explain the increasing effects of ticagrelor on hemostasis even beyond doses at which platelet $P2Y_{12}$ receptor inhibition is almost maximal.[43]

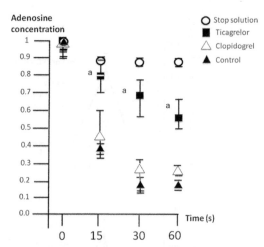

Fig. 2. Effects of ticagrelor on adenosine uptake by red blood cells. After addition of adenosine in vitro, the uptake of adenosine by red blood cells over 60 seconds is delayed in whole blood from patients receiving ticagrelor (*solid squares*) compared with blood from clopidogrel-treated patients (*open triangles*) or control subjects (*solid triangles*). Open circles = stop solution. [a] $P<.001$ ticagrelor group versus clopidogrel group. (*Adapted from* Bonello L, Laine M, Kipson N, et al. Ticagrelor increases adenosine plasma concentration in patients with an acute coronary syndrome. J Am Coll Cardiol 2014;63(9):876; with permission.)

As discussed previously, ticagrelor increases levels of anti-inflammatory molecule IL-10 in a human model of sepsis.[25] This is potentially mediated through the inhibition of adenosine uptake, as adenosine stimulates IL-10 production through macrophage $A_{2B}R$ receptors.[44]

Several side effects of ticagrelor might potentially be explained by its effect on adenosine uptake. Ticagrelor can induce a sensation of dyspnea that is usually mild or moderate and often well-tolerated.[45–49] In the PLATO trial, ticagrelor compared with clopidogrel significantly increased the incidence of dyspnea adverse events (13.8% vs 7.8%, $P<.001$).[6] This effect might be mediated by adenosine, as adenosine induces dyspnea through stimulation of vagal nerve C fibers.[50] However, there are weaknesses in this hypothesis that have not yet been addressed. Other reversibly binding $P2Y_{12}$ antagonists, cangrelor and elinogrel, also have been reported to cause dyspnea despite being of different chemical classes to ticagrelor. Although cangrelor does not inhibit ENT1, its principal inactive metabolite does have a weak inhibitory effect on this adenosine transporter.[40] On the other hand, dipyridamole is a stronger inhibitor of adenosine uptake than ticagrelor or cangrelor inactive metabolite, but is not

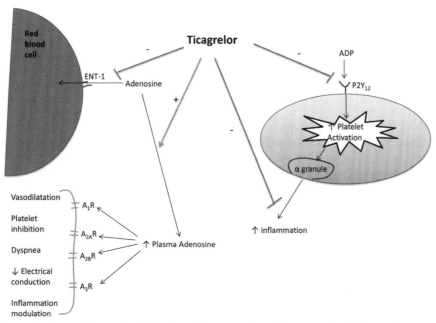

Fig. 3. Pleiotropic effects of ticagrelor. Ticagrelor reduces vascular inflammation by inhibiting the activation of the $P2Y_{12}$ receptor pathway by ADP, thereby reducing the proinflammatory effects of platelet α-granule release. In addition, ticagrelor increases extracellular adenosine concentrations by weakly inhibiting ENT-1, leading to numerous potential positive or adverse effects mediated via adenosine receptors (A_1R, $A_{2A}R$, $A_{2B}R$, A_3R).

reported to cause dyspnea.[40,51] Despite these weaknesses in the adenosine-dyspnea hypothesis, ticagrelor-related dyspnea shares the characteristics of dyspnea induced by adenosine infusion and ticagrelor has also been shown to exacerbate adenosine-induced dyspnea.[38]

Ventricular pauses also were more frequent during the first week of ticagrelor treatment compared with clopidogrel (5.8% vs 3.6%, $P = .01$), predominantly as a result of more sino-atrial pauses.[6,52] Theoretically, these effects also could be adenosine-mediated, as adenosine is known to inhibit cardiac pacemaker automaticity through A_1R inhibition.[34]

TICAGRELOR AND ENDOTHELIAL FUNCTION

Ticagrelor has been shown to have favorable effects on endothelial function. In a study of 127 patients with history of ACS, patients treated with ticagrelor had improved endothelial function compared with prasugrel, clopidogrel, or no $P2Y_{12}$ antagonist using peripheral arterial tonometry as a marker of endothelial function.[53] It has been hypothesized that this effect is mediated by a reduction in platelet-endothelial cell interaction through a reduction in P-selectin expression[14] or that increased extracellular adenosine concentration causes vascular smooth muscle relaxation

through A_{2A} receptor activation.[54] Ticagrelor also has been shown to inhibit vasoconstriction in response to vasopressors in rats as compared with other $P2Y_{12}$ inhibitors or placebo.[55]

SUMMARY

Ticagrelor is a potent reversibly binding $P2Y_{12}$ receptor antagonist that, through platelet inhibition, is able to positively modulate inflammation and its subsequent prothrombotic effects. Ticagrelor also blocks the ENT-1 transporter, thereby inhibiting adenosine cellular uptake at clinically relevant concentrations. This potentially contributes toward the effects of ticagrelor on platelet inhibition and modulation of inflammation, as well as some of the adverse effects observed with ticagrelor, such as dyspnea and ventricular pauses.

REFERENCES

1. Coughlin SR. Protease-activated receptors and platelet function. Thromb Haemost 1999;82(2):353–6.
2. Storey RF. Biology and pharmacology of the platelet P2Y12 receptor. Curr Pharm Des 2006; 12(10):1255–9.
3. Leger AJ, Covic L, Kuliopulos A. Protease-activated receptors in cardiovascular diseases. Circulation 2006;114(10):1070–7.

4. Roffi M, Patrono C, Collet JP, et al. 2015 ESC guidelines for the management of acute coronary syndromes in patients presenting without persistent ST-segment elevation: task force for the management of acute coronary syndromes in patients presenting without persistent ST-segment elevation of the European Society of Cardiology (ESC). Eur Heart J 2016;37(3):267–315.

5. Amsterdam EA, Wenger NK, Brindis RG, et al. 2014 AHA/ACC guideline for the management of patients with non-ST-elevation acute coronary syndromes: a report of the American College of Cardiology/American Heart Association Task Force on practice guidelines. J Am Coll Cardiol 2014; 64(24):e139–228.

6. Wallentin L, Becker RC, Budaj A, et al. Ticagrelor versus clopidogrel in patients with acute coronary syndromes. N Engl J Med 2009;361(11):1045–57.

7. Yusuf S, Zhao F, Mehta SR, et al. Effects of clopidogrel in addition to aspirin in patients with acute coronary syndromes without ST-segment elevation. N Engl J Med 2001;345(7):494–502.

8. Wiviott SD, Braunwald E, McCabe CH, et al. Prasugrel versus clopidogrel in patients with acute coronary syndromes. N Engl J Med 2007;357(20):2001–15.

9. Varenhorst C, Alstrom U, Scirica BM, et al. Factors contributing to the lower mortality with ticagrelor compared with clopidogrel in patients undergoing coronary artery bypass surgery. J Am Coll Cardiol 2012;60(17):1623–30.

10. Varenhorst C, Alstrom U, Braun OO, et al. Causes of mortality with ticagrelor compared with clopidogrel in acute coronary syndromes. Heart 2014; 100(22):1762–9.

11. Storey RF, James SK, Siegbahn A, et al. Lower mortality following pulmonary adverse events and sepsis with ticagrelor compared to clopidogrel in the PLATO study. Platelets 2014;25(7):517–25.

12. Thomas MR, Storey RF. The role of platelets in inflammation. Thromb Haemost 2015;114(3):449–58.

13. Blair P, Flaumenhaft R. Platelet alpha-granules: basic biology and clinical correlates. Blood Rev 2009;23(4):177–89.

14. Mine S, Fujisaki T, Suematsu M, et al. Activated platelets and endothelial cell interaction with neutrophils under flow conditions. Intern Med 2001; 40(11):1085–92.

15. Evangelista V, Manarini S, Sideri R, et al. Platelet/polymorphonuclear leukocyte interaction: P-selectin triggers protein-tyrosine phosphorylation-dependent CD11b/CD18 adhesion: role of PSGL-1 as a signaling molecule. Blood 1999;93(3):876–85.

16. Caplain H, Donat F, Gaud C, et al. Pharmacokinetics of clopidogrel. Semin Thromb Hemost 1999;25(Suppl 2):25–8.

17. Stone GW, Witzenbichler B, Weisz G, et al. Platelet reactivity and clinical outcomes after coronary artery implantation of drug-eluting stents (ADAPT-DES): a prospective multicentre registry study. Lancet 2013;382(9892):614–23.

18. Heitzer T, Rudolph V, Schwedhelm E, et al. Clopidogrel improves systemic endothelial nitric oxide bioavailability in patients with coronary artery disease: evidence for antioxidant and antiinflammatory effects. Arterioscler Thromb Vasc Biol 2006; 26(7):1648–52.

19. Xiao Z, Theroux P. Clopidogrel inhibits platelet-leukocyte interactions and thrombin receptor agonist peptide-induced platelet activation in patients with an acute coronary syndrome. J Am Coll Cardiol 2004;43(11):1982–8.

20. Chen YG, Xu F, Zhang Y, et al. Effect of aspirin plus clopidogrel on inflammatory markers in patients with non-ST-segment elevation acute coronary syndrome. Chin Med J (Engl) 2006;119(1):32–6.

21. Vivekananthan DP, Bhatt DL, Chew DP, et al. Effect of clopidogrel pretreatment on periprocedural rise in C-reactive protein after percutaneous coronary intervention. Am J Cardiol 2004;94(3):358–60.

22. Gurbel PA, Bliden KP, Butler K, et al. Randomized double-blind assessment of the ONSET and OFFSET of the antiplatelet effects of ticagrelor versus clopidogrel in patients with stable coronary artery disease: the ONSET/OFFSET study. Circulation 2009;120(25):2577–85.

23. Silvain J, Storey RF, Cayla G, et al. P2Y12 receptor inhibition and effect of morphine in patients undergoing primary PCI for ST-segment elevation myocardial infarction. The PRIVATE-ATLANTIC study. Thromb Haemost 2016;116(2):369–78.

24. Storey RF, Angiolillo DJ, Patil SB, et al. Inhibitory effects of ticagrelor compared with clopidogrel on platelet function in patients with acute coronary syndromes: the PLATO (PLATelet inhibition and patient outcomes) PLATELET substudy. J Am Coll Cardiol 2010;56(18):1456–62.

25. Thomas MR, Outteridge SN, Ajjan RA, et al. Platelet P2Y12 inhibitors reduce systemic inflammation and its prothrombotic effects in an experimental human model. Arterioscler Thromb Vasc Biol 2015;35(12):2562–70.

26. Linden J. Molecular approach to adenosine receptors: receptor-mediated mechanisms of tissue protection. Annu Rev Pharmacol Toxicol 2001;41: 775–87.

27. Molina-Arcas M, Casado FJ, Pastor-Anglada M. Nucleoside transporter proteins. Curr Vasc Pharmacol 2009;7(4):426–34.

28. Plagemann PG. Transport and metabolism of adenosine in human erythrocytes: effect of transport inhibitors and regulation by phosphate. J Cell Physiol 1986;128(3):491–500.

29. Headrick JP, Ashton KJ, Rose'meyer RB, et al. Cardiovascular adenosine receptors: expression,

actions and interactions. Pharmacol Ther 2013; 140(1):92–111.

30. Ham J, Evans BA. An emerging role for adenosine and its receptors in bone homeostasis. Front Endocrinol (Lausanne) 2012;3:113.

31. Mustafa SJ, Morrison RR, Teng B, et al. Adenosine receptors and the heart: role in regulation of coronary blood flow and cardiac electrophysiology. Handb Exp Pharmacol 2009;(193):161–88.

32. Johnston-Cox HA, Yang D, Ravid K. Physiological implications of adenosine receptor-mediated platelet aggregation. J Cell Physiol 2011;226(1):46–51.

33. Barletta KE, Ley K, Mehrad B. Regulation of neutrophil function by adenosine. Arterioscler Thromb Vasc Biol 2012;32(4):856–64.

34. Belardinelli L, Shryock JC, Song Y, et al. Ionic basis of the electrophysiological actions of adenosine on cardiomyocytes. FASEB J 1995;9(5):359–65.

35. Burki NK, Lee LY. Blockade of airway sensory nerves and dyspnea in humans. Pulm Pharmacol Ther 2010;23(4):279–82.

36. Li L, Mizel D, Huang Y, et al. Tubuloglomerular feedback and renal function in mice with targeted deletion of the type 1 equilibrative nucleoside transporter. Am J Physiol Renal Physiol 2013;304(4):F382–9.

37. van Giezen JJ, Sidaway J, Glaves P, et al. Ticagrelor inhibits adenosine uptake in vitro and enhances adenosine-mediated hyperemia responses in a canine model. J Cardiovasc Pharmacol Ther 2012; 17(2):164–72.

38. Wittfeldt A, Emanuelsson H, Brandrup-Wognsen G, et al. Ticagrelor enhances adenosine-induced coronary vasodilatory responses in humans. J Am Coll Cardiol 2013;61(7):723–7.

39. Bonello L, Laine M, Kipson N, et al. Ticagrelor increases adenosine plasma concentration in patients with an acute coronary syndrome. J Am Coll Cardiol 2014;63(9):872–7.

40. Armstrong D, Summers C, Ewart L, et al. Characterization of the adenosine pharmacology of ticagrelor reveals therapeutically relevant inhibition of equilibrative nucleoside transporter 1. J Cardiovasc Pharmacol Ther 2014;19(2):209–19.

41. Alexopoulos D, Moulias A, Koutsogiannis N, et al. Differential effect of ticagrelor versus prasugrel on coronary blood flow velocity in patients with non-ST-elevation acute coronary syndrome undergoing percutaneous coronary intervention: an exploratory study. Circ Cardiovasc Interv 2013;6(3):277–83.

42. Nylander S, Femia EA, Scavone M, et al. Ticagrelor inhibits human platelet aggregation via adenosine in addition to P2Y12 antagonism. J Thromb Haemost 2013;11(10):1867–76.

43. Storey RF, Angiolillo DJ, Bonaca MP, et al. Platelet inhibition with Ticagrelor 60 mg versus 90 mg twice daily in the PEGASUS-TIMI 54 trial. J Am Coll Cardiol 2016;67(10):1145–54.

44. Nemeth ZH, Lutz CS, Csoka B, et al. Adenosine augments IL-10 production by macrophages through an A2B receptor-mediated posttranscriptional mechanism. J Immunol 2005;175(12):8260–70.

45. Cannon CP, Husted S, Harrington RA, et al. Safety, tolerability, and initial efficacy of AZD6140, the first reversible oral adenosine diphosphate receptor antagonist, compared with clopidogrel, in patients with non-ST-segment elevation acute coronary syndrome: primary results of the DISPERSE-2 trial. J Am Coll Cardiol 2007;50(19):1844–51.

46. Storey RF, Bliden KP, Patil SB, et al. Incidence of dyspnea and assessment of cardiac and pulmonary function in patients with stable coronary artery disease receiving ticagrelor, clopidogrel, or placebo in the ONSET/OFFSET study. J Am Coll Cardiol 2010;56(3):185–93.

47. Storey RF, Becker RC, Harrington RA, et al. Characterization of dyspnoea in PLATO study patients treated with ticagrelor or clopidogrel and its association with clinical outcomes. Eur Heart J 2011; 32(23):2945–53.

48. Unverdorben M, Parodi G, Pistolesi M, et al. Dyspnea related to reversibly-binding P2Y12 inhibitors: a review of the pathophysiology, clinical presentation and diagnostics. Int J Cardiol 2016;202:167–73.

49. Parodi G, Storey RF. Dyspnoea management in acute coronary syndrome patients treated with ticagrelor. Eur Heart J Acute Cardiovasc Care 2015; 4(6):555–60.

50. Burki NK, Sheatt M, Lee LY. Effects of airway anesthesia on dyspnea and ventilatory response to intravenous injection of adenosine in healthy human subjects. Pulm Pharmacol Ther 2008;21(1):208–13.

51. Cattaneo M, Faioni EM. Why does ticagrelor induce dyspnea? Thromb Haemost 2012;108(6):1031–6.

52. Scirica BM, Cannon CP, Emanuelsson H, et al. The incidence of bradyarrhythmias and clinical bradyarrhythmic events in patients with acute coronary syndromes treated with ticagrelor or clopidogrel in the PLATO (platelet inhibition and patient outcomes) trial: results of the continuous electrocardiographic assessment substudy. J Am Coll Cardiol 2011; 57(19):1908–16.

53. Torngren K, Ohman J, Salmi H, et al. Ticagrelor improves peripheral arterial function in patients with a previous acute coronary syndrome. Cardiology 2013;124(4):252–8.

54. Sato A, Terata K, Miura H, et al. Mechanism of vasodilation to adenosine in coronary arterioles from patients with heart disease. Am J Physiol Heart Circ Physiol 2005;288(4):H1633–40.

55. Grzesk G, Kozinski M, Navarese EP, et al. Ticagrelor, but not clopidogrel and prasugrel, prevents ADP-induced vascular smooth muscle cell contraction: a placebo-controlled study in rats. Thromb Res 2012;130(1):65–9.

Protease-Activated Receptor-1 Antagonists Post-Percutaneous Coronary Intervention

Pierluigi Tricoci, MD, MHS, PhD

KEYWORDS

- Antiplatelet therapy • Coronary artery disease • Protease-activated receptors • Vorapaxar
- Myocardial infarction • Percutaneous coronary intervention

KEY POINTS

- Thrombin is the most potent platelet activator and acts through the protease-activated receptors (PARs).
- PAR-1 is the main thrombin receptor on human platelet.
- Vorapaxar is an oral, selective PAR-1 antagonist.
- The TRACER trial and TRA 2P-TIMI 50 trial are the 2 phase 3 clinical trials testing vorapaxar in addition to standard of care.
- In the absence of dedicated clinical trials in percutaneous coronary intervention patients, subgroup analyses from the large phase 3 trial provide helpful insights in patients with coronary stents.

INTRODUCTION

Thrombin is not only the final enzyme of the coagulation cascade, but it is also the most potent platelet agonist. The protease-activated receptors (PAR) mediate the effect of thrombin on platelets. Given the role of thrombin on platelet activation, PARs, and in particular, PAR-1 antagonist have been developed aiming at the reduction of platelet-mediated thrombotic events. Vorapaxar is the only PAR-1 antagonist evaluated in phase III clinical trials and the only agent currently available for clinical use. In this review, the author introduces the rationale of PAR-1 antagonism as a therapeutic target and reviews the key clinical trial results of vorapaxar, highlighting the available evidence on efficacy and safety in the context of percutaneous coronary interventions (PCI).

PROTEASE-ACTIVATED RECEPTORS

Platelets are activated by multiple pathways, and their inner mechanism of amplification leads to the expansion of initial platelet thrombus.[1] Collagen-induced platelet activation is key in maintaining normal hemostasis.[2] Secretion of agonists, such as ADP and thromboxane A2 from activated platelets, leads to the amplification of platelet activation.[1] Thrombin-mediated activation is another important mechanism of platelet activation exerting its effects at very low concentrations.[1]

The receptors of thrombin in human platelets are known as "protease-activated receptor" or PAR, and there are the 2 main PAR receptors on human platelets: the PAR-1 and the PAR-4.[3,4] PAR-1 and PAR-4 can each independently transmit thrombin signaling, but the PAR-1 is thought to be the main thrombin receptor because it is activated

Disclosure Statement: Research Grant and Advisory Board from Merck.
Division of Cardiology, Duke Clinical Research Institute, Duke University Medical Center, 2400 Pratt Street, 0311 Terrace Level, Box 3850 DUMC, Durham, NC 27705, USA
E-mail address: pierluigi.tricoci@duke.edu

Intervent Cardiol Clin 6 (2017) 57–66
http://dx.doi.org/10.1016/j.iccl.2016.08.005
2211-7458/17/© 2016 Elsevier Inc. All rights reserved.

by low thrombin concentrations (Fig. 1)[5] The PAR-4 is activated by higher concentration of thrombin, and it is unclear if it is mainly a "backup" receptor or if it is only active in conditions with a higher concentration of thrombin.[3] PAR-1 is a G-protein–coupled receptor and interacts with thrombin as a substrate for the protease action of thrombin (Fig. 2).[6] Thrombin removes the N-terminus of the PAR-1 receptor, unmasking a tethered ligand (SFLLRN), which is the actual "agonist" of the PAR-1.[7] Because of this mechanism, PARs can only be activated once, which is different from typical receptors, and requires deactivation, which occurs through phosphorylation and arrestin binding and lysosomal degradation.[6,8]

Roles of Protease-Activated Receptors in Hemostasis

Mice have been the primary model to understand the function of PARs in hemostasis and have laid the foundation to formulate the translational hypothesis of PAR-antagonism as therapeutic strategy.[3,9]

Mice platelets express PAR-3 and PAR-4. PAR-4 is the main receptor in mice, whereas PAR-3 is purely a cofactor for PAR-4, yet it is necessary at low thrombin concentrations.[10] PAR-3-deficient mice (PAR-3−/−) are a model for PAR-1 antagonism in humans. In fact, in PAR-3-deficient mice platelet activation can only occur with high concentration of thrombin, which is what happens in humans when PAR-1 is antagonized (ie, thrombin-mediated response depends on PAR-4).

The PAR-4-deficient (PAR-4−/−) mouse platelet is unresponsive to thrombin, which theoretically is what would occur in humans if both PAR-1 and PAR-4 were concomitantly blocked.[10] Despite the fact that PAR-4-deficient mice platelets cannot be activated by thrombin, those animals do not have a bleeding tendency, and the female mouse can support pregnancies.[10] The formation of an initial PAR-4 hemostatic thrombus at the site of vascular injury is not impaired in PAR-4-deficient mice, but further growth of the thrombus is inhibited.[11]

PAR-3-deficient mice do not have an increase in bleeding time, except when a P2Y12 deficiency is concomitantly present. In the cynomolgus monkey surgical blood loss model, a vorapaxar intravenous analogue SCH 530348 did not cause an increase in bleeding time unless it also received a P2Y12 inhibitor.[12]

PAR-4-deficient mice have a reduced thrombus formation in response to arterial wall

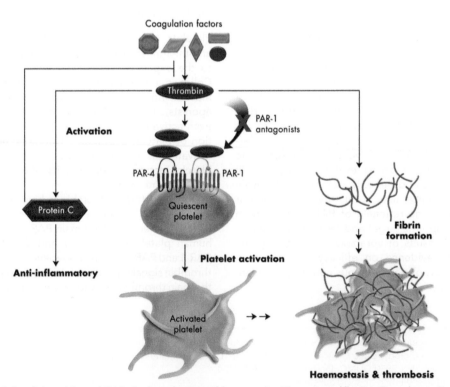

Fig. 1. Role of thrombin and PARs in thrombosis and hemostasis. (*From* Angiolillo DJ, Capodanno D, Goto S. Platelet thrombin receptor antagonism and atherothrombosis. Eur Heart J 2010;31:18; with permission.)

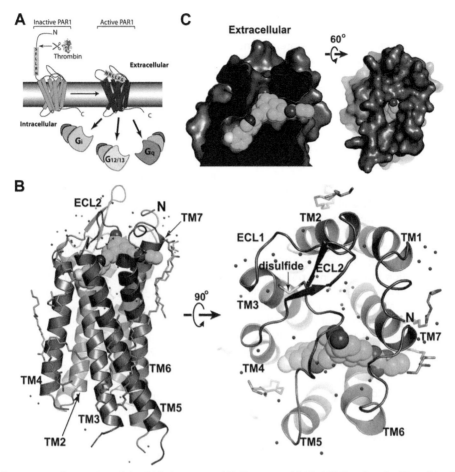

Fig. 2. Structure and activation of the PAR-1 receptor. (*A*) Cleavage of PAR-1-N-Terminus by Thrombin. (*B*) PAR-1 structure and extracellular surface. (*C*) Ligand binding pocket vorapaxar is shown as green spheres. (*From* Zhang C, Srinivasan Y, Arlow DH, et al. High-resolution crystal structure of human protease-activated receptor 1. Nature 2012;492:387; with permission.)

injury.[9] At a low level of vascular injury (4% $FeCl_3$), PAR-3-deficient mice (ie, comparable to PAR-1 inhibition in human) showed similar impairment in thrombus formation as PAR-4-deficient mice and a higher degree of impairment than P2Y12-deficient mice. However, at a higher level of vascular injury, PAR-3 did not show significant reduction in thrombus formation, unlike PAR-4- and PY12-deficient mice.[9] These results suggest that the decreased response to thrombin caused by pharmacologic PAR-1 antagonism may be effective at a lower degree vascular injury, like in spontaneous coronary plaque rupture and less so in extensive plaque rupture, like during PCI.

Based on these animal models, it was hypothesized that thrombin-mediated platelet activation is not critical to normal hemostasis. Thus, the working hypothesis in developing PAR antagonists was that by blocking thrombin receptors could it be possible to achieve an antithrombotic effect without significant impairment of hemostasis, and thus, an bleeding increase would be minimized.

VORAPAXAR

Pharmacodynamics and Pharmacokinetic

Vorapaxar is an oral competitive PAR-1 antagonist and is highly selective for the PAR-1 receptor, with no effect on PAR-4.[6,13,14] Vorapaxar binds the PAR-1 in a reversible fashion, but the very slow off-rate due to the structure of binding pocked makes the interaction virtually irreversible.[6] Vorapaxar does not have any effect on the PAR-4-mediated response to thrombin. Vorapaxar is rapidly absorbed and reaches a peak plasma concentration in 1 to 2 hours during fasting. The vorapaxar metabolism is mainly mediated by the liver cytochromes, CYP3A4 and CYP2J2, and metabolites are largely eliminated through feces, and only 25% are renally excreted.[15] Therefore, potent CYP3A4 inhibitors and inducer significantly affect exposure. One of the main pharmacologic features of vorapaxar is its long duration of action, with a terminal elimination half-life of 8 days and 50% of platelet inhibitor effect still seen after 4 weeks (https://www.merck.com/product/usa/pi_circulars/z/zontivity/zontivity_pi.pdf).

Antiplatelet effect
Loading doses of vorapaxar 20 mg or 40 mg result in a greater than 80% inhibition of thrombin receptor activating peptide (TRAP)-induced platelet aggregation within 1 hour.[15] Daily maintenance doses of 1 and 3 mg/d achieved nearly complete inhibition of 15 µg TRAP-induced platelet aggregation at day 7. In a phase II trial among patients undergoing PCI, a 40-mg loading dose achieved, within 2 hours, an 80% inhibition of TRAP (15 µg)-induced platelet aggregation in nearly all patients.[16] The maintenance doses of 1 mg and 2.5 mg daily yielded greater than the 80% platelet inhibition to TRAP in all patients at 30 and 60 days. These results were confirmed in the Thrombin Receptor Antagonist for Clinical Event Reduction in Acute Coronary Syndrome (TRACER) Pharmacodynamic Substudy, among non-ST elevation acute coronary syndrome (NSTE-ACS). A 97% (94%–98% interquartile range) inhibition of maximum platelet aggregation to TRAP were observed at 2 hours with a 40-mg loading dose and maintained until the end of the 2.5 mg/dy maintenance treatment.[17]

CLINICAL TRIALS OF VORAPAXAR
Phase II Trial in Percutaneous Coronary Intervention Patients
Vorapaxar was studied in the phase II Thrombin Receptor Antagonist (TRA)-PCI trial among 1030 patients undergoing elective coronary angiography with the intention to perform a PCI.[16] Patients were randomized to 3 loading doses of vorapaxar (10 mg, 20 mg, or 40 mg), or placebo before the coronary angiography. Those who actually underwent PCI (n = 573) were randomized to 3 daily maintenance doses (0.5 mg, 1.0 mg, or 2.5 mg) or placebo for 60 days. Patients undergoing PCI also received concomitant aspirin and clopidogrel. Thrombolysis in myocardial infarction (TIMI), major or minor bleeding, was not significantly different between vorapaxar and placebo (3.3% placebo vs 2.8% vorapaxar; odds ratio [OR] 0.86, 95% confidence interval [CI] 0.30–2.47), although a numerical trend suggesting more bleeding with the

highest dose of vorapaxar was seen. The rate of death, major cardiac event, or stroke was numerically lower in the vorapaxar group (all doses), when compared with placebo (6% vs 9%, OR 0.67, 95% CI 0.33–1.34).

The Thrombin Receptor Antagonist for Clinical Event Reduction in Acute Coronary Syndrome Trial
The TRACER study is a phase III, double-blind, multicenter clinical trial of patients with NSTE-ACS comparing vorapaxar (40-mg loading dose followed by 2.5 mg daily maintenance) versus placebo in addition to the standard medical therapy according to treating physician's recommendations, including dual antiplatelet therapies.[18] A total of 12,944 patients were randomized, mostly (>90%) with elevated biomarkers (CK-MB or troponin). The loading dose had to be administered at least 1 hour before any revascularization procedure. The duration of the 2.5-mg daily maintenance dose was for the entire duration of the study and a minimum of 1 year. One of the most important features of the trial is that it was largely conducted on a background of dual antiplatelet therapy with 91.8% receiving clopidogrel during the initial ACS hospitalization. Randomized patients were followed for a median of 502 days. After enrollment was completed and 5 months before the planned end of the study, the Data Safety Monitoring Board (DSMB) recommended the early termination of the study based on the increased rate of intracranial hemorrhages (ICHs) with vorapaxar and the fact that the study had already achieved the minimum number of primary endpoint events.

The TRACER trial had as a primary endpoint a complex, quintuple component outcome that should be kept in mind when interpreting the results (ie, a composite of cardiovascular death, myocardial infarction [MI], stroke, rehospitalization for ischemia, or urgent coronary revascularization).

The study prespecified a key secondary endpoint (meaning the study was powered to assess that outcome) of cardiovascular death, MI, or stroke. This triple endpoint is a more standard measure of outcomes in cardiovascular clinical trials.

The 2-year rate of the primary endpoint was 18.5% in the vorapaxar group and 19.9% in the placebo group (hazard ratio [HR] 0.92, 95% CI 0.85–0.98; P = .07); thus, the study failed to meet its primary objective. Cardiovascular death, MI, or stroke was reduced with vorapaxar (14.5% at 2 years) compared with the placebo

(16.4% at 2 years) (HR 0.89, 95% CI 0.81–0.98; *P* = .02), driven by a reduction in the MI rate (11.1% vs 12.5%; HR 0.88, 95% CI 0.79–0.98; *P* = .02), especially type 1 MI.[19] Despite the "positive" finding on the triple endpoint, because of the hierarchical statistical analysis, superiority on the key secondary endpoint could not be declared.

The overall modest efficacy signal was largely offset by an increase in bleeding.

GUSTO moderate and severe bleeding were significantly increased with vorapaxar (7.2% vorapaxar vs 5.2% placebo, 95% CI 1.16–1.58; *P*<.001) as well as clinically significant bleeding by TIMI criteria (20.2% vorapaxar vs 14.6% placebo; HR 1.43, 95% CI 1.31–1.57; *P*<.001). In particular, vorapaxar resulted in an increase of intracranial bleeding (1.1% vs 0.2%, HR 3.39, 95% CI 1.78–6.45; *P*<.0001).

The results of TRACER need to be read as reflecting the efficacy and safety of vorapaxar in the setting of a triple therapy with aspirin and thienopyridine. Also, the fact that the trial failed to meet the primary endpoint is likely due to the choice of the quintuple endpoint, including unstable angina with negative biomarkers and physician-driven coronary revascularization that are unlikely modified by an additional antiplatelet medication. The results of TRACER overall support the biological effect of PAR-1 blockade in ACS patients, as indicated by a reduction of the triple endpoint and the reduction observed in MI, especially type 1.

In the context of TRACER, the significant increase in bleeding, including severe bleeding and ICH, makes the potential benefit observed non-clinically viable. Other studies with triple

therapies have shown similar bleeding increases, such as the ATLAS-2 with rivaroxaban or APPRAISE-2 with apixaban.[20,21] In TRACER, there was an additional 20% of patients who received concomitant glycoprotein IIb/IIIa inhibitors. Future studies are needed to reassess vorapaxar in ACS and PCI in the context of a more selective and prudent concomitant antiplatelet strategy, that is, as single- or dual-antiplatelet therapy.

Insights on Percutaneous Coronary Intervention Patients from the Thrombin Receptor Antagonist for Clinical Event Reduction in Acute Coronary Syndrome Trial

The TRACER trial included an "all-comer" NSTE-ACS population with high-risk features that were randomized upfront before cardiac catheterization, thus before final treatment was established.[18] A total of 88% of patients underwent coronary angiography during the index hospitalization and approximately 58% of the population underwent index PCI. In general, PCI occurred quite expeditiously after treatment, with a median of 3.5 hours between loading those administration and PCI, a time sufficient to allow full effect of the loading dose. Of patients who underwent PCI, 56% received at least one drug-eluting stent (DES).[22] Overall, the results in patients undergoing PCI was consistent with the main study results on both the primary (*P* for interaction = 0.54) and the key secondary endpoint (*P* for interaction = 0.55). Interestingly, differences in the efficacy of vorapaxar were noted according to the type of stent implanted. Patients having a bare metal stent (BMS) implanted seemingly had a better efficacy of vorapaxar (Fig. 3). The rate of the primary

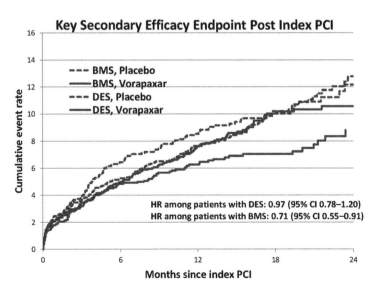

Key Secondary Efficacy Endpoint Post Index PCI

- --- BMS, Placebo
- ——— BMS, Vorapaxar
- --- DES, Placebo
- ——— DES, Vorapaxar

HR among patients with DES: 0.97 (95% CI 0.78–1.20)
HR among patients with BMS: 0.71 (95% CI 0.55–0.91)

Cumulative event rate — Months since index PCI

Fig. 3. Cardiovascular death, myocardial infarction, or stroke with vorapaxar or placebo according to stent type during index PCI. (*From* Valgimigli M, Tricoci P, Huang Z, et al. Usefulness and safety of vorapaxar in patients with non-ST-segment elevation acute coronary syndrome undergoing percutaneous coronary intervention (from the TRACER trial). Am J Cardiol 2014;114:668; with permission.)

endpoint in patients who had BMS was 14.1% of patients with vorapaxar versus 16.6% of patients with the placebo at 2 years (adjusted HR 0.82; 95% CI 0.66–1.02). In DES patients, there was not a reduction in ischemic outcomes observed with vorapaxar (2-year event rate 15.5% vorapaxar vs 16.4% placebo; adjusted HR 1.05, 95% CI 0.87, 1.28). Nonetheless, the interaction between type of stent and treatment effects was not statistically significant (interaction P value = 0.233). Similar trends were observed on the key secondary endpoint. Cardiovascular death, MI, or stroke occurred in 8.8% of patients in the vorapaxar group versus 12.2% of patients in the placebo group (adjusted HR: 0.86 [0.64, 1.14]). In the DES group, 10.6% of patients with vorapaxar and 12.8% of patients with placebo experienced the triple endpoint at 2 years (adjusted HR 0.96, 95% CI 0.74, 1.25). A trend for interaction between type of stents and vorapaxar on the key secondary endpoint was noted (P value = .069), which was attenuated after adjustment for baseline characteristics and treatments (P value = .543). Because it is unlikely that the type of stent would affect the efficacy of vorapaxar, the investigators hypothesized that the type of stent was only a marker of different patient selection and concomitant treatment. For example, patients with BMS received a shorter duration of clopidogrel and therefore a shorter duration of vorapaxar treatment in the context of triple therapy. The investigators formally tested baseline and treatment cofactors resulting in treatment effect modification, but none was statistically significant and the strongest association was with clopidogrel treatment duration (P = .09). In another analysis, however, assessing the association between persistence in clopidogrel treatment and efficacy and safety of vorapaxar, there was not any interaction between use of clopidogrel over time and vorapaxar.[23] Interestingly, in patients who were on chronic thienopyridine before the index ACS, there appeared to be less bleeding when vorapaxar was used compared with thienopyridine-naive patients, in which antiplatelet medications were started at the time of hospitalization.[24] This finding suggests that vorapaxar was safer in patients who were already able to tolerate chronic clopidogrel (ie, a patient who had a significant bleeding while on clopidogrel would have been excluded from TRACER).

Vorapaxar did not show a significant effect on peri-PCI MI.[19] The phase II trial had shown a dose-dependent trend toward less peri-PCI MI, but in TRACER, with a much larger cohort (353 peri-PCI MI observed in TRACER), the difference between vorapaxar and placebo was not statistically significant (HR 0.90; 95% CI 0.73–1.12; P = .350). Of note, the definition of TRACER was a modified version of the Second Universal MI definition (CK-MB elevation greater than 3 times the upper limit of normal in the setting or stable or falling pre-PCI biomarkers), and no symptoms of recurrent ischemia, ECG changes, or angiographic complication were required. The lack of a significant effect seen in peri-PCI MI, but a marked decrease in spontaneous MI with vorapaxar, is consistent with the preclinical models, suggesting that impaired PAR function may be protective in the setting of small vascular injuries, like in the case of a coronary plaque tear or erosion (ie, spontaneous plaque rupture), but less in the setting of major vascular injury, like in the case of plaque disruption during balloon inflation/coronary.[9]

In TRACER, definite stent thrombosis, according to the Academic Research Consortium definition, was not significantly reduced by vorapaxar among those patients who had a coronary stent implanted during the index ACS hospitalization (HR 1.12; 95% CI 0.78–1.62).[18] Stent thrombosis was adjudicated by the clinical event committee (CEC) using source documents provided by the sites, which included catheterization laboratory reports but not angiograms, as it is the standard for large cardiovascular trials. In an angiographic substudy of TRACER, serial angiograms of 329 patients with possible stent thrombosis (ie, stent thrombosis reported by the investigator or admitted with acute MI confirmed by the CEC) were reviewed by a central angiographic core laboratory for the detection of stent thrombosis.[25] Of the 108 stent thromboses identified by the core laboratory, only 61 (56%) were captured by the CEC, which was due to the fact stent thromboses were not reported in the catheterization laboratory reports. When vorapaxar treatment effect was analyzed based on angiographic core laboratory–defined stent thrombosis only, a trend toward reduction of stent thrombosis with vorapaxar was observed (HR 0.82 95% CI 0.56–1.20).

The Thrombin Receptor Antagonist in Secondary Prevention of Atherothrombotic Ischemic Events 50 Trial

Vorapaxar was studied for secondary prevention among stable patients with documented atherosclerotic disease in the Thrombin Receptor Antagonist in Secondary Prevention of Atherothrombotic Ischemic Events (TRA 2P-TIMI 50) trial, the trial that ultimately lead to the US Food and Drug Administration (FDA) and European Medicines Agency (EMA) marketing approval and current label of the drug.[26] The trial randomized 26,449 patients to vorapaxar or placebo, in addition to the standard of care. Similar to TRACER, the TRA 2P-TIMI 50 trials allowed the use of dual antiplatelet therapy according to treating physician choice and thus resulted in a high proportion of patients receiving vorapaxar on top of aspirin and clopidogrel. There were 3 populations included in the TRA 2P study. The largest (about 67% of trial population) comprised patients with recent (2 weeks to 12 months) MI. Patients with documented peripheral arterial disease (PAD), about 18% of the sample, represented the second group included, and the third group were patients with recent (2 weeks to 12 months post-MI) stroke. Patients were randomized to receive a maintenance dose of vorapaxar 2.5 mg daily (without loading dose) or placebo. Following a DSMB review, due to significantly higher rate of intracranial bleeding with vorapaxar in patients who had a prior stroke, the safety monitoring committee recommended the interruption of the study in patients with prior stroke (including those who had a stroke during the course of the study) and the continuation in post-MI and PAD patients. The primary endpoint of the TRA 2P-TIMI 50 was the composite of cardiovascular death, MI, or stroke, which was updated after the TRACER results were released, while the original primary endpoint also included urgent coronary revascularization. However, the quadruple endpoint was the main end point used for regulatory submission. The use of thienopyridine in the TRA 2P-TIMI 50 trial was high in the post-MI group (78%) and lower, but still substantial, in the PAD group (37%).

Vorapaxar significantly reduced the primary endpoint compared with placebo (3-year rates 9.3% vorapaxar vs 10.5% placebo, HR 0.87, 95% CI 0.80–0.94; $P<.001$). The composite of cardiovascular death, MI, stroke, or urgent coronary revascularization (ie, the primary endpoint used for the FDA submission) was 11.2% in the vorapaxar group and 12.4% in the placebo group (HR 0.88, 95% CI 0.82–0.95; $P = .001$). On the individual components of the primary endpoint, the strongest reduction was observed on MI (5.2% vs 6.1%, HR 0.83, 95% CI 0.74–0.93; $P = .001$), and no significant differences were seen on cardiovascular (2.7% vorapaxar vs 3.0% placebo; $P = .15$) and all-cause (5.0% vorapaxar vs 5.3% placebo; $P = .41$) mortality.

Vorapaxar significantly increased major bleeding. GUSTO moderate or severe bleeding

events were increased by 66% with vorapaxar (4.2% vs 2.5%, HR 1.66, 95% CI 1.43–1.93; $P<.001$), and TIMI clinically significant bleeding was increased by 46% (15.8% in the vorapaxar group vs 11.1% in the placebo group, HR 1.46, 95% CI 1.36–1.57; $P<.001$). There was also a significant increase in intracranial bleeding with vorapaxar (1.0% vs 0.5%, HR 1.94, 95% CI 1.39–2.70; $P<.001$). However, the increase in intracranial bleeding with vorapaxar strongly correlated with a prior history of stroke. In fact, patients with prior stroke had a 2.5-fold increase in the risk when treated with vorapaxar (2.4% vs 0.9%, HR 2.55, 95% CI 1.52–4.28; $P<.001$), whereas the increased risk in patients without history of stroke was more modest (0.6% vs 0.4%; $P = .049$).

Of the 3 populations included in the TRA 2P trial, the post-MI cohort derived the most remarkable benefits from vorapaxar.[27] There were 17,779 patients who were included based on a recent MI, and those had a 20% reduction in cardiovascular death, MI, or stroke (8.1% vs 9.7%; HR 0.80, 95% CI 0.72–0.89; $P<.0001$). There was an increase in the rate of GUSTO moderate or severe bleeding with vorapaxar (HR 1.61, 95% CI 1.31–1.97; $P<.0001$), whereas the difference in intracranial bleeding was not statistically significant (0.6% vs 0.4%, $P = .076$).

Based on the results of the TRA 2P-TIMI 50 study, vorapaxar was approved by the FDA for secondary prevention in patients with history of MI or with PAD (ie, the TRA 2P population minus the stroke group) and with history of MI (EMA). Because of the increasing rate of intracranial bleeding, the drug is contraindicated in patients with previous stroke or transient ischemic attack.

Insights on Percutaneous Coronary Intervention Patients from the Thrombin Receptor Antagonist in Secondary Prevention of Atherothrombotic Ischemic Events 50 Trial

In the TRA 2P-TIMI 50 trial, 14,042 of the randomized patients had a history of coronary stent before randomization, 93% of these qualified into the study with history of MI, and 83% were on a thienopyridine at randomization.[28] An additional 449 patients received a coronary stent during the trial. The efficacy of vorapaxar in patients who had a coronary stent implanted was consistent with the main trial results, indicating a 17% reduction in the primary endpoint of cardiovascular death, MI, or stroke with vorapaxar (HR: 0.83, 95% CI: 0.74–0.93; $P = .001$), due mainly to a reduction in MI (HR: 0.82, 95% CI: 0.72–0.94; $P = .003$). Similarly, GUSTO

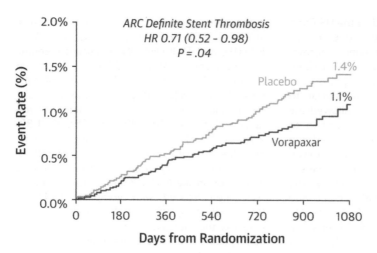

Fig. 4. Effect of vorapaxar on definite stent thrombosis in the TRA 2P-TIMI 50 study. (*From* Bonaca MP, Scirica BM, Braunwald E, et al. Coronary stent thrombosis with vorapaxar versus placebo: results from the TRA 2°P-TIMI 50 Trial. J Am Coll Cardiol 2014;64:2314; with permission.)

moderate or severe bleeding was increased with vorapaxar (HR 1.57, 95% CI1.26–1.94). The rate of ICH was low and not significantly different between vorapaxar (0.5% at 3 year) versus placebo (0.4%). The analysis from the TRA 2P-TIMI 50 on patients with a coronary stent is of particular interest regarding the effect of vorapaxar on stent thrombosis. Vorapaxar significantly reduced by 29%, the occurrence of definite stent thrombosis according to the ARC definition (1.1% vs 1.4%, HR: 0.71, 95% CI 0.51–0.98; $P = .037$) (Fig. 4). Reductions were observed in acute, late, and very late stent thrombosis. There was no heterogeneity noted according to the duration of thienopyridine therapy, which is consistent with the lack of interaction between vorapaxar and thienopyridine observed in the main study, and similar to the TRACER observation.

SUMMARY

PAR-1 antagonism represents a novel approach to reduce atherothrombotic events in patients with atherosclerosis. Vorapaxar is the most largely studied PAR-1 antagonist and is currently approved for use in secondary prevention in patients with prior MI and PAD. Although the TRA 2P-TIMI 50 study met its primary endpoint, overall, the results of phase III trials have had mixed results, with more robust efficacy seen in the TRA 2P than in TRACER and an increase in bleeding observed in both trials. In part, this is due to the fact that the drug was tested in the setting of triple therapy, with most patients receiving aspirin and thienopyridine (nearly all clopidogrel).

In the absence of new studies indicating a marked benefit, especially in the acute,

high-risk ACS patient setting, it is unlikely that the drug will see large uptake in the treatment of coronary artery disease.

To date, there are not dedicated phase III trials specifically assessing PCI patients; thus all that is known derives from the subgroups of patients included in TRACER and TRA 2P who underwent PCI during the trial (58% of TRACER patients) or largely before randomization (TRA 2P). Overall, the studies suggest a consistency of the results in the PCI subgroup compared with the main trial results, with no statistically significant heterogeneity seen. Consequently, the benefit observed in TRACER in PCI patients was modest, whereas the benefit was quite robust in TRA 2P. In TRACER, intriguing findings, yet with unclear explanation were seen, indicating a stronger benefit in patients who received BMS only compared with patients who underwent DES placement. In TRA 2P, the most clinically relevant result observed was the 29% reduction in definite stent thrombosis, which indicate a possible role of PAR-1 antagonism in addition to P2Y12 following stent implantation.

Despite the mixed results, the phase III trials of vorapaxar clearly demonstrate a biological and clinical efficacy on PAR-1 antagonism. Therefore, the author thinks that vorapaxar, or other PAR-1 antagonist, may still have a role in the treatment of patients with coronary disease, including those undergoing coronary stent placement. However, a larger adoption of vorapaxar in clinical practice will require more trials, especially in higher-risk patients, such as those with ACS. Moreover, dedicated trials in patients undergoing coronary stents may clarify the role of PAR-1 antagonism in this important population. Of particular interest would be studies assessing vorapaxar in combination with P2Y12 compared with current standard dual antiplatelet therapy, including aspirin. In fact, we still must learn how vorapaxar performs in a true "head-to-head" comparison with current standard antiplatelet treatments. Another interesting aspect to clarify is whether chronic therapy with vorapaxar as a monotherapy may provide similar or enhanced efficacy and better safety compared with prolonged DAPT or chronic aspirin monotherapy, once the "mandatory" dual antiplatelet therapy period following stent implantation has been completed. These and other hypotheses may further clarify the role of vorapaxar and other PAR-1 antagonists in the treatment of patients with cardiovascular disease.

REFERENCES

1. Jennings LK. Mechanisms of platelet activation: need for new strategies to protect against platelet-mediated atherothrombosis. Thromb Haemost 2009;102:248–57.

2. Farndale RW, Sixma JJ, Barnes MJ, et al. The role of collagen in thrombosis and hemostasis. J Thromb Haemost 2004;2:561–73.

3. Coughlin SR. Thrombin signalling and protease-activated receptors. Nature 2000;407:258–64.

4. Macfarlane SR, Seatter MJ, Kanke T, et al. Proteinase-activated receptors. Pharmacol Rev 2001;53:245–82.

5. Angiolillo DJ, Capodanno D, Goto S. Platelet thrombin receptor antagonism and atherothrombosis. Eur Heart J 2010;31:17–28.

6. Zhang C, Srinivasan Y, Arlow DH, et al. High-resolution crystal structure of human protease-activated receptor 1. Nature 2012;492:387–92.

7. Chen J, Ishii M, Wang L, et al. Thrombin receptor activation. Confirmation of the intramolecular tethered liganding hypothesis and discovery of an alternative intermolecular liganding mode. J Biol Chem 1994;269:16041–5.

8. Arora P, Ricks TK, Trejo J. Protease-activated receptor signalling, endocytic sorting and dysregulation in cancer. J Cell Sci 2007;120:921–8.

9. Cornelissen I, Palmer D, David T, et al. Roles and interactions among protease-activated receptors and P2ry12 in hemostasis and thrombosis. Proc Natl Acad Sci U S A 2010;107:18605–10.

10. Coughlin SR. Protease-activated receptors in hemostasis, thrombosis and vascular biology. J Thromb Haemost 2005;3:1800–14.

11. Vandendries ER, Hamilton JR, Coughlin SR, et al. Par4 is required for platelet thrombus propagation but not fibrin generation in a mouse model of thrombosis. Proc Natl Acad Sci U S A 2007;104:288–92.

12. Chintala M, Strony J, Yang B, et al. SCH 602539, a protease-activated receptor-1 antagonist, inhibits thrombosis alone and in combination with cangrelor in a Folts model of arterial thrombosis in cynomolgus monkeys. Arterioscler Thromb Vasc Biol 2010;30:2143–9.

13. Chackalamannil S, Xia Y, Greenlee WJ, et al. Discovery of potent orally active thrombin receptor (protease activated receptor 1) antagonists as novel antithrombotic agents. J Med Chem 2005;48:5884–7.

14. Judge HM, Jennings LK, Moliterno DJ, et al. PAR1 antagonists inhibit thrombin-induced platelet activation whilst leaving the PAR4-mediated response intact. Platelets 2015;26:236–42.

15. Kosoglou T, Reyderman L, Tiessen RG, et al. Pharmacodynamics and pharmacokinetics of the novel PAR-1 antagonist vorapaxar (formerly SCH 530348) in healthy subjects. Eur J Clin Pharmacol 2012;68:249–58.

16. Becker RC, Moliterno DJ, Jennings LK, et al. Safety and tolerability of SCH 530348 in patients undergoing non-urgent percutaneous coronary intervention: a randomised, double-blind, placebo-controlled phase II study. Lancet 2009;373:919–28.

17. Storey RF, Kotha J, Smyth SS, et al. Effects of vorapaxar on platelet reactivity and biomarker expression in non-ST-elevation acute coronary syndromes. The TRACER Pharmacodynamic Substudy. Thromb Haemost 2014;111:883–91.

18. Tricoci P, Huang Z, Held C, et al. Thrombin-receptor antagonist vorapaxar in acute coronary syndromes. N Engl J Med 2012;366:20–33.

19. Leonardi S, Tricoci P, White HD, et al. Effect of vorapaxar on myocardial infarction in the thrombin receptor antagonist for clinical event reduction in acute coronary syndrome (TRA.CER) trial. Eur Heart J 2013;34:1723–31.

20. Alexander JH, Lopes RD, James S, et al. Apixaban with antiplatelet therapy after acute coronary syndrome. N Engl J Med 2011;365:699–708.

21. Mega JL, Braunwald E, Wiviott SD, et al. Rivaroxaban in patients with a recent acute coronary syndrome. N Engl J Med 2012;366:9–19.

22. Valgimigli M, Tricoci P, Huang Z, et al. Usefulness and safety of vorapaxar in patients with non–ST-segment elevation acute coronary syndrome undergoing percutaneous coronary intervention (from the TRACER trial). Am J Cardiol 2014;114:665–73.

23. Tricoci P, Lokhnygina Y, Huang Z, et al. Vorapaxar with or without clopidogrel after non-ST-segment elevation acute coronary syndromes: results from the thrombin receptor antagonist for clinical event reduction in acute coronary syndrome trial. Am Heart J 2014;168:869–77.e1.

24. Harskamp RE, Clare RM, Ambrosio G, et al. Use of thienopyridine prior to presentation with non-ST-segment elevation acute coronary syndrome and association with safety and efficacy of vorapaxar: insights from the TRACER trial. Eur Heart J Acute Cardiovasc Care 2016. [Epub ahead of print].

25. Popma CJ, Sheng S, Korjian S, et al. Lack of concordance between local investigators, angiographic core laboratory, and clinical event committee in the assessment of stent thrombosis: results from the tracer angiographic substudy. Circ Cardiovasc Interv 2016;9(5).

26. Morrow DA, Alberts MJ, Mohr JP, et al. Efficacy and safety of vorapaxar in patients with prior ischemic stroke. Stroke 2013;44:691–8.

27. Scirica BM, Bonaca MP, Braunwald E, et al. Vorapaxar for secondary prevention of thrombotic events for patients with previous myocardial infarction: a prespecified subgroup analysis of the TRA 2 degrees P-TIMI 50 trial. Lancet 2012; 380:1317–24.

28. Bonaca MP, Scirica BM, Braunwald E, et al. Coronary stent thrombosis with vorapaxar versus placebo: results from the TRA 2°P-TIMI 50 trial. J Am Coll Cardiol 2014;64:2309–17.

Switching P2Y$_{12}$ Receptor Inhibiting Therapies

Fabiana Rollini, MD*, Francesco Franchi, MD, Dominick J. Angiolillo, MD, PhD

KEYWORDS

- P2Y$_{12}$ receptor inhibitors • Switching • Clopidogrel • Prasugrel • Ticagrelor • Cangrelor

---

KEY POINTS

- Antiplatelet therapy with aspirin and a P2Y$_{12}$ receptor inhibitor (clopidogrel, prasugrel, ticagrelor, or cangrelor) represents the cornerstone of acute and long-term treatment of patients with atherothrombotic disease manifestations.
- Switching between P2Y$_{12}$ inhibitors is common in clinical practice and attributed to multiple factors, including individual risk of bleeding and ischemic events, occurrence of adverse events, socioeconomic factors, and pharmacodynamic/genetic profiles.
- Pharmacologic properties of P2Y$_{12}$ inhibiting therapies (competitive vs noncompetitive binding and onset and offset of actions) and timing of clinical presentation (acute vs chronic) are key to define switching strategies.
- Drug interactions have been described when transitioning between P2Y$_{12}$ receptor inhibiting agents of different pharmacologic classes, raising concerns as to optimal switching strategies.
- Clinical trials evaluating the safety and efficacy of switching antiplatelet agents are lacking, and the only available data derive from pharmacodynamic studies and registries.

Dual antiplatelet therapy (DAPT) with aspirin and a platelet P2Y$_{12}$ receptor antagonist represents the keystone of treatment of acute coronary syndrome (ACS) patients and those undergoing percutaneous coronary intervention (PCI).[1–4] Although clopidogrel is still the most commonly used P2Y$_{12}$ receptor inhibitor,[5,6] the newer generation agents, prasugrel and ticagrelor, provide more rapid, consistent, and potent antiplatelet effects, which lead to a greater reduction in ischemic recurrences, including stent thrombosis, compared with clopidogrel in patients with ACS.[7–9] These agents are associated with increased risk of bleeding and higher costs, however, compared with clopidogrel.[7,8] For all these reasons, the treatment of choice for an individual patient takes into account a multitude of factors, which include clinical presentation, patient characteristics, and socioeconomic issues. In an acute setting, such as patients presenting with an ACS, when DAPT is started, information on patient risk for ischemic and bleeding events, socioeconomic status, medication adherence, and preferences may not be available. Moreover, patients may develop adverse effects or contraindications to the used agent during the treatment period. In all these scenarios, switching to another antiplatelet agent may be necessary. Switching between P2Y$_{12}$ agents is, therefore, not uncommon in clinical practice and represents a challenge due to potential drug interactions, which may lead to ineffective platelet inhibition, thus increasing the risk of thrombotic complications or, on the contrary, potential

---

Disclosures: D.J. Angiolillo: has received payment as an individual for (1) consulting fee or honorarium from Sanofi, Eli Lilly, Daiichi-Sankyo, The Medicines Company, AstraZeneca, Merck, Abbott Vascular, and PLx Pharma; (2) participation in review activities from CeloNova, Johnson & Johnson, and St. Jude Medical. Institutional payments for grants from GlaxoSmithKline, Eli Lilly, Daiichi-Sankyo, The Medicines Company, AstraZeneca, Janssen Pharmaceuticals, Osprey Medical, Inc, Novartis, CSL Behring, and Gilead. Other authors have no conflict of interest to report..
University of Florida College of Medicine-Jacksonville, Jacksonville, FL, USA
* Corresponding author. Division of Cardiology, University of Florida College of Medicine-Jacksonville, ACC Building 5th Floor, 655 West 8th Street, Jacksonville, FL 32209.
E-mail address: Fabiana.Rollini@jax.ufl.edu

overdosing due to overlap in drug therapy, which might cause excessive platelet inhibition and increased bleeding.[9,10] These considerations are further enhanced by the recent introduction into clinical practice of intravenous P2Y$_{12}$ inhibitors (eg, cangrelor).[11,12] This article provides an overview of the literature on switching antiplatelet treatment strategies with P2Y$_{12}$ receptor inhibitors and provides practical considerations for switching therapies in the acute and chronic phases of presentation in patients requiring DAPT.

PHARMACOLOGIC PROPERTIES

Differences in the pharmacologic properties of ADP-P2Y$_{12}$ receptor inhibitors have a key role in the potential for drug interactions when switching from one agent to another, in particular with regard to their binding site to the P2Y$_{12}$ receptor (competitive vs noncompetitive), drug half-life, and speeds of onset and offset of action (Table 1).[9,11,13] Clopidogrel, a second-generation thienopyridine, is a prodrug that is up to 85% hydrolyzed into an inactive acid metabolite by human carboxylesterase-1 after intestinal absorption. The remaining 15% of the prodrug requires a 2-step oxidation process using multiple hepatic cytochrome P-450 (CYP) isoenzymes, mainly CYP2C19, to generate an active metabolite. Afterward, clopidogrel's active metabolite irreversibly blocks the ADP binding site on the P2Y$_{12}$ receptor.[9,14] Because ADP-induced P2Y$_{12}$ receptor activation plays a pivotal role in pathologic thrombosis, a clopidogrel-based antiplatelet regimen has represented for more than a decade the mainstay of secondary prevention in patients with ACS or PCI.[5,6,14]

Prasugrel is a third-generation thienopyridine with a more favorable pharmacologic profile compared with clopidogrel. In particular, metabolism of prasugrel is more efficient than that of clopidogrel given that it requires only a single-step hepatic oxidation to generate the active metabolite. Therefore, although prasugrel's active metabolite is equipotent to that derived from clopidogrel, the available plasma concentration is higher, which translates into more prompt, potent, and predictable platelet inhibitory effects compared with clopidogrel.[9,14] The active metabolites of thienopyrdines, however, are unstable, with a short half-life and thus are rapidly eliminated if they do not bind to the P2Y$_{12}$ receptor.[14,15] Given the irreversible binding, recovery time after treatment discontinuation is approximately equivalent to the life span of platelets, although it is longer after prasugrel discontinuation (7 days) compared with clopidogrel (5 days) due to the more profound level of platelet inhibition achieved.[14–16]

Reversibly binding inhibitors available for clinical use are ticagrelor and cangrelor. Ticagrelor is an oral cyclopentyl-triazolopyrimidine, which

Table 1
Pharmacologic properties of P2Y$_{12}$ receptor inhibitors

	Clopidogrel	Prasugrel	Ticagrelor	Cangrelor
Receptor blockade	Irreversible	Irreversible	Reversible	Reversible
Prodrug	Yes	Yes	No	No
Half-life	~6 h	~7 h	7 h	3–5 min
Competitive binding	Competitive	Competitive	Noncompetitive	Undetermined[a]
Administration route	Oral	Oral	Oral	Intravenous
Frequency	Once daily	Once daily	Twice daily	Bolus plus infusion
Onset of action	2–8 h	30 min–4 h	30 min–4 h	~2 min
Offset of action	7–10 d	7–10 d	3–5 d	30–60 min
CYP drug interaction	CYP2C19	No	CYP3A	No
Approved settings	ACS (invasive and noninvasively managed) and stable CAD PCI	ACS undergoing PCI	ACS (invasive or noninvasively managed)	PCI in patients with or without ACS

[a] The binding site of cangrelor at the P2Y$_{12}$ receptor level is not clearly defined; nevertheless, cangrelor is associated with high levels of receptor occupancy preventing ADP signaling.

From Rollini F, Franchi F, Angiolillo DJ. Switching P2Y$_{12}$-receptor inhibitors in patients with coronary artery disease. Nat Rev Cardiol 2016;13:13; with permission.

reversibly binds the P2Y$_{12}$ receptor. It is a direct-acting agent that does not require hepatic metabolism to exert its effect, although approximately 30% of ticagrelor effects derive from active metabolites (mainly AR-C124910XX) generated through CYP3A4-5 enzymes.[9,14,17] Due to its reversible binding to the receptor and the half-life of 7 to 12 hours, ticagrelor requires twice-daily dosing. Unlike the active metabolites of thienopyridines, which directly block the ADP binding site on the P2Y$_{12}$ receptor, ticagrelor reversibly binds to a distinct site on the receptor and acts through an allosteric mechanism to prevent G-protein–mediated signal transduction after ADP binding in a noncompetitive fashion.[9,14,17] Due to its rapid absorption and direct activity, ticagrelor is characterized by more prompt, potent, and predictable pharmacodynamic effects compared with clopidogrel. Because of its reversible binding and relatively short half-life, ticagrelor has a faster offset of antiplatelet effect (approximately 3 days) compared with prasugrel and clopidogrel.[14,17,18] Cangrelor is an intravenous analog of ATP, which is able to exert its effect without needing metabolic biotransformation and reversibly inhibits in a dose-dependent manner the P2Y$_{12}$ receptor, achieving rapid and potent platelet inhibition. Although its binding site at the P2Y$_{12}$ receptor level is not clearly defined, cangrelor is associated with high levels of receptor occupancy, preventing ADP signaling. In addition, because cangrelor is promptly inactivated through dephosphorylation and has a short plasma half-life (3–6 minutes), recovery of platelet function is rapid (30–60 minutes) after discontinuation of infusion.[10,11]

SWITCHING FROM CLOPIDOGREL TO PRASUGREL OR TICAGRELOR

Given the results of large-scale clinical trials showing overall better clinical outcomes in ACS patients treated with prasugrel or ticagrelor compared with clopidogrel, these new-generation oral P2Y$_{12}$ receptor antagonists now represent the first line of treatment in patients presenting with ACS.[1–4,7,8] Therefore, switching from clopidogrel to a more potent agent is commonly applied in clinical practice for patients experiencing an ACS while on clopidogrel treatment. Most of the data, however, available on this topic derive from registries and pharmacodynamic (PD) studies, because no specifically designed clinical trial has been conducted so far. In particular, in the Trial to Assess Therapeutic Outcomes by Optimizing

Platelet Inhibition with Prasugrel–Thrombolysis in Myocardial Infarction 38 (TRITON-TIMI 38), prior exposure to a P2Y$_{12}$ receptor inhibitor represented an exclusion criteria for the study and, therefore, the clinical impact of switching from clopidogrel to prasugrel was not explored.[8] In the Targeted Platelet Inhibition To Clarify the Optimal Strategy To Medically Manage Acute Coronary Syndromes (TRILOGY ACS) trial, however, assessing the clinical impact of long-term use of prasugrel compared with clopidogrel in patients with non-ST elevation myocardial infarction–ACS selected for medical management without revascularization, patients who were not randomized within 72 hours (approximately 95% of the trial population), required to be treated with clopidogrel before randomization; therefore, 70% of patients randomized to prasugrel had been treated with a loading dose (LD) of clopidogrel. Although results need to be interpreted with caution as within the context of a trial that did not reach its primary endpoint, there were no differences in the primary safety endpoint of major bleeding complications.[19]

The Platelet Inhibition and Patient Outcomes (PLATO) trial allowed for patients who had been pretreated with clopidogrel to be enrolled and approximately 50% of patients randomized to ticagrelor were pretreated with clopidogrel. The efficacy and safety of ticagrelor were consistent irrespective of prior clopidogrel exposure, which provide reassuring clinical data on switching from clopidogrel to ticagrelor.[7] Overall, the absence of clinical trials specifically evaluating the effects of switching P2Y$_{12}$ inhibiting therapies have prompted to the design of several PD studies and registries focused on this topic.

Pharmacodynamic Studies of Switching from Clopidogrel to New-Generation P2Y$_{12}$ Receptor Inhibitors

Studies exploring the PD profiles of switching from clopidogrel to a new-generation P2Y$_{12}$ receptor inhibitor are summarized in **Tables 2** and **3**.[20–39] All these studies have consistently shown enhanced platelet inhibitory effects of both prasugrel and ticagrelor over clopidogrel, irrespective of clinical setting (healthy volunteers, stable coronary artery disease [CAD], or ACS) as well as a reduction in rates of high on-treatment platelet reactivity (HPR),[20–43] a well-defined marker of risk of ischemic recurrences, including stent thrombosis.[44]

The Switching Anti Platelet (SWAP) study was a PD investigation specifically designed to assess the effects of switching from clopidogrel to prasugrel and to evaluate how these were affected

Table 2
Pharmacodynamic studies of switching from clopidogrel to prasugrel

Study (Acronym)	Study Design	Study Population (N)	Pharmacodynamic Test	Key Pharmacodynamic Switching Findings	Clinical Outcomes (Exploratory)
Payne et al,[20] 2008	Open-label, randomized, fixed sequence	Healthy subjects (N = 35)	LTA	MPA 37% on C → 5% 1 h after P 60 mg; MPA 37% on C → 28% 1 h after P 10 mg	Outcomes at 22 d: no differences in bleeding episodes or other adverse events.
Wiviott et al,[21] 2007 (PRINCIPAL TIMI44)	Multicenter, randomized, double-blind, double-dummy, active comparator-controlled, crossover	Planned PCI (N = 201)	LTA VASP VN P2Y12	IPA 45.4% on C 150 mg → 60.8% after 15 d on P 10 mg; PRI 39.7% on C 150 mg → 25.1% after 15 d on P 10 mg; VN: consistent finding (data not reported)	Outcomes at 29 d: bleeding occurred in 4 subjects switching from C to P.
Montalescot et al,[22] 2010 (ACAPULCO)	Double-blind, randomized, crossover	UA/non-STEMI (N = 56)	LTA VN P2Y12 VASP	MPA 38.6% after C 900 mg → 28.9% after 15 d on P 10 mg; MPA 38.6% after C 900 mg → 38.2% after 15 d on C 150 mg → 25% after 15 d on C 150 mg → 25% after 15 d on P 10 mg. PRU 96.3 ± 67.6 on C 150 mg → 47.1 ± 32.4 after 15 d on P 10 mg; PRI 40.6 ± 22.5% on C 150 mg → 22.8 ± 15.7% after 15 d on P 10 mg	Outcomes at 60 d: there were no differences in any non–CABG-related TIMI major or GUSTO severe/life-threatening bleeding events. Five subjects (3 P and 2 C) experienced bleeding during MD treatment.
Angiolillo et al,[23] 2010 (SWAP)	Multicenter, randomized, double-blind, double-dummy, active control	Prior ACS (30–330 d) (N = 139)	LTA VN P2Y12 VASP	MPA 60.2% on C 75 mg → 41.1% after 7 d on P 10 mg; MPA 55.5% on C 75 mg → 41% after a dose of P 60 mg + 7 d of P 10 mg; MPA 53.8% on C 75 mg → 55% after 7 d on C 75 mg; VN and VASP: consistent finding (data not reported)	Outcomes at 15 d: bleeding by TIMI criteria was reported in 12.5% of the C, 75 mg MD group, 8.5% of the P 10 mg MD group, and 13.6% of the P LD + MD group

Study	Design	Population	Test method	Results	Outcomes
Trenk et al,[24] 2012 (TRIGGER-PCI)	Randomized, parallel-assignment, double-blind	Stable CAD with HPR undergoing PCI (N = 212)	VN P2Y$_{12}$	Observed a substantial decrease in PRU in the P arm compared with C 176 (94.1%) patients of the P arm reached a PRU ≤208.	Outcomes at 6 mo: TIMI major noncoronary artery bypass graft bleeding occurred in 3 patients on P and 1 patient on C.
Diodati et al,[25] 2013 (TRIPLET)	Randomized, double-blind, double-dummy, 3-arm, parallel, active comparator controlled	ACS undergoing planned PCI (N = 282)	VN P2Y$_{12}$	PRU 57.9, 6 h after placebo/P 60 mg; PRU 35.6, 6 h after C 600 mg/P 60 mg; PRU 53.9, 6 h after C 600 mg/P 30 mg	Outcomes at 72 h: treatment-emergent adverse events were 3 in the placebo LD/P 60 mg group; 4 in the C 600 mg LD/P 60 mg LD group; and 7 in the C 600 mg LD/P 30 mg. There were 2 deaths in the placebo/P 60 mg LD treatment group.
Rollini et al,[26] 2016	Prospective, randomized, parallel design, open-label	CAD (N = 110)	LTA VN P2Y$_{12}$ VASP	MPA 52.3 ± 5% on C → 32 ± 6% 30 min after P 60 mg, → 18.8 ± 4% 2 h after P 60 mg, → 16.6 ± 2% 24 h after P 60 mg, → 28.6 ± 4% 1 wk after P 60 mg PRU 182 ± 19 on C → 105 ± 23 30 min after P 60 mg, → 33 ± 13 2 h after P 60 mg, → 15 ± 11 24 h after P 60 mg, → 73 ± 14 1 wk after P 60 mg PRI 60.8 ± 7% on C → 33.6 ± 7% 30 min after P 60 mg, → 13.4 ± 6% 2 h after P 60 mg, → 14.2 ± 4% 24 h after P 60 mg, → 32.1 ± 5% 1 wk after P 60 mg	Outcomes at 1 wk: 2 minor bleeding
Sardella et al,[27] 2012 (RESET GENE)	Open-label, crossover randomized	Stable CAD with HPR undergoing PCI (N = 32)	MEA	AUC 576 on C→180.5 after 15 d on P 10 mg AUC 380.5 on C 150 mg→ 256 after 15 d on P 10 mg	Outcomes at 3 mo: 3 minor bleedings in patients initially treated with P and 1 minor bleeding while on C

(continued on next page)

Study (Acronym)	Study Design	Study Population (N)	Pharmacodynamic Test	Key Pharmacodynamic Switching Findings	Clinical Outcomes (Exploratory)
Lhermusier et al,[28] 2014	Prospective, open-label, randomized	ACS (N = 48)	VN P2Y$_{12}$ VASP	PRU 143 (53–199) after C 600 mg → 111 (7–127) 4 h after P 10 mg → 97 (41–145) 24 h after initial P dose PRU 122 (82–149) after C 600 mg → 7 (6–31) 4 h after P 30 mg → 27 (7–20) 24 h after initial P dose PRI 44 (29–58)%, after C 600 mg → 35 (16–41)%, 4 h after P 10 mg → 21 (19–58)%, 24 h after initial P dose. PRI 59 (16–68)%, after C 600 mg → 15 (2–30)%, 4 h after P 30 mg → 10 (7–20)%, 24 h after initial P dose	N/A
Alexopoulos et al,[29] 2012	Randomized, single-center, single-blind, crossover	ACS with HPR (N = 44)	VN P2Y$_{12}$	PRU 280.3 on C → 90.8 after 15 d on P 10 mg → 32.1 after 15 d on T 90 mg/twice a day	Outcomes at 30 d: no patient exhibited a major adverse cardiovascular event or a major bleeding event; 4 patients (2 P and 2 T) reported minimal bleeding events. Allergic reactions (n = 2), dyspepsia, (n = 2), dyspnea (n = 4) occurred with T
Koul et al,[30] 2014	Prospective, observational registry	STEMI undergoing PCI (N = 223)	VASP	PRI 79% after C 600 (pre-PCI) mg → 74% after P 60 mg (after PCI) → 17% 1 day after PCI	Outcomes in-hospital: 1.1% major bleeding

Study	Study design	Population	Assay	Results	Outcomes
Cuisset et al,[31] 2013	Prospective, observational registry	NSTE ACS with DM undergoing PCI (N = 107)	VASP	PRI 47 ± 21% after C 600 mg → 31 ± 13% after 1 mo on P 10 mg On C HPR 50% LPR 13% On P HPR 8% LPR 22%	Outcomes at 30 d: 1 stent thrombosis; 10 BARC bleeding complications
Nührenberg et al,[32] 2013	Nonrandomized, observational	STEMI undergoing PCI (N = 47)	VN P2Y$_{12}$ LTA MEA	PRU 10 (8–31) after C 600 mg + P 60 mg MPA 1 after C 600 mg + P 60 mg AU*min 214 (184–250) after C 600 mg + P 60 mg	N/A
Parodi et al,[33] 2014	Nonrandomized, observational	CAD undergoing PCI (N = 454)	LTA	HPR group MPA 72 ± 11% on C → 43 ± 16% on P	Outcomes in hospital and at 6 mo: there were no differences in major or minor TIMI bleeding rates or in BARC bleeding rates or ischemic events between the patients switching and naïve.
Aradi et al,[34] 2014	Prospective, observational registry	ACS undergoing PCI (N = 741)	MEA	P 60 mg/10 mg provided significantly more potent platelet inhibition than the repeated LD of C 600 mg. 86% of the P MD treated patients remained below the cut point for HPR	Outcomes at 1 y: rates of thrombotic complications in HPR group were similar to those in the no HPR group without any difference in all-cause death, myocardial infarction, stent thrombosis, or stroke. No excess of major bleeding after switching to P in HPR group compared with those without HPR.

(continued on next page)

Study (Acronym)	Study Design	Study Population (N)	Pharmacodynamic Test	Key Pharmacodynamic Switching Findings	Clinical Outcomes (Exploratory)
Mayer et al,[35] 2014 (ISAR-HPR)	Prospective observational registry	ACS with HPR undergoing PCI (N = 428)	MEA	AU*min 651 (543–780) after C 600 mg→ 156 (88–261) after P 60 mg	Outcomes at 30 d: 2 (1.7%) combined death/stent thrombosis and 10 (8.7%) TIMI major bleeding
Lhermusier et al,[36] 2014	Open-label, multicenter, nonrandomized observational	ACS with planned invasive strategy (N = 75)	VN P2Y$_{12}$ VASP	PRU 234 (164–267) after C 600 mg→ 23 (5–71), 4 h after P 60 mg→ 9 (5–47) at discharge on P 10 mg PRI 68.4 (31.53–79.61)% after C 600 mg→ 8.67 (4.51–16.85)%, 4 h after P 60 mg → 8.05 (5.12–13.38% at discharge on P 10 mg	Outcomes at discharge: no differences in bleeding between groups (3 in the C to P group and 3 in the P-only group)

Abbreviations: ACAPULCO, Prasugrel Compared with High-Dose Clopidogrel in Acute Coronary Syndrome; AUC, area under the aggregation curve; AU*min, aggregation unit * minutes; BARC, Bleeding Academic Research Consortium; C, clopidogrel; GP IIb/IIIa inhibitor, glycoprotein IIb/IIIa inhibitors; GUSTO, global use of strategies to open occluded arteries; IPA, inhibition of platelet aggregation; ISAR-HPR, A Comparative Cohort Study on Personalised Antiplatelet Therapy in PCI-Treated Patients with High On-Clopidogrel Platelet Reactivity; LPR, low on-treatment platelet reactivity; LTA, light transmission aggregometry; MEA, multiple electrode platelet aggregometry; MPA, maximal platelet aggregation; N/A, not applicable; POBA, Predictor of Bleeding with Antiplatelet Drugs; P, prasugrel; PRI, platelet reactivity index; PRINCIPAL TIMI44, Prasugrel in Comparison to Clopidogrel for Inhibition of Platelet Activation and Aggregation—Thrombolysis in Myocardial Infarction 44; PRU, P2Y$_{12}$ reaction units; RESET GENE, Pharmacodynamic Effects Of Switching Therapy in Patients With High On-Treatment Platelet Reactivity And Genotype Variation: High Clopidogrel Dose Versus Prasugrel; T, ticagrelor; TIMI, Thrombolysis in Myocardial Infarction; UA, unstable angina; VASP, vasodilator-stimulated phosphoprotein; VN P2Y$_{12}$, VerifyNow P2Y$_{12}$.

From Rollini F, Franchi F, Angiolillo DJ. Switching P2Y$_{12}$-receptor inhibitors in patients with coronary artery disease. Nat Rev Cardiol 2016;13:15; with permission.

Table 3
Pharmacodynamic studies of switching from clopidogrel to ticagrelor

Study (Acronym)	Study Design	Study Population (N)	Pharmacodynamic Test	Key Pharmacodynamic Switching Findings	Clinical Outcomes (Exploratory)
Gurbel et al,[37] 2010 (RESPOND)	Randomized, double-blind, double-dummy crossover	Stable CAD (N = 98)	LTA VN P2Y$_{12}$ VASP	Nonresponder cohort MPA 59 ± 9% on C → 35 ± 11%, 4 h after T 180 mg Responder cohort MPA 47 ± 15% on C → 32 ± 8%, 4 h after T 180 mg VN and VASP: consistent finding (data not reported)	Outcomes at 30 d: 4 patients (2 nonresponders and 2 responders) experienced the 5 serious adverse events, and all events occurred during or after T therapy. One major and 3 minor bleeding events occurred during T treatment, and no bleeding events occurred during C treatment. Dyspnea was reported in 13 and 4 patients receiving T and C, respectively. Two nonresponder patients had dyspnea during switching.
Caiazzo et al,[38] 2014 (SHIFT-OVER)	Randomized, single-blind	ACS (N = 50)	MEA LTA	AU 34.4 ± 1.3 on C → 17.6 ± 7.2, 2 h after T 90 mg AU 41.7 ± 2 on C → 18.1 ± 6, 2 h after T 180 mg MPA 24 ± 17% on C → 9 ± 4%, 2 h after T 90 mg MPA 25 ± 14% on C → 9 ± 3%, 2 h after T 180 mg	Outcomes at 30 d: no deaths nor strokes were reported after switch. A total of 2 patients underwent a new hospitalization within the shift to T.

(continued on next page)

Study (Acronym)	Study Design	Study Population (N)	Pharmacodynamic Test	Key Pharmacodynamic Switching Findings	Clinical Outcomes (Exploratory)
Lhermusier et al,[28] 2014	Prospective, open-label, randomized	ACS (N = 48)	VN P2Y$_{12}$ VASP	PRU 146 (97–236) after C 600 mg → 12 (4–46), 4 h after T 90 mg → 9 (5–10), 24 h after initial T dose PRU 92 (33–143) after C 600 mg → 4 (2–6) 4 h after T 180 mg → 4 (3–5), 24 h after initial T dose PRI 57 (18–80)%, after C 600 mg → 3 (2–6)%, 4 h after T 90 mg → 4 (2–11)%, 24 h after initial T dose PRI 47 (10–65)%, after C 600 mg → 2 (0–5)%, 4 h after T 180 mg → 3 (0–4)%, 24 h after initial T dose	Outcomes at 24 h: 1 bleeding event following switch to T 90 mg
Rollini et al,[26] 2016	Prospective, randomized, parallel design, open-label	CAD (N = 110)	LTA VN P2Y$_{12}$ VASP	MPA 50.2 ± 6% on C → 42 ± 6% 30 min after T 180 mg, → 21.9 ± 4% 2 h after T 180 mg, → 18.9 ± 1.1% 24 h after T 180 mg (12 h after T 90 mg), → 34 ± 4% 1 wk after T 180 mg (12 h after T 90 mg) PRU 170 ± 24 on C → 125 ± 25 30 min after T 180 mg, → 28 ± 15 2 h after T 180 mg, → 20 ± 10 24 h after T 180 mg (12 h after T 90 mg), → 58 ± 15 1 wk after T 180 mg (12 h after T 90 mg) PRI 57.6 ± 9% on C → 41.1 ± 8% 30 min after T 180 mg, → 15.6 ± 6% 2 h after T 180 mg, → 19.7 ± 5% 24 h after T 180 mg (12 h after T 90 mg), → 32.6 ± 5% 1 wk after T 180 mg (12 h after T 90 mg)	Outcomes at 1 wk: 1 minor bleeding, 26 dyspnea

Study	Design	Population	Assay	Results	Outcomes
Alexopoulos et al,[29] 2012	Prospective, randomized, single-blind, crossover	ACS with HPR (N = 44)	VN P2Y$_{12}$	PRU 277.4 on C → 34.1 after 15 d on T 90 mg/twice a day → 111.4 after 15 d on P 10 mg	Outcomes at 30 d: no patient exhibited a major adverse cardiovascular event or a major bleeding event; 4 patients (2 P and 2 T) reported minimal bleeding events. Allergic reactions (n = 2), dyspepsia, (n = 2), dyspnea (n = 4) occurred with T.
Hibbert et al,[39] 2014 (CAPITAL RELOAD)	Prospective, observational	STEMI (N = 52)	VN P2Y$_{12}$	PRU 252 (233–280) naïve patients → 220(82–269) 2 h after T 180 mg PRU 255 (233–304) after C 600 mg → 90 (5–205) 2 h after T 180 mg	N/A
Koul et al,[30] 2014	Prospective registry	STEMI undergoing PCI (N = 223)	VASP	PRI 64% after C 600 (pre-PCI) mg → 53% after P 60 mg (after PCI) → 29% 1 d after PCI	In-hospital outcomes: the rate of major in-hospital bleeding was 3.3% in this cohort.

Abbreviations: AU, aggregation unit; C, clopidogrel; CAPITAL RELOAD, A Comparative Pharmacodynamic Study of Ticagrelor versus Clopidogrel and Ticagrelor in Patients Undergoing Primary Percutaneous Coronary Intervention; LTA, light transmission aggregometry; MEA, multiple electrode platelet aggregometry; MPA, maximal platelet aggregation; P, prasugrel; PRI, platelet reactivity index; PRU, P2Y$_{12}$ reaction units; SHIFT-OVER, Administration of a Loading Dose Has No Additive Effect on Platelet Aggregation During the Switch from Ongoing Clopidogrel Treatment to Ticagrelor in Patients With Acute Coronary Syndrome; T, ticagrelor; VASP, vasodilator-stimulated phosphoprotein; VN P2Y$_{12}$, VerifyNow P2Y$_{12}$.
Adapted from Rollini F, Franchi F, Angiolillo DJ. Switching P2Y$_{12}$-receptor inhibitors in patients with coronary artery disease. Nat Rev Cardiol 2016;13:16–17; with permission.

by the administration of an LD. The study was conducted in patients with a prior (>30 days) ACS and showed that switching from clopidogrel to prasugrel provides further platelet inhibition and reduces HPR rates, with an effect that can be achieved more rapidly (within 2 hours) if a 60-mg LD of prasugrel is administered compared with switching with a 10-mg maintenance dose (MD).[23] The PD effects of switching were tested, however, in patients who were already stabilized on clopidogrel therapy after their ACS, while in clinical practice the need to switch to a more potent agent may occur in the acute setting. This led to the design of the Transferring from Clopidogrel Loading Dose to Prasugrel Loading Dose in Acute Coronary Syndrome Patients (TRIPLET) study, which was conducted in patients with ACS undergoing PCI. This study confirmed enhanced platelet inhibition by prasugrel and showed that the effect of adding prasugrel (60-mg LD) within 24 hours after clopidogrel (600-mg LD) was not significantly different compared with prasugrel (60-mg LD) alone, demonstrating no additive PD effect of clopidogrel pretreatment.[25] The pivotal PD investigation exploring the switch from clopidogrel to ticagrelor is the Response to Ticagrelor in Clopidogrel Nonresponders and Responders and Effect of Switching Therapies (RESPOND) study, conducted in patients with stable CAD. This study showed that ticagrelor therapy was able to overcome HPR while on clopidogrel and that its antiplatelet effect was similar regardless of clopidogrel responsiveness.[37]

Overall, PD studies of adding prasugrel or ticagrelor to patients previously exposed to clopidogrel did not show any type of drug interaction or concerns of overdosing. After a clopidogrel LD, a substantial number of $P2Y_{12}$ receptors remains uninhibited, allowing for additional blockade by administering an LD of prasugrel or ticagrelor. After inhibition of all the $P2Y_{12}$ receptors available on the platelet surface, further blockade cannot be achieved and, thus, the degree of $P2Y_{12}$ receptor blockade after prasugrel or ticagrelor administration is similar regardless prior exposure to clopidogrel.[10]

Registry Findings on Switching from Clopidogrel to New-Generation $P2Y_{12}$ Receptor Inhibitors

A vast majority of registries on switching from clopidogrel to a new-generation $P2Y_{12}$ receptor inhibitor report data on the transition from clopidogrel to prasugrel. This is mainly because prasugrel became clinically available before

ticagrelor. Although a large number of post hoc observational analyses on switching have been reported,[45–53] which are summarized in Table 4, the major prospective registries collecting data on switching strategies include Treatment with ADP Receptor Inhibitors: Longitudinal Assessment of Treatment Patterns and Events After Acute Coronary Syndrome (TRANSLATE-ACS),[45] Greek Antiplatelet Registry (GRAPE),[46] Employed Antithrombotic Therapies in Patients With Acute Coronary Syndromes Hospitalized in Italian Cardiac Care Units (EYESHOT),[47] and Multinational Non-Interventional Study of Patients With ST-Segment Elevation Myocardial Infarction Treated With Primary Angioplasty And Concomitant Use of Upstream Antiplatelet Therapy With Prasugrel or Clopidogrel (European MULTIPRAC).[48]

Overall, the prevalence of switching from clopidogrel to either prasugrel or ticagrelor reported in these registries varies from 5% to 50%, which differs depending on the clinical setting and the period of observation (in-hospital vs after discharge) (see Table 4).[45–53] The reasons for switching included mostly clinical factors, such as ST-segment elevation myocardial infarction (STEMI) presentation, in-hospital reinfarction, high-risk angiographic characteristics, younger age, higher body weight, and gender as well as socioeconomic factors, such as being employed or having private health insurance coverage.[45–53] In a majority of cases, the switch occurred in the catheterization laboratory (Cath-lab) at the time of or immediately after PCI, and switching with an LD was more common with ticagrelor than with prasugrel. Although these registries did not highlight any major safety concerns associated with switching (ie, bleeding events), this should be interpreted with caution because the studies were not designed nor powered to assess clinical outcomes.[45–53]

SWITCHING FROM PRASUGREL OR TICAGRELOR TO CLOPIDOGREL

Despite the evidence for sustained efficacy and safety of prasugrel and ticagrelor with long-term treatment, many physicians limit treatment duration with these agents to the early phases after an ACS (weeks or months).[45–50] Reduced costs associated with a generic formulation of clopidogrel as well as concerns of increased risk of bleeding or the presence of dyspnea with ticagrelor therapy remain important reasons for switching to clopidogrel.[10] Overall, registry data indicate that the prevalence of in-hospital switching from a new-generation P2Y$_{12}$ receptor inhibitor to clopidogrel ranges from 5.0% to 13.6%.[45–50] These patients are less likely to be privately insured and have risk factors associated with increased bleeding risk, such as older age, lower body weight, prior transient ischemic attack/stroke, in-hospital treatment with coronary artery bypass graft (CABG), atrial fibrillation/flutter, and use of oral anticoagulants.[45–50] Although rates of switching after hospital discharge are not reported in the literature, this switch is likely to occur in a considerable number of patients who realize the financial burden associated with the use of the novel P2Y$_{12}$ receptor inhibitors only after discharge. These drugs are often used for only the first month after an ACS in patients with economic restraints, who might use a voucher or temporary financial assistance provided by the pharmaceutical manufacturers of these agents. In addition, despite the ischemic benefit of long-term treatment with prasugrel and ticagrelor, major bleeding events also tend to increase over time and may lead to switch to a less potent antiplatelet agent.[7,8,54,55] Discontinuation of ticagrelor treatment of adverse events is also common, primarily driven by mild to moderate dyspnea and nonmajor bleeding, with rates of dyspnea occurring in 13.8% to 19% of patients and leading to discontinuation in 0.9% to 6.5% of patients.[7,56] To date, however, there are no randomized trials that have assessed the clinical outcomes of such a switching strategy, and most information on this issue derives from PD investigations.

The PD effects of transitioning from a new-generation P2Y$_{12}$ receptor inhibitor to clopidogrel have mainly been studied with prasugrel in several crossover studies in various clinical settings as well as in other small cohort studies (Table 5).[21,22,27,37,57–59] These studies have consistently shown an increase in platelet reactivity and HPR rates associated with this strategy. Some of these studies have reported lower bleeding events when switching to clopidogrel; however, these findings, as well as the absence of increased thrombotic events despite a higher rate of patients developing HPR, should be interpreted with caution because none of these studies was powered for clinical outcomes.[21,22,27,37,57–59] The Optimizing Crossover from Ticagrelor to Clopidogrel in Patients with Acute Coronary Syndrome: The CAPITAL OPTI-CROSS Randomized Trial (CAPITAL OPTI-CROSS) is the only reported study exploring the PD of switching from ticagrelor to clopidogrel. The study showed that switching to

clopidogrel with an LD is associated with greater platelet inhibition at 48 hours than switching with an MD, although no difference was found at 72 hours, which was the study primary end point.[57] The ongoing SWAP-4 (NCT02287909) study is specifically designed to better understand the optimal strategy, in terms of dosing and timing, of switching from ticagrelor to clopidogrel based on PD measures. The Testing Responsiveness to Platelet Inhibition on Chronic Antiplatelet Treatment for Acute Coronary Syndromes (TRIOUCAK-ACS) trial will provide information on the safety and efficacy of switching from prasugrel to clopidogrel if patients have levels of platelet reactivity below thresholds associated with ischemic risk (NCT01959451).

SWITCHING BETWEEN PRASUGREL AND TICAGRELOR

To date there is limited information on switching between the new-generation P2Y$_{12}$ receptor inhibitors prasugrel and ticagrelor, and the few available registry data indicate that the switching between these agents ranges from 2% to 4% (see Table 4).[45–48] Although there is also limited information on factors associated with this switching, several reasons may prompt a transition between prasugrel and ticagrelor. Reasons for switching may include both patient and physician preference as a result of drug access (eg, depending on health care system or medical insurance). Although ticagrelor can be administered in ACS patients upstream prior to knowing coronary anatomy, physicians may want to consider switching to prasugrel because it is administered once daily, which may improve compliance. Another reason to consider switching from ticagrelor to prasugrel is to overcome dyspnea, which occurs more frequently with ticagrelor and which has also shown to affect drug compliance.[7,56] In clinical practice, several reasons may lead to a switch from prasugrel to ticagrelor. These include ticagrelor's mortality benefit during the first year after an ACS[7] as well as the recent demonstration of ischemic benefits, albeit at the expense of increased bleeding, associated with prolonging ticagrelor therapy beyond 1 year post-ACS.[55] Moreover, data from real-world clinical practice show that some patients may be treated with prasugrel, despite having a contraindication, and are candidates for ticagrelor therapy. These include ACS patients who get pretreated with prasugrel prior to defining coronary anatomy but do not undergo PCI or those who have a prior cerebrovascular event.[45,48,50]

Table 4
Switching oral P2Y$_{12}$ receptor inhibitors: registry findings

Name (Acronym)	Study Population (N)	Switch from Clopidogrel to New P2Y$_{12}$ Receptor Inhibitors (Prevalence)	Switch from New P2Y$_{12}$ Receptor Inhibitors to Clopidogrel	Switch Between New P2Y$_{12}$ Receptor Inhibitors	Clinical Outcomes (Exploratory)
Alexopoulos et al,[46] 2014 (GRAPE)	ACS undergoing PCI (N = 1794)	C → P: 40.1% C → T: 50.3%	P → C: 1% T → C: 4.3%	Between P and T: 4.3%[a]	Outcomes at 1 mo: higher risk of bleeding and less MACE in patients switched from C to P or T compared with those treated with C only. No differences in MACE and bleeding when compared with those initially treated with P or T.
Clemmensen et al,[48] 2015 (European MULTIPRAC)	STEMI (N = 2053)	C → P: 48.7% C → T: 11.6%	P → C: 8.3% T → C: N/A	P → T: 2.8% T → P: N/A	In-hospital outcomes: no differences in MACE and non-CABG related bleeding in patients switched from C to P vs patients on P only.
Bagai et al,[45] 2015 (TRANSLATE-ACS)	NSTEMI, STEMI (N = 11,999)	C → P: 10.4% C → T: 1%	P → C: 11.5% T → C: 2.1%	P → T: 0.3% T → P: 3.4%	Outcomes at 6 mo: no significant differences in MACE and bleeding in switched (any switching) vs nonswitched patients.
Schiele et al,[49] 2016 (FAST-MI)	NSTEMI, STEMI (N = 4101)	C → P: 16.5% C → T: N/A	P → C: 4.6% T → C: N/A	N/A	N/A
De Luca et al,[47] 2015 (EYESHOT)	NSTE-ACS STEMI (N = 2585)	In cath-lab switch: C → P/T: 3% At discharge switch C → P/T: 9.6% Switch in medically managed patients C → P/T: 2%	In cath-lab switch: P/T → C: 0.3% At discharge switch P/T → C: 3.2% Switch in medically managed patients P/T → C: 3.4%	In cath-lab switch: Between P and T: 0.3% At discharge switch Between P and T: 1.3% Switch in medically managed patients Between P and T: 0.3%	N/A

Study	Population				Outcomes
Bagai et al,[50] 2014 (ACTION Registry—GWTG and CathPCI)	NSTEMI and STEMI undergoing PCI (N = 47,040)	C → P: 5.2% C → T: N/A	P → C: 11.5% T → C: N/A	N/A	N/A
De Luca et al,[51] 2014	NSTEMI, STEMI, UA underwent PCI (N = 450)	150 patients switched from C to P matched with 300 C-only treated patients	N/A	N/A	Outcomes at 30 days: no differences in MACE, NACE and bleeding between groups.
Loh et al,[52] 2013	ACS undergoing PCI (N = 606)	C → P: 14.8% C → T: N/A	N/A	N/A	In-hospital outcomes: no differences in bleeding between patients who switched to P compared those on P only. MACE were greater in patients who switched to P compared woth those on P only.
Almendro-Delia et al,[53] 2015	ACS (N = 468)	C → P: 25% C → T: N/A	N/A	P → T: 0.3% T → P: N/A	In-hospital outcomes: no difference in bleeding and MACCE between patients who switched to P compared with those on C only.

Abbreviations: ACTION Registry—GWTG and CathPCI, National Cardiovascular Data Registry Acute Coronary Treatment and Intervention Outcomes Network Registry—Get With the Guidelines and National Cardiovascular Data Registry CathPCI Registry; C, clopidogrel; MACCE, major adverse cardiac and cerebrovascular event; MACE, major adverse cardiac events; NACE, net adverse clinical events; NSTEMI, non-ST-elevation myocardial infarction; P, prasugrel; T, ticagrelor; UA, unstable angina.

a Cumulative rate only available.

Adapted from Rollini F, Franchi F, Angiolillo DJ. Switching P2Y$_{12}$-receptor inhibitors in patients with coronary artery disease. Nat Rev Cardiol 2016;13:18; with permission.

Table 5
Pharmacodynamic studies of switching from novel P2Y$_{12}$ receptor inhibitors to clopidogrel

Study (Acronym)	Study Design	Study Population (N)	Pharmacodynamic Test	Key Pharmacodynamic Switching Findings	Clinical Outcomes (Exploratory)
Gurbel et al,[37] 2010 (RESPOND)	Randomized, double-blind, double-dummy crossover	Stable CAD (N = 98)	LTA VN P2Y$_{12}$ VASP	Nonresponder cohort MPA 36 ± 14% on T → 56 ± 9% 4 h after C 600 mg Responder cohort MPA 25 ± 11% on T → 45 ± 8% 4 h after C 600 mg VN and VASP: consistent finding (data not reported)	Outcomes at 30 d: 4 patients (2 nonresponders and 2 responders) experienced the 5 serious adverse events, and all events occurred during or after T therapy. One major and 3 minor bleeding events occurred during T treatment, and no bleeding events occurred during C treatment. Dyspnea was reported in 13 and 4 patients receiving T and C, respectively. Two nonresponder patients had dyspnea during switching.
Wiviott et al,[21] 2007 (PRINCIPAL TIMI44)	Multicenter, randomized, double-blind, double-dummy, active comparator-controlled, crossover	Planned PCI (N = 201)	LTA VASP VN P2Y$_{12}$	IPA 61.9% on P 10 mg → 46.8% after 15 d on C 150 mg PRI 21.7% on P 10 mg → 48% after 15 d on C 150 mg VN: consistent finding (data not reported)	Outcomes at 29 d: no bleeding events in subject switching from P to C.
Montalescot et al,[22] 2010 (ACAPULCO)	Double-blind, randomized, crossover	UA/non-STEMI (N = 56)	LTA VN P2Y$_{12}$ VASP	MPA 28.9% on P 10 mg → 42.5% after 15 d on C 150 mg PRU 41.3 ± 43.8 on P 10 mg → 101.3 ± 60.8 after 15 d on C 150 mg PRI 21.5± 13.4% on P 10 mg → 38.1± 19.8% after 15 d on C 150 mg	Outcomes at 60 d: there were no differences in any non–CABG-related TIMI major or GUSTO severe/life-threatening bleeding events. Five subjects (3 P and 2 C) experienced bleeding during MD treatment.
Sardella et al,[27] 2012 (RESET GENE)	Open-label, crossover randomized	Stable CAD with HPR undergoing PCI (N = 32)	MEA	AUC 180.5 after 15 on P 10 mg →330 after 15 d on C 150 mg	Outcomes at 3 mo: 3 minor bleedings in patients initially treated with P and 1 minor bleeding while on C.

Pourdjabbar et al,[57] 2015 (CAPITAL OPTI-CROSS)	Prospective, randomized, open-label	ACS (N = 60)	VN P2Y$_{12}$	PRU ~40 on T^a → 114 ± 73.1, 48 h after C 600 mg; PRU ~40 on T^a → 165.1 ± 70.5, 48 h after C 75 mg; PRU ~40 on T^a → 165.8 ± 71, 72 h after C 600 mg; PRU ~40 on T^a → 184.1 ± 68, 72 h after C 75 mg; HPR rate after C 600 mg: 27%; HPR rate after C 75 mg: 57%	Outcomes at 30 d: No differences in MACE, TIMI major bleeding or stent thrombosis between groups.
Kerneis et al,[58] 2013	Prospective, observational registry	ACS (N = 31)	LTA VN P2Y$_{12}$ VASP	MPA 21.01 ± 10.47% on P 10 mg → 43.84 ± 15.19% after 15 on C 75 mg; PRU 14.23 ± 27.98 on P 10 mg → 155 ± 87.24 after 15 d on C 75 mg; PRI 12.55 ± 11.9% on P 10 mg → 43.63 ± 21.82% after 15 d on C 75 mg	Outcomes at 30 d: no major bleedings
Deharo et al,[59] 2013 (POBA)	Prospective, observational	ACS with LPR (N = 20)	VASP	PRI 7 ± 2% on P → 37.8 ± 15.6% on C	Outcomes at 30 d: no bleeding events after switching to C.

Abbreviations: ACAPULCO, Prasugrel Compared with High-Dose Clopidogrel in Acute Coronary Syndrome; BARC, Bleeding Academic Research Consortium; C, clopidogrel; GP IIb/IIIa inhibitor, glycoprotein IIb/IIIa inhibitors; GUSTO, Global Use of Strategies to Open Occluded Arteries; IPA, inhibition of platelet aggregation; LPR, low platelet reactivity; LTA, light transmission aggregometry; MPA, maximal platelet aggregation; P, prasugrel; POBA, Predictor of Bleeding with Antiplatelet Drugs; PRI, platelet reactivity index; PRINCIPAL TIMI44, Prasugrel in Comparison to Clopidogrel for Inhibition of Platelet Activation and Aggregation—Thrombolysis in Myocardial Infarction 44; PRU, P2Y$_{12}$ reaction units; RESET GENE, Pharmacodynamic Effects of Switching Therapy in Patients With High On-Treatment Platelet Reactivity And Genotype Variation: High Clopidogrel Dose Versus Prasugrel; T, ticagrelor; TIMI, Thrombolysis in Myocardial Infarction; UA, unstable angina; VASP, vasodilator-stimulated phosphoprotein; VN P2Y$_{12}$, VerifyNow P2Y$_{12}$.

^{a} Value estimated from the figure.

Adapted from Rollini F, Franchi F, Angiolillo DJ. Switching P2Y$_{12}$-receptor inhibitors in patients with coronary artery disease. Nat Rev Cardiol 2016;13:23; with permission.

The PD effects of switching from ticagrelor to prasugrel have been investigated in the SWAP-2 study. In this study, patients were switched to prasugrel (with or without a 60-mg LD) 12 hours after the last ticagrelor MD. Platelet reactivity was higher in prasugrel-treated patients compared with the ticagrelor-treated at 7 days, not meeting the noninferiority primary endpoint. Moreover, at 24 and even more so at 48 hours, platelet reactivity increased in patients switched to prasugrel compared with preswitch levels, and the use of an LD of prasugrel seemed essential to mitigate the increase in platelet reactivity after switching.[60] These data also suggest that this potential drug-drug interaction could have been attributed to the presence of ticagrelor or its major metabolite on the $P2Y_{12}$ receptor when prasugrel was administered after 12 hours from the last MD of ticagrelor. This also suggested that switching should occur after a later time frame post-MD (eg, after 24 hours) to enable more time for the receptor to be unbounded by ticagrelor or its metabolite to allow more optimal switching.

The recently published SWAP-3 study investigated the PD effects of switching from prasugrel to ticagrelor. The study showed that transitioning to ticagrelor patients who were on standard of care maintenance treatment with prasugrel, on a background of aspirin, after PCI in the setting of an ACS, was associated with a reduction in levels of platelet reactivity. These PD findings were observed as early as 2 hours after switching therapy, without any signs of drug interactions during the entire study time course, and no increase in HPR rates. These findings were observed when switching to ticagrelor irrespective of the use of an LD.[61]

SWITCHING BETWEEN ORAL AGENTS AND CANGRELOR

Given the different pharmacologic properties of cangrelor and oral $P2Y_{12}$ receptor inhibitors, several studies have investigated the potential for drug interactions when these agents are concomitantly administered,[62–67] which could result in reduced platelet inhibition and lack of protection from thrombotic complications in the early phase during or after PCI. Studies performed among healthy volunteers showed that administering clopidogrel during the infusion of cangrelor is associated with impaired clopidogrel-induced antiplatelet effects.[62] This is likely because clopidogrel cannot bind to the $P2Y_{12}$ receptors while these are almost entirely occupied by cangrelor. On the other hand,

clopidogrel's antiplatelet effects are not diminished when it is administered after cangrelor infusion, because of the fast offset of action of cangrelor.[62] Similar findings were observed when platelets were incubated with cangrelor before the addition of the active metabolites of either prasugrel or clopidogrel, where the ability of thienopyridines to inhibit platelet aggregation was strongly reduced.[63] Conversely, in blood preincubated with the active metabolites of clopidogrel or prasugrel, as well as in blood from patients treated with these agents, addition of cangrelor led to more profound platelet inhibition.[63,64] PD studies conducted in patients with stable CAD have been performed to define the ideal transition strategies between cangrelor and oral agents.[65–67] These studies showed no interaction when cangrelor is administered on top of prasugrel or ticagrelor, which leads to enhanced antiplatelet effect.[65,66] No interaction was also showed when transitioning from cangrelor to ticagrelor, which can be administered at any time during cangrelor infusion or immediately after discontinuation.[65] On the other end, transitioning from cangrelor to a thienopyridine was associated with drug interactions.[66,67] The transition from cangrelor to prasugrel was associated with transient recovery of platelet reactivity, in particular within 1 hour after cangrelor discontinuation. It was observed, however, that the recovery of platelet function was attenuated when prasugrel was administered 30 minutes before stopping cangrelor.[66] Conversely, administration of clopidogrel 30 minutes or 1 hour before cangrelor infusion discontinuation did not prevent recovery of platelet reactivity more effectively than administration at the end of the infusion.[67]

The presence of an interaction between thienopyridines and cangrelor, but not between ticagrelor and cangrelor, is probably the result of different half-lives of these drugs as well as the different sites and types of binding to the $P2Y_{12}$ receptor.[9,10] During cangrelor infusion, almost all $P2Y_{12}$ receptors are occupied by cangrelor. Therefore, the active metabolites of thienopyridines cannot bind to the receptors and are very unstable with rapid clearance from systemic circulation. After stopping cangrelor infusion, receptors become available for binding but most of the thienopyridines' active metabolite has already been hydrolyzed. Therefore, they should be administered after discontinuation of cangrelor infusion. Ticagrelor does not bind to the $P2Y_{12}$ receptor when occupied by cangrelor. Given its half-life of 10 to 12 hours, however, it will be available for binding once cangrelor has been cleared. Moreover, ticagrelor reversibly binds the P2Y$_{12}$ receptor at a site distinct from the ADP-binding site. Therefore, ticagrelor can be administered before, during or after cangrelor infusion.[68]

Given these PD observations, in the Cangrelor versus Standard Therapy to Achieve Optimal Management of Platelet Inhibition (CHAMPION) PHOENIX trial, the pivotal study leading to the clinical approval of cangrelor for patients undergoing PCI, clopidogrel was administered immediately after discontinuation of cangrelor infusion to avoid a drug interaction.[69,70] To date, no clinical study has investigated the effects of cangrelor in addition to the new-generation P2Y$_{12}$ receptor inhibitors prasugrel and ticagrelor.

PRACTICAL CONSIDERATIONS FOR SWITCHING

In the absence of dedicated trials specifically designed for assessing the safety and efficacy of switching strategies, the choice on the best modality of switching is based on analyses of clinical trials and PD studies. The strategy to switch antiplatelet agents may differ depending on the clinical scenario where switching occurs, in terms of being in the acute or chronic phase after an ACS (Fig. 1). To this extent, the acute phase could be defined as the first 7 to 30 days after the acute ACS event, because this is the period where stent thrombosis is more likely to occur in case of lack of protection from DAPT.[71]

Switching from clopidogrel to ticagrelor occurred in approximately half of the patients enrolled in PLATO using a 180-mg LD irrespective of timing of last dose of clopidogrel followed by a 90-mg MD administered 12 hours after LD.[7] Accordingly, in the acute phase, a parallel approach should be applied whenever switching from clopidogrel to ticagrelor. Because clinical trials testing ticagrelor in patients with more stable clinical presentations started treatment directly with the MD regimen (without LD),[55] it is reasonable to consider a 90-mg twice-a-day MD when switching in the chronic phase after an ACS and to initiate treatment at the timing of the next scheduled MD,

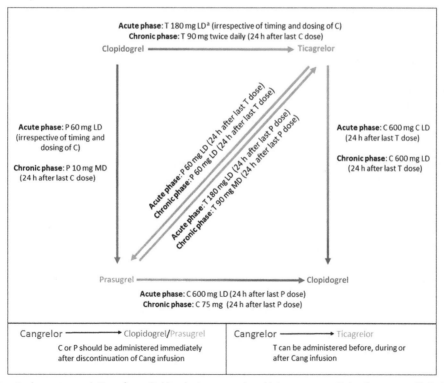

Fig. 1. Practical recommendations for switching between oral and intravenous antiplatelet agents. Switching from an oral agent (*upper panel*) and switching from an intravenous agent (*lower panel*). [a] Followed by ticagrelor, 90 mg twice daily, with first MD administered 12 h after the LD. C, clopidogrel; Cang, cangrelor; P, prasugrel; T, ticagrelor. (*Adapted from* Rollini F, Franchi F, Angiolillo DJ. Switching P2Y$_{12}$-receptor inhibitors in patients with coronary artery disease. Nat Rev Cardiol 2016;13:11–27; with permission.)

which is approximately 24 hours from last dose of clopidogrel.

Switching from clopidogrel to prasugrel was not explored in the TRITON-TIMI 38.[8] Based on results of PD studies, switching from clopidogrel to prasugrel in the acute phase of patients' clinical presentation should occur with the use of 60-mg LD irrespective of timing of last dose of clopidogrel, because fast and potent platelet inhibition is required in this setting. The use of a 10-mg MD approximately 24 hours from last dose of clopidogrel seems, however, a reasonable option when switching is required in the chronic phase.

Based on the limited available PD data and on PD considerations, whenever switching from prasugrel or ticagrelor to clopidogrel is required, clopidogrel should be administered with a 600-mg LD, given its unpredictable platelet inhibitory profile.[14,44] Although the optimal timing of switching after the last dose of ticagrelor or prasugrel is unknown, waiting 24 hours after the last MD should be considered, because this may prevent drug interactions with ticagrelor and allow for new platelets to be released into circulation and be exposed to clopidogrel's active metabolite. In the chronic phase after an ACS, it may be reasonable to switch from prasugrel to clopidogrel, 75 mg/d MD, without an LD, because no drug interaction has been described when switching between thienopyridines.

PD data suggest that when switching from ticagrelor to prasugrel there is a potential for a drug interaction, which can be mitigated with the use of a 60-mg LD of prasugrel, whereas switching to a 10-mg MD should be avoided.[60] In addition, waiting 24 hours after the last MD of ticagrelor to administer the 60-mg LD of prasugrel should be considered, because this allows ticagrelor and its metabolite to be eliminated. Switching from prasugrel to ticagrelor is associated with transiently higher levels of platelet inhibition.[61] Therefore, this switching can be performed without any concerns about drug interactions by transitioning to a standard 90-mg twice-a-day MD dose regimen, without the need for an LD. The use of an LD, however, can be considered when switching occurs at the time of PCI in patients with ACS, because this always ensures $P2Y_{12}$ receptor blockade.

In cases of transition strategies involving cangrelor, when transitioning from any oral $P2Y_{12}$ receptor inhibitor to cangrelor, the infusion can be started at any time. When switching from cangrelor to a thienopyridine (clopidogrel or prasugrel), these should be administered immediately after discontinuation of cangrelor to avoid a PD interaction, whereas ticagrelor can be administered before, during, or after cangrelor infusion.

SUMMARY

Switching antiplatelet therapies is a common occurrence in clinical practice. The current availability of different oral $P2Y_{12}$ receptor antagonists allows for multiple treatment options and has raised the question on the optimal approach for switching among these therapies if needed. The clinical impact of most switching strategies, however, is not fully determined given the lack of trials adequately powered or designed to test for safety and efficacy. Therefore, most of the available data on switching with currently approved therapies derive from registries and PD studies, which have been helpful to define switching approaches associated with more favorable measures using surrogate markers of platelet reactivity. Although no signals of harm have been identified from the small studies performed so far, before deciding how to switch agents, it is pivotal for the clinicians to ensure that switching is clinically required.

REFERENCES

1. Levine GN, Bates ER, Blankenship JC, et al. 2011 ACCF/AHA/SCAI guideline for percutaneous coronary intervention. A report of the American College of Cardiology Foundation/American Heart Association Task Force on Practice Guidelines and the Society for Cardiovascular Angiography and Interventions. Circulation 2011;124:e574–651.

2. O'Gara PT, Kushner FG, Ascheim DD, et al. 2013 ACCF/AHA guideline for the management of ST-elevation myocardial infarction: executive summary: a report of the American College of Cardiology Foundation/American Heart Association Task Force on Practice Guidelines. Circulation 2013; 127:529–55.

3. Amsterdam EA, Wenger NK, Brindis RG, et al. 2014 AHA/ACC guideline for the management of patients with non-ST-elevation acute coronary syndromes: a report of the American College of Cardiology/American Heart Association Task Force on Practice Guidelines. Circulation 2014;130:e344–426.

4. Authors/Task Force Members, Windecker S, Kolh P, et al. 2014 ESC/EACTS guidelines on myocardial revascularization: the task force on myocardial revascularization of the European Society of Cardiology (ESC) and the European Association for Cardio-Thoracic Surgery (EACTS) Developed with the special contribution of the

European Association of Percutaneous Cardiovascular Interventions (EAPCI). Eur Heart J 2014;35:2541–619.

5. Sherwood MW, Wiviott SD, Peng SA, et al. Early clopidogrel versus prasugrel use among contemporary STEMI and NSTEMI patients in the US: insights from the National Cardiovascular Data Registry. J Am Heart Assoc 2014;3:e000849.

6. Bueno H, Sinnaeve P, Annemans L, et al. Opportunities for improvement in anti-thrombotic therapy and other strategies for the management of acute coronary syndromes: Insights from EPICOR, an international study of current practice patterns. Eur Heart J Acute Cardiovasc Care 2016;5:3–12.

7. Wallentin L, Becker RC, Budaj A, et al. Ticagrelor versus clopidogrel in patients with acute coronary syndromes. N Engl J Med 2009;361:1045–57.

8. Wiviott SD, Braunwald E, McCabe CH, et al. Prasugrel versus clopidogrel in patients with acute coronary syndromes. N Engl J Med 2007;357:2001–15.

9. Franchi F, Angiolillo DJ. Novel antiplatelet agents in acute coronary syndrome. Nat Rev Cardiol 2015;12:30–47.

10. Rollini F, Franchi F, Angiolillo DJ. Switching P2Y12-receptor inhibitors in patients with coronary artery disease. Nat Rev Cardiol 2016;13:11–27.

11. Franchi F, Rollini F, Muñiz-Lozano A, et al. Cangrelor: a review on pharmacology and clinical trial development. Expert Rev Cardiovasc Ther 2013;11:1279–91.

12. Cangrelor United States full prescribing information. Available at: http://www.kengreal.com/pdfs/kengreal-us-prescribing-information.pdf. Accessed July 30, 2016.

13. Angiolillo DJ, Ueno M, Goto S. Basic principles of platelet biology and clinical implications. Circ J 2010;74:597–607.

14. Angiolillo DJ. The evolution of antiplatelet therapy in the treatment of acute coronary syndromes: from aspirin to the present day. Drugs 2012;72:2087–116.

15. Farid NA, Kurihara A, Wrighton SA. Metabolism and disposition of the thienopyridine antiplatelet drugs ticlopidine, clopidogrel, and prasugrel in humans. J Clin Pharmacol 2010;50:126–42.

16. Price MJ, Walder JS, Baker BA, et al. Recovery of platelet function after discontinuation of prasugrel or clopidogrel maintenance dosing in aspirin-treated patients with stable coronary disease: the recovery trial. J Am Coll Cardiol 2012;59:2338–43.

17. Husted S, van Giezen JJ. Ticagrelor: the first reversibly binding oral P2Y12 receptor antagonist. Cardiovasc Ther 2009;27:259–74.

18. Gurbel PA, Bliden KP, Butler K, et al. Randomized double-blind assessment of the ONSET and OFFSET of the antiplatelet effects of ticagrelor versus clopidogrel in patients with stable coronary artery disease: the ONSET/OFFSET study. Circulation 2009;120:2577–85.

19. Roe MT, Armstrong PW, Fox KA, et al. Prasugrel versus clopidogrel for acute coronary syndromes without revascularization. N Engl J Med 2012;367:1297–309.

20. Payne CD, Li YG, Brandt JT, et al. Switching directly to prasugrel from clopidogrel results in greater inhibition of platelet aggregation in aspirin-treated subjects. Platelets 2008;19:275–81.

21. Wiviott SD, Trenk D, Frelinger AL, et al. Prasugrel compared with high loading- and maintenance-dose clopidogrel in patients with planned percutaneous coronary intervention: the Prasugrel in Comparison to Clopidogrel for Inhibition of Platelet Activation and Aggregation-Thrombolysis in Myocardial Infarction 44 trial. Circulation 2007;116:2923–32.

22. Montalescot G, Sideris G, Cohen R, et al. Prasugrel compared with high-dose clopidogrel in acute coronary syndrome. The randomised, double-blind ACAPULCO study. Thromb Haemost 2010;103:213–23.

23. Angiolillo DJ, Saucedo JF, Deraad R, et al, SWAP Investigators. Increased platelet inhibition after switching from maintenance clopidogrel to prasugrel in patients with acute coronary syndromes: results of the SWAP (SWitching Anti Platelet) study. J Am Coll Cardiol 2010;56:1017–23.

24. Trenk D, Stone GW, Gawaz M, et al. A randomized trial of prasugrel versus clopidogrel in patients with high platelet reactivity on clopidogrel after elective percutaneous coronary intervention with implantation of drug-eluting stents: results of the TRIGGER-PCI (Testing Platelet Reactivity In Patients Undergoing Elective Stent Placement on Clopidogrel to Guide Alternative Therapy With Prasugrel) study. J Am Coll Cardiol 2012;59:2159–64.

25. Diodati JG, Saucedo JF, French JK, et al. Effect on platelet reactivity from a prasugrel loading dose after a clopidogrel loading dose compared with a prasugrel loading dose alone: Transferring From Clopidogrel Loading Dose to Prasugrel Loading Dose in Acute Coronary Syndrome Patients (TRIPLET): a randomized controlled trial. Circ Cardiovasc Interv 2013;6:567–74.

26. Rollini F, Franchi F, Cho JR, et al. A head-to-head pharmacodynamic comparison of prasugrel vs. ticagrelor after switching from clopidogrel in patients with coronary artery disease: results of a prospective randomized study. Eur Heart J 2016 [pii:ehv744].

27. Sardella G, Calcagno S, Mancone M, et al. Pharmacodynamic effect of switching therapy in patients with high on-treatment platelet reactivity and genotype variation with high clopidogrel Dose versus prasugrel: the RESET GENE trial. Circ Cardiovasc Interv 2012;5:698–704.

28. Lhermusier T, Voisin S, Murat G, et al. Switching patients from clopidogrel to novel P2Y12 receptor inhibitors in acute coronary syndrome: comparative effects of prasugrel and ticagrelor on platelet reactivity. Int J Cardiol 2014;174:874–6.

29. Alexopoulos D, Galati A, Xanthopoulou I, et al. Ticagrelor versus prasugrel in acute coronary syndrome patients with high on-clopidogrel platelet reactivity following percutaneous coronary intervention: a pharmacodynamic study. J Am Coll Cardiol 2012;60:193–9.

30. Koul S, Andell P, Martinsson A, et al. A pharmacodynamic comparison of 5 anti-platelet protocols in patients with ST-elevation myocardial infarction undergoing primary PCI. BMC Cardiovasc Disord 2014;14:189.

31. Cuisset T, Gaborit B, Dubois N, et al. Platelet reactivity in diabetic patients undergoing coronary stenting for acute coronary syndrome treated with clopidogrel loading dose followed by prasugrel maintenance therapy. Int J Cardiol 2013;168:523–8.

32. Nührenberg TG, Trenk D, Leggewie S, et al. Clopidogrel pretreatment of patients with ST-elevation myocardial infarction does not affect platelet reactivity after subsequent prasugrel-loading: platelet reactivity in an observational study. Platelets 2013; 24:549–53.

33. Parodi G, De Luca G, Bellandi B, et al. Switching from clopidogrel to prasugrel in patients having coronary stent implantation. J Thromb Thrombolysis 2014;38:395–401.

34. Aradi D, Tornyos A, Pintér T, et al. Optimizing P2Y12 receptor inhibition in patients with acute coronary syndrome on the basis of platelet function testing: impact of prasugrel and high-dose clopidogrel. J Am Coll Cardiol 2014;63:1061–70.

35. Mayer K, Schulz S, Bernlochner I, et al. A comparative cohort study on personalised antiplatelet therapy in PCI-treated patients with high on-clopidogrel platelet reactivity. Results of the ISAR-HPR registry. Thromb Haemost 2014;112: 342–51.

36. Lhermusier T, Lipinski MJ, Drenning D, et al. Switching patients from clopidogrel to prasugrel in acute coronary syndrome: impact of the clopidogrel loading dose on platelet reactivity. J Interv Cardiol 2014;27:365–72.

37. Gurbel P, Bliden KP, Butler K, et al. Response to ticagrelor in clopidogrel nonresponders and responders and effect of switching therapies: the RESPOND study. Circulation 2010;121:1188–99.

38. Caiazzo G, De Rosa S, Torella D, et al. Administration of a loading dose has no additive effect on platelet aggregation during the switch from ongoing clopidogrel treatment to ticagrelor in patients with acute coronary syndrome. Circ Cardiovasc Interv 2014;7:104–12.

39. Hibbert B, Maze R, Pourdjabbar A, et al. A comparative pharmacodynamic study of ticagrelor versus clopidogrel and ticagrelor in patients undergoing primary percutaneous coronary intervention: the CAPITAL RELOAD study. PLoS One 2014;9:e92078.

40. Michelson AD, Frelinger AL 3rd, Braunwald E, et al, TRITON-TIMI 38 Investigators. Pharmacodynamic assessment of platelet inhibition by prasugrel vs. clopidogrel in the TRITON-TIMI 38 trial. Eur Heart J 2009;30:1753–63.

41. Saucedo JF, Angiolillo DJ, DeRaad R, et al. Decrease in high on-treatment platelet reactivity (HPR) prevalence on switching from clopidogrel to prasugrel: insights from the switching antiplatelet (SWAP) study. Thromb Haemost 2013; 109:347–55.

42. Bliden KP, Tantry US, Storey RF, et al. The effect of ticagrelor versus clopidogrel on high on-treatment platelet reactivity: combined analysis of the ONSET/OFFSET and RESPOND studies. Am Heart J 2011;162:160–5.

43. Storey RF, Angiolillo DJ, Patil SB, et al. Inhibitory effects of ticagrelor compared with clopidogrel on platelet function in patients with acute coronary syndromes: the PLATO (PLATelet inhibition and patient Outcomes) PLATELET substudy. J Am Coll Cardiol 2010;56:1456–62.

44. Tantry US, Bonello L, Aradi D, et al. Consensus and update on the definition of on-treatment platelet reactivity to adenosine diphosphate associated with ischemia and bleeding. J Am Coll Cardiol 2013;62:2261–73.

45. Bagai A, Peterson ED, Honeycutt E, et al. In-hospital switching between adenosine diphosphate receptor inhibitors in patients with acute myocardial infarction treated with percutaneous coronary intervention: Insights into contemporary practice from the TRANSLATE-ACS study. Eur Heart J Acute Cardiovasc Care 2015;4:499–508.

46. Alexopoulos D, Xanthopoulou I, Deftereos S, et al. In-hospital switching of oral P2Y12 inhibitor treatment in patients with acute coronary syndrome undergoing percutaneous coronary intervention: prevalence, predictors and short-term outcome. Am Heart J 2014;167:68–76.e2.

47. De Luca L, Leonardi S, Cavallini C, et al. Contemporary antithrombotic strategies in patients with acute coronary syndrome admitted to cardiac care units in Italy: The EYESHOT Study. Eur Heart J Acute Cardiovasc Care 2015;4:441–52.

48. Clemmensen P, Grieco N, Ince H, et al. MULTInational non-interventional study of patients with ST-segment elevation myocardial infarction treated with PRimary Angioplasty and Concomitant use of upstream antiplatelet therapy with prasugrel or clopidogrel - the European MULTIPRAC

Registry. Eur Heart J Acute Cardiovasc Care 2015; 4:220–9.

49. Schiele F, Puymirat E, Bonello L, et al. Switching between thienopyridines in patients with acute myocardial infarction and quality of care. Open Heart 2016;3:e000384.

50. Bagai A, Wang Y, Wang TY, et al. In-hospital switching between clopidogrel and prasugrel among patients with acute myocardial infarction treated with percutaneous coronary intervention: insights into contemporary practice from the national cardiovascular data registry. Circ Cardiovasc Interv 2014;7:585–93.

51. De Luca G, Verdoia M, Schaffer A, et al. Switching from high-dose clopidogrel to prasugrel in ACS patients undergoing PCI: a single-center experience. J Thromb Thrombolysis 2014;38:388–94.

52. Loh JP, Pendyala LK, Kitabata H, et al. Safety of reloading prasugrel in addition to clopidogrel loading in patients with acute coronary syndrome undergoing percutaneous coronary intervention. Am J Cardiol 2013;111:841–5.

53. Almendro-Delia M, Blanco Ponce E, Gomez-Domínguez R, et al. Safety and efficacy of in-hospital clopidogrel-to-prasugrel switching in patients with acute coronary syndrome. An analysis from the 'real world'. J Thromb Thrombolysis 2015;39:499–507.

54. Mauri L, Kereiakes DJ, Yeh RW, et al. Twelve or 30 months of dual antiplatelet therapy after drug-eluting stents. N Engl J Med 2014;371:2155–66.

55. Bonaca MP, Bhatt DL, Cohen M, et al. Long-term use of ticagrelor in patients with prior myocardial infarction. N Engl J Med 2015;372:1791–800.

56. Bonaca MP, Bhatt DL, Ophuis TO, et al. Long-term tolerability of ticagrelor for the secondary prevention of major adverse cardiovascular events a secondary analysis of the PEGASUS-TIMI 54 trial. JAMA Cardiol 2016;1:425–32.

57. Pourdjabbar A, Hibbert B, Simard T, et al. Optimizing crossover from ticagrelor to clopidogrel in patients with acute coronary syndrome: the CAPITAL OPTI-CROSS randomized trial. J Am Coll Cardiol 2015;65(10 Suppl).

58. Kerneis M, Silvain J, Abtan J, et al. Switching acute coronary syndrome patients from prasugrel to clopidogrel. JACC Cardiovasc Interv 2013;6: 158–65.

59. Deharo P, Pons C, Pankert M, et al. Effectiveness of switching 'hyper responders' from Prasugrel to Clopidogrel after acute coronary syndrome: the POBA (Predictor of Bleeding with Antiplatelet drugs) SWITCH study. Int J Cardiol 2013;168:5004–5.

60. Angiolillo DJ, Curzen N, Gurbel P, et al. Pharmacodynamic evaluation of switching from ticagrelor to prasugrel in patients with stable coronary artery disease: results of the SWAP-2 study (switching anti platelet-2). J Am Coll Cardiol 2014;63:1500–9.

61. Franchi F, Faz GT, Rollini F, et al. Pharmacodynamic effects of switching from prasugrel to ticagrelor: results of the prospective, randomized SWAP-3 study. JACC Cardiovasc Interv 2016;9:1089–98.

62. Steinhubl SR, Oh JJ, Oestreich JH, et al. Transitioning patients from cangrelor to clopidogrel: pharmacodynamic evidence of a competitive effect. Thromb Res 2008;121:527–34.

63. Dovlatova NL, Jakubowski JA, Sugidachi A, et al. The reversible P2Y antagonist cangrelor influences the ability of the active metabolites of clopidogrel and prasugrel to produce irreversible inhibition of platelet function. J Thromb Haemost 2008;6: 1153–9.

64. Rollini F, Franchi F, Tello-Montoliu A, et al. Pharmacodynamic effects of cangrelor on platelet P2Y12 receptor-mediated signaling in prasugrel-treated patients. JACC Cardiovasc Interv 2014;7:426–34.

65. Schneider DJ, Agarwal Z, Seecheran N, et al. Pharmacodynamic effects during the transition between cangrelor and ticagrelor. JACC Cardiovasc Interv 2014;7:435–42.

66. Schneider DJ, Seecheran N, Raza SS, et al. Pharmacodynamic effects during the transition between cangrelor and prasugrel. Coron Artery Dis 2015; 26:42–8.

67. Schneider DJ, Agarwal Z, Seecheran N, et al. Pharmacodynamic effects when clopidogrel is given before cangrelor discontinuation. J Interv Cardiol 2015;28:415–9.

68. Franchi F, Rollini F, Park Y, et al. A safety evaluation of cangrelor in patients undergoing PCI. Expert Opin Drug Saf 2016;15:275–85.

69. Bhatt DL, Stone GW, Mahaffey KW, et al. Effect of platelet inhibition with cangrelor during PCI on ischemic events. N Engl J Med 2013;368:1303–13.

70. Angiolillo DJ, Schneider DJ, Bhatt DL, et al. Pharmacodynamic effects of cangrelor and clopidogrel: the platelet function substudy from the cangrelor versus standard therapy to achieve optimal management of platelet inhibition (CHAMPION) trials. J Thromb Thrombolysis 2012;34:44–55.

71. Mehran R, Baber U, Steg PG, et al. Cessation of dual antiplatelet treatment and cardiac events after percutaneous coronary intervention (PARIS): 2 year results from a prospective observational study. Lancet 2013;382:1714–22.

Antiplatelet and Antithrombotic Therapy in Patients with Atrial Fibrillation Undergoing Coronary Stenting

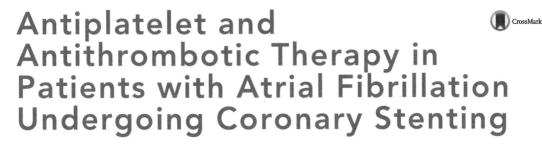

Mikhail S. Dzeshka, MD[a,b], Richard A. Brown, MD[a],
Davide Capodanno, MD, PhD[c], Gregory Y.H. Lip, MD[a,d],*

KEYWORDS

- Atrial fibrillation • Stroke • Coronary artery disease • Acute coronary syndrome
- Percutaneous coronary intervention • Stenting • Oral anticoagulation • Antiplatelet therapy

---

KEY POINTS

- Prognosis in atrial fibrillation (AF) is determined by ischemic stroke risk, the prevention of which is the main priority.
- Many patients with AF have associated coronary artery disease (CAD) requiring percutaneous coronary intervention (PCI).
- The major challenge is how to balance risks of stroke, coronary ischemic events, and major bleeding in patients with AF referred for PCI.
- Different thrombotic mechanisms necessitate initial triple antithrombotic therapy with oral anticoagulation (OAC) plus dual antiplatelet therapy (DAPT) of shortest possible duration (depending on the clinical setting, CHA_2DS_2-VASc and HAS-BLED scores and the type of stent), followed by dual antithrombotic therapy of OAC plus single antiplatelet agent, followed by OAC alone after 12 months.
- For OAC, a lower intensity is recommended with either vitamin K antagonists or non–vitamin K OAC.

INTRODUCTION

Atrial fibrillation (AF) is the most prevalent sustained arrhythmia. Ischemic stroke is a devastating and debilitating complication of AF associated with a poor prognosis. Stroke prevention is therefore a major priority in the management of patients with AF. The vast majority have at least one additional stroke risk factor and therefore require chronic oral anticoagulation (OAC) as the only means of effective stroke prevention.[1]

Twenty percent to 35% of patients with AF also have coronary artery disease (CAD) that may cause AF. Furthermore, development of acute coronary syndrome (ACS) can be precipitated by AF paroxysms.[2] Percutaneous coronary

---

Disclosure Statement: G.Y.H. Lip has served as a consultant for Bayer/Janssen, Astellas, Merck, Sanofi, BMS/Pfizer, Biotronik, Medtronic, Portola, Boehringer Ingelheim, Microlife; and Daiichi-Sankyo; and as a speaker for Bayer, BMS/Pfizer, Medtronic, Boehringer Ingelheim, Microlife, Roche, and Daiichi-Sankyo. D. Capodanno has served as a consultant for speaker for Abbott Vascular, Cordis and The Medicine Company; and as a speaker for Aspen, AstraZeneca, Cordis, and Daiichi-Sankyo. M.S. Dzeshka and R.A. Brown have nothing to disclose.
[a] University of Birmingham Institute of Cardiovascular Sciences, City Hospital, Dudley Road, Birmingham, West Midlands B18 7QH, UK; [b] Department of Internal Medicine I, Grodno State Medical University, Gorkogo 80, Grodno 230009, Belarus; [c] Cardio-Thoracic-Vascular Department, Ferrarotto Hospital, University of Catania, Via Salvatore Citelli 6, CT 95124, Italy; [d] Department of Clinical Medicine, Aalborg Thrombosis Research Unit, Aalborg University, Aalborg Hospital Science and Innovation Center, Søndre Skovvej 15, Aalborg 9100, Denmark
* Corresponding author.
E-mail address: g.y.h.lip@bham.ac.uk

intervention (PCI) with stenting is standard of care for patients with ACS and is also frequently used for myocardial revascularization in stable CAD. Prevention of recurrent cardiac ischemia and stent thrombosis necessitates DAPT that has to be administered for up to 12 months.[3]

The challenge is how to balance the risks of stroke and systemic embolism (SE), coronary ischemic events, and major bleeding. Increasing AF prevalence means that interventional cardiologist will encounter more patients with AF in the cardiac catheterization laboratory but there is little evidence from randomized controlled trials (RCTs) addressing antithrombotic management in this complex cohort, because patients with indications for chronic OAC were largely excluded from trials involving PCI.[4]

A joint consensus document of the European Society of Cardiology (ESC) Working Group on Thrombosis, European Heart Rhythm Association, European Association of Percutaneous Cardiovascular Interventions, and European Association of Acute Cardiac Care endorsed by the Heart Rhythm Society and Asia-Pacific Heart Rhythm Society was published, providing detailed recommendations on managing these patients based on best available data.[5]

THROMBOEMBOLIC RISKS IN ATRIAL FIBRILLATION

It has been widely acknowledged for decades that AF carries an increased probability of thromboembolic complications with the ischemic stroke considered to be the most devastating with respect to quality of life, hospitalizations, and survival. It is also known that not all patients with AF are similar in terms of their thromboembolic risk. The latter is characterized by the presence of comorbid conditions (eg, hypertension, heart failure with left ventricular dysfunction, diabetes mellitus, previous history of stroke or transient ischemic attacks [TIA], vascular disease including peripheral disease and also history of myocardial infarction [MI] or coronary revascularization) and patient-independent factors, such as increasing age and female gender. These factors were incorporated in the CHA_2DS_2-VASc (congestive heart failure, hypertension, age $\geq$75 years, diabetes, stroke, vascular disease, age 65-74 years, sex category) stroke score (Table 1), which provides the best discrimination between low stroke risk patients (ie, those without an additional stroke risk factor) and all the others (ie, those with at least one stroke risk factor).[6,7] The risk of stroke also may depend on other factors, such as left atrial size and function,

inflammation and cytokines, fibrosis and ischemia, epicardial fat and endothelial dysfunction, AF burden, and obesity and obstructive sleep apnea, but these variables are not easily measured in routine clinical practice.[8–10]

According to current ESC guidelines, the presence of a single CHA_2DS_2-VASc stroke risk factor (apart from female gender that should appear in conjunction with one other stroke risk factor) mandates initiation of OAC, because stroke and SE rates are increased threefold[11] compared with those without additional risk factors (ie, CHA_2DS_2-VASc = 0 or 1 for male and female patients, respectively).[12,13] This was shown in a large Danish nationwide cohort study comprising 39,400 patients discharged with nonvalvular AF with a CHA_2DS_2-VASc, score of 0 or 1. Such patients had a stroke rate of 0.49 per 100 person-years at 1 year compared with 1.55 per 100 person-years in patients with one CHA_2DS_2-VASc risk factor beyond female gender if left untreated. An increase in mortality rate was also observed.[14] An analysis performed in the same cohort revealed a hazard ratio of 3.8 for stroke/TIA/SE embolism in patients with one or more risk factors compared with those with none.[15]

These differences in embolic event rate created the positive net clinical benefit seen with warfarin therapy compared with no treatment or aspirin (ie, risks of bleeding with warfarin are outweighed significantly by stroke prevention).[16] Of note, the American Heart Association/American College of Cardiology/Heart Rhythm Society (AHA/ACC/HRS) guidelines recommend that the choice of no treatment, aspirin, or OAC in patients with moderate stroke risk lies with the treating physician. This is in contrast to the ESC guidelines.[11,17]

The risk of major bleeding is a common reason for clinicians to withdraw OAC in cases in which it may be indicated despite accumulating evidence on effectiveness and safety of warfarin as well as non–vitamin K oral anticoagulants (NOACs) when appropriately controlled. There is a trend toward higher adherence to current guidelines, but OAC remains underused with significant proportion of patients with AF at stroke risk treated with aspirin.[18]

IMPACT OF ATRIAL FIBRILLATION ON CLINICAL COURSE OF CORONARY ARTERY DISEASE

CAD is the second (with arterial hypertension being the first) most common comorbidity in patients with AF. In the EURObservational Research Programme–Atrial Fibrillation Pilot

Table 1
Stroke and bleeding risk stratification with the CHA_2DS_2-VASc and HAS-BLED scores, and choice of OAC with the SAMe-TT_2R_2 score

CHA_2DS_2-VASc	Score	HAS-BLED	Score	SAMe-TT_2R_2	Score
CHF (moderate-to-severe LV systolic dysfunction with LV EF $\leq$40% or recent decompensated heart failure requiring hospitalization)	1	Hypertension (systolic blood pressure >160 mm Hg)	1	Sex category (ie, female gender)	1
Hypertension	1	Abnormal renal or liver function	1 or 2	Age <60 y	1
Age $\geq$75 y	2	Stroke	1	Medical history ($\geq$2 of the following: hypertension, diabetes mellitus, CAD/MI, PAD, CHF, previous stroke, pulmonary, hepatic or renal disease)	1
Diabetes mellitus	1	Bleeding tendency or predisposition	1	Treatment with interacting drugs (eg, amiodarone)	1
Stroke/TIA/SE	2	Labile INRs (if on warfarin)	1	Tobacco use (within 2 y)	2
Vascular disease (prior MI, PAD, or aortic plaque)	1	Age (eg, >65, frail condition)	1	Race (ie, not white)	2
Aged 65–74 y	1	Drugs (eg, concomitant antiplatelets or NSAIDs) or alcohol excess/abuse	1 or 2	Maximum score	8
Sex category (ie, female gender)	1				
Maximum score	9	Maximum score	9		

Abbreviations: CAD, coronary artery disease; CHF, congestive heart failure; EF, ejection fraction; INR, international normalized ratio; LV, left ventricular; MI, myocardial infarction; NSAIDs, nonsteroidal anti-inflammatory drugs; PAD, peripheral artery disease; TIA/SE, transient ischemic attack/systemic embolism.
   Data from Refs.[82–84]

General Registry (EORP-AF), with participants from 9 ESC member countries, there were 36.4% of patients with AF suffering from CAD, of which 44.8% of patients also had a history of MI.[19] Similar data were derived from the Outcomes Registry for Better Informed Treatment for Atrial Fibrillation (ORBIT-AF) project in the United States: 36.3% patients with AF had CAD.[20] In the phase II Global Registry on Long-Term Oral Antithrombotic Treatment in Patients with Atrial Fibrillation (GLORIA-AF) registry with more than 10,000 patients from 5 geographic areas worldwide (Europe, North and Latin America, Africa/Middle East, and Asia), there were 20.6% and 10.5% of patients with CAD and MI, respectively.[18] Broadly similar prevalence of CAD was observed in another international registry addressing management of patients with AF: the Global Anticoagulant Registry in the FIELD (GARFIELD), which reported 19.2% of patients with AF to have CAD and 10.0% of patients to have history of ACS (including cases of unstable angina).[21]

CAD also may cause AF. Indeed, major pathways associated with structural atrial remodeling in AF, for example, oxidative stress, subclinical vascular inflammation, tissue hypoxia, and renin-angiotensin system activation, can all be triggered by coronary atherosclerosis and reduction of coronary blood flow.[9] These changes accumulate with chronic stable disease, but AF also may occur in the setting of ACS due to coronary thrombosis. For example, an analysis of the Framingham Heart Study original and offspring cohorts involved more than 1400 patients with secondary AF following acute MI, which appeared to be among the most common causes of secondary AF (in line with cardiothoracic or noncardiothoracic surgery and acute infectious diseases; eg, respiratory infection).[22] Moreover, these patients, despite having reversible cause(s), are prone to developing recurrent arrhythmia with approximately twofold higher risk compared with patients with AF not precipitated by acute MI.[22] Sharing of the common cardiovascular risk factors between patients with AF and those with CAD is also illustrated by applicability of the CHA_2DS_2-VASc stroke assessment scheme to the non-AF population. For example, among individuals after acute MI and with no history of AF, increase by 1 point according to the score resulted in 41% increase in stroke risk and 23% increase in mortality rate.[23]

What risk does co-presentation of AF and CAD carry? Due to extensive overlap between AF and CAD, patients presenting with both conditions are likely to appear in a higher-risk population.[24] That was illustrated in a pooled analysis of 10 clinical trials on STEMI and NSTE-ACS involving more than 120,000 patients. Patients with AF were found to be older, more often diabetic, with higher Killip class and more likely to have a history of MI or vascular disease.[25] Similar results were obtained in the cohort of the Atherosclerosis Risk in Communities Study (ARIC), in which there were more patients in the AF subgroup who were smokers, obese, hypertensive, and diabetic, and rates of heart failure, CAD, and lower creatinine-based estimated glomerular filtration were more common.[26]

Although AF can be merely a reflection of more advanced disease, it has been found to be an independent predictor of adverse cardiovascular and cerebrovascular outcomes (MACCE) in patients presenting with stable CAD or ACS treated pharmacologically or with PCI (Table 2).

PCI with stent implantation is now the most prevalent treatment option for patients with CAD. This, however, poses them at risk of serious ischemic complications (eg, stent thrombosis) and requires DAPT for prevention. Triple

antithrombotic therapy in turn increases the probability of bleeding complications. AF amplifies the risk, because patients with CAD are now also at elevated risk of thromboembolic events (eg, ischemic stroke), that due to different mechanisms of thrombosis require oral anticoagulation.[1,5,27]

Thrombi that develop under high-flow conditions adjacently to the arterial wall lesion at the place of endothelial denudation, plaque rupture, or stent implantation, are due to platelet activation, adhesion to vessel wall, and aggregation; that is, platelet-rich referring to white thrombi. Platelets are particularly predominant during the early hours of thrombus formation in the coronary artery, whereas coagulation cascade with thrombin generation and fibrin formation are activated later on. Thrombi collected within 3 hours since onset of ischemic symptoms were found to include 48.4% of fibrin and 24.9% of platelets, whereas those collected after 6 hours had passed show an increase of fibrin content to 66.9% and decrease in platelets to 9.1%.[28] This leads to development of occlusive thrombi in coronary arteries (clinically manifests as MI with ST elevation) or propagation of white thrombi with red fibrin-reach tail (clinically manifests as ACS without persistent ST-segment elevation).[4]

On the contrary, SE in AF more closely resembles venous thrombosis, developing frequently under low-flow conditions in the left atrial appendage. Histologic analysis showed random fibrin fibers mixed with platelet deposits with a marked heterogeneity, but most thrombi obtained from patients with stroke were fibrin-dominant and relatively platelet-poor with fibrin constituting approximately 60% of the thrombi.[4,28]

These differences in clot properties mean that some period of time after stent implantation needs to be covered by both antiplatelet agents (preferably DAPT of aspirin and a $P2Y_{12}$ inhibitor) and OAC (either well-adjusted warfarin dose or one of NOACs); that is, triple antithrombotic therapy, as neither OAC alone is sufficient.[2,5]

TRIPLE ANTITHROMBOTIC THERAPY IN CURRENT PRACTICE

Who Benefits from Triple Antithrombotic Therapy?

Combining antithrombotic agents improves protection from ischemic and embolic events, but elevates bleeding risk. A number of studies have shown this but none so far have adequately addressed the effectiveness of triple therapy in

Table 2
Studies on impact of AF on prognosis of patients with CAD

Study	No. of Patients	Study Design	Follow-up	Population	Death, %	CV Death, %	MI, %	Clinical Outcomes[a]			MACE or Other Composite Endpoint, %[b]	Major Bleeding, %[b]
								TVR, %	Stent Thrombosis, %	Ischemic Stroke, %		
Almendro-Delia et al,[24] 2014	39,237	Retrospective, multicenter, ARIAM registry	Duration of hospital stay	ACS, STEMI 59.9% AF 4.2% (new-onset), 3.2% (prior)	New-onset AF 14.0/5.2 1.62 (1.09–2.89)c Prior AF 11.6/5.2	NR	New onset 2.9/1.6c Prior AF 1.4/1.6	NR	NR	New onset 3.0/2.4 Prior AF 2.6/2.4	NR	New onset 12.0/14.5 Prior AF 14.0/14.5
Chan et al,[85] 2012	3307	Prospective, multicenter	1 mo	PCI AF 4.9% (prior) ACS 64.7%	9.9/2.2c 2.78 (1.35–5.72)	8/1.7c	3.7/2.3	1.2/2.2	0.6/0.9	0.6/0.2c	13/5.5c	5/2.1c,d
Gizurarson et al,[86] 2015	35,232	Retrospective, multicenter, RIKS-HIA registry	1 y	CCU pts IHD or chest pain 81.8% AF 15.3% (prior)	6.4/2.7 1.32 (1.16-1.50)c	NR	NR	NR	NR	NR	NR	NR
Jabre et al,[87] 2011	3220	Retrospective, Rochester Epidemiology Project	6.6 y	MI AF 9.4% (prior), 22.6% (new-onset)	Prior AF: 1.46 (1.26–1.70)c New-onset AF: Early 1.63 (1.37–1.93)c Intermediate 1.81 (1.45–2.27)c Late 2.58 (2.21–3.00)c	Prior AF: 1.55 (1.22–1.98)c,e New-onset AF: Early 1.72 (1.32–2.25)c,e Intermediate 1.94 (1.40–2.68)c,e Late 2.70 (2.17–3.36)c,e	NR	NR	NR	NR	NR	NR
Lau et al,[88] 2009	3393	Prospective, multicenter, Acute Coronary Syndrome Prospective Audit registry	1 y	STEMI, NSTE-ACS AF 4.4% (new-onset), 11.4% (prior)	New-onset AF 1.36 (0.84–2.20) Prior AF 1.42 (1.01–1.99)c	NR	New-onset AF 1.80 (1.13–2.86)c Prior AF 0.82 (0.54–1.24)	NR	NR	Prior AF 1.01 (0.21–4.78)	New-onset AF 1.66 (1.18–2.33)c Prior AF 1.13 (0.86–1.49)	New-onset AF 5.8 (3.1–10.6)c,d Prior AF 0.2 (0.1–0.9)c,d

(continued on next page)

Study	No. of Patients	Study Design	Follow-up	Population	Clinical Outcomes[a]							
					Death, %	CV Death, %	MI, %	TVR, %	Stent Thrombosis, %	Ischemic Stroke, %	MACE or Other Composite Endpoint, %[b]	Major Bleeding, %[b]
Lopes et al,[89] 2009	5745	Post hoc analysis of the APEX-AMI trial (prospective, double-blind, multicenter RCT)	90 d	STEMI, PCI AF 6.3% (new-onset)	1.81 (1.06–3.09)[c]	NR	NR	NR	NR	2.98 (1.47–6.04)[c]	NR	13.8/4.6[f] 1.95 (0.93–4.09)[d]
Lopes et al,[25] 2008	120566	Pooled database of ACS clinical trials[g]	8 d (short-term), 1 y (long-term)	ACS AF 7.5% (new-onset, in total): 8.0% in STEMI, 6.4% in NSTE-ACS	STEMI: 5.4/1.8 1.65 (1.44–1.90)[c] (short-term), 8.4/2.1 2.37 (1.79–3.15)[c] (long-term) NSTE-ACS: 4.2/1.2, 2.30 (1.83–2.90)[c] (short-term), 14.2/5.6, 1.67 (1.41–1.99)[c] (long-term)	NR	NR	NR	NR	STEMI: 2.1/1.1 1.46 (1.17–1.82)[c,h] (short-term), 2.3/0.5 3.60 (1.51–8.52)[c,h] (long-term) NSTE-ACS: 1.8/0.4 3.45 (2.41–4.95)[c,h] (short-term), 1.5/0.3 2.90 (1.62–5.20)[c,h] (long-term)	STEMI: 11.1/4.8 1.91 (1.70–2.14)[c,d] NSTE-ACS: 15.0/6.7, 2.06 (1.81–2.34)[c,d]	STEMI: 22.0/8.3, 2.36 (2.19–2.54)[c,i] NSTE-ACS: 39.2/10.8, 4.67 (4.26–5.13)[c,i]
Lopes et al,[90] 2012	69,255	Retrospective, multicenter, ACTION registry	In-hospital stay	STEMI, NSTEMI AF 7.1% (prior) PCI 68.7%	9.9/4.2[c]	NR	1.2/1.0	NR	NR	1.3/0.7[c]	NR	14.6/9.9[c]
Meyer et al,[91] 2016	1028	Prospective, 2-center	13 y	CHD AF 2.6% (new-onset)	NR	NR	NR	NR	NR	NR	71.2/24.3 2.6 (1.6–4.3)[c]	NR
Pilgrim et al,[92] 2013	6308	Prospective, single-center	4 y	PCI, DES AF 5.3% (prior) ACS 54.5%	22.5/9.6 1.67 (1.27–2.20)[c]	11.8/4.7 1.84 (1.26–2.71)[c]	6.5/4.8 1.37 (0.81–2.3)	16.3/14.8 1.07 (0.77–1.48)	6.8/6.5 1.17 (0.75–1.84)	3.4/0.8 3.08 (1.45–6.56)[c]	NR	3.7/1.7 1.59 (0.81–3.09)[c]
Rene et al,[93] 2014	3281	Post hoc analysis of the HORIZONS-AMI (prospective, open-label, multicenter RCT)	3 y	STEMI, PCI AF 4.5% (new-onset)	11.9/6.3 1.91 (1.16–3.14)[c]	6.3/3.7 1.7 (0.86–3.34)[c]	16.4/7.0 2.56 (1.66–3.94)[c]	24.2/14.0 1.90 (1.34–2.70)[c]	10.2/4.8 2.22 (1.26–3.91)[c]	5.8/1.3 4.49 (2.10–9.60)[c]	38.4/21.2 2.05 (1.56–2.69)[c]	20.9/8.2 2.67 (1.83–3.89)[c]

Rohla et al,[94] 2015	2890	Retrospective, single-center	Stable CAD 56 ± 29 mo; ACS 57 ± 28 mo	PCI ACS 50.4% AF 10.2% (stable CAD), 6.4% (ACS)	Stable CAD: 12.7, 1.95 (1.27–2.99)[c]; ACS: 40.9/13.5, 1.95 (1.23–3.11)[c]	Stable CAD: 41.1/ NR	NR	NR	NR	NR	NR	Stable CAD: 0.9/0.2; ACS: 4.7/2.2
Ruff et al,[95] 2014	44,518	Retrospective, multicenter, REACH registry	4 y	Stable outpatients with multiple risk factors for atherosclerosis, verified CAD, CVD, or PAD AF 10.3%	NR	10.6/3.5[c]	NR	4.9/3.6	NR	7.7/4.1[c]	18.9/9.4[c]	NR

Abbreviations: ACS, acute coronary syndrome; ACTION, the National Cardiovascular Data Registry's Acute Coronary Treatment and Intervention Outcomes Network Registry—Get With the Guidelines; AF, atrial fibrillation; APEX-AMI, Assessment of Pexelizumab in Acute Myocardial Infarction; ARIAM, Análisis del Retraso en el Infarto Agudo de Miocardio (Analysis of Delay in Acute Myocardial Infarction); CV, cardiovascular; CVD, cerebrovascular disease; HORIZONS-AMI, Harmonizing Outcomes With Revascularization and Stents in Acute Myocardial Infarction; MACE, major adverse cardiac events; MI, myocardial infarction; NR, not reported; NSTEMI, myocardial infarction without ST-segment elevation; PAD, peripheral arterial disease; PCI, percutaneous coronary intervention; RCT, randomized controlled trial; REACH, Reduction of Atherothrombosis for Continued Health; RIKS-HIA, Register of Information and Knowledge about Swedish Heart Intensive Care Admissions; STEMI, myocardial infarction with ST-segment elevation; TVR, target vessel revascularization.

a Event rate in patients with AF versus patients with sinus rhythm, adjusted hazard ratios (95% confidence interval) for significant associations when available.
b Definitions vary across the studies.
c Significant difference in event rates.
d In-hospital event rate.
e Among 30-day survivors.
f Trend toward between-groups difference.
g The STEMI population involved patients from the Global Utilization of Streptokinase and t-PA For Occluded Coronary Arteries (GUSTO I), Global Use of Strategies to Open Occluded Arteries in Acute Coronary Syndromes (GUSTO IIb), Global Use of Strategies to Open Occluded Coronary Arteries (GUSTO III), Assessment of the Safety and Efficacy of a New Thrombolytic Regimen-3 (ASSENT 3), and Assessment of the Safety and Efficacy of a New Thrombolytic Regimen-3 Plus (ASSENT 3 Plus). The NSTE-ACS population involved patients from the Global Use of Strategies to Open Occluded Arteries in Acute Coronary Syndromes (GUSTO IIb); Platelet IIb/IIIa in Unstable Angina: Receptor Suppression Using Integrilin Therapy (PURSUIT); Platelet IIb/IIIa Antagonist for the Reduction of Acute Coronary Syndrome Events in a Global Organization Network A (PARAGON-A); Platelet IIb/IIIa Antagonist for the Reduction of Acute Coronary Syndrome Events in a Global Organization Network B (PARAGON-B); and Superior Yield of the New Strategy of Enoxaparin, Revascularization and Glycoprotein IIb/IIIa Inhibitors (SYNERGY).
h Any stroke.
i Moderate or severe bleeding.

comparison with DAPT in patients with CAD presenting with AF and undergoing PCI due to being observational, retrospective, or underpowered (Table 3).

Meta-analyses of these studies have consistently shown (Table 4) significantly higher rates of major bleeding. These are costs for reducing the risk of ischemic stroke. However, all-cause mortality and ischemic endpoints, such as MI and stent thrombosis, are not affected by adding OAC to DAPT, because the latter alone is standard of care for prevention of ischemic events after PCI.[3]

Nevertheless, bleeding risks can be attenuated with appropriate precautions. The HAS-BLED score (≥3 high risk) (see Table 1) can be used for this purpose. It is important to emphasize that a high HAS-BLED score does not rule out OAC but rather highlights modifiable risk factors that can be further controlled; for example, high blood pressure, use of nonsteroidal anti-inflammatory drugs, or labile international normalized ratios (INRs).

The HAS-BLED score can also be used to inform pharmacologic strategy in terms of combination and duration of antithrombotic and antiplatelet treatment. Where bleeding risk is higher, a shorter duration of triple antithrombotic therapy, particularly if associated with moderate stroke risk, is used. Depending on the clinical scenario various approaches to initial antithrombotic therapy, ranging from DAPT (ie, no OAC used additionally) to 6 months triple therapy of OAC plus DAPT, have been proposed (Tables 5 and 6).

Patients with AF by virtue of presenting with CAD and stent implantation get at least 1 point on the CHA_2DS_2-VASc score. When more than 1 year has passed since stent implantation, the risk of stent thrombosis is minimal, as most are endothelialized. The probability of coronary ischemic events then becomes similar to that in patients with stable (and pharmacologically treated) CAD. In the latter group of patients, the extent of platelet activation is relatively low, and, thus, OAC for stroke prevention allows prevention of ischemic events without the need for antiplatelet agents on top of OAC.

In the large Danish nationwide cohort study, addition of antiplatelet therapy to OAC was not associated with any advantage in terms of efficacy outcomes, but there was a significant increase of serious bleeds (see Table 3). Administration of either of antiplatelet agent alone or DAPT did not increase bleeding risks, but nonuse of OAC was associated with a marked increased risk of stroke and thromboembolism, MI/coronary death, and all-cause death.[29]

Beyond 1 year, single or DAPT is commonly administered instead of OAC, or antiplatelet agents are concomitantly prescribed with OAC.[30,31] In the EuroObservational Research Programme-Atrial Fibrillation (EORP-AF) Pilot General Registry, presentation of the AF patient with CAD was one of the major independent predictors of nonadherence to antithrombotic management (odds ratio [OR] 4.53, 95% confidence interval [CI] 3.49–5.88), which translated into poorer outcomes; for example, all-cause mortality plus any thromboembolism in patients (OR 1.68, 95% CI 1.20–2.35 for undertreatment, and OR 1.62, 95% CI 1.17–2.24 for overtreatment).[30]

Is Triple Antithrombotic Therapy Always Better than Dual Therapy?

Thus far, most of the evidence comes from the observational data and meta-analyses of various smaller studies. The WOEST (What is the Optimal antiplatElet and anticoagulant therapy in patients with oral anticoagulation and coronary StenTing) trial was an open-label, intention-to-treat randomized controlled trial,[32] which showed that after 1 year of follow-up there was no excess of thromboembolic events with dual therapy of OAC plus clopidogrel, whereas mortality and bleeding rates were lower with dual antithrombotic therapy compared with triple therapy (see Table 3).[32] The primary endpoint was "all bleeding" and the excess with triple therapy was largely driven by minor rather than major bleeds. Many aspects of the WOEST trial design were also criticized with regard to definition of bleeding, recruitment of patients with various indications for OAC referred to elective PCI mostly, vascular access selection, extended duration of triple therapy, and underuse of proton pump inhibitors, all of which might affect efficacy and safety outcomes.[2]

In the Danish nationwide registry, the cumulative endpoint of coronary death, MI, and ischemic stroke after MI or PCI was similar in both dual and triple therapy groups (19.4% and 20.1%, respectively), whereas fatal and nonfatal bleeds developed less commonly with dual antithrombotic therapy (9.7% vs 14.2%, respectively).[33] OAC plus clopidogrel was not associated with an increase in risk of all-cause mortality, whereas both OAC plus aspirin and DAPT resulted in 52% to 60% elevated risk, respectively.[34]

In the AFCAS (Management of Patients With Atrial Fibrillation Undergoing Coronary Artery

Table 3

Summary of studies comparing triple antithrombotic therapy with dual antiplatelet therapy or OAC plus single antiplatelet therapy

Study	n	Design	Follow-up	Population	Compared Regimens	Major Bleeding	Minor Bleeding	Any Bleeding	Death	Clinical Outcomes[a]						
										CV Death	MI	TVR	Stent Thrombosis	Stroke	SE	MAC(C)E Overall
Bernard et al,[96] 2013	417	Retrospective single-center	650 d	AF, PCI-S ACS 61.9%	OAC/no OAC at discharge	4.3/3.4	NR	NR	5.2/11.9	NR	20.6/25.0	5.2/3.4	NR	5.2/9.1[b]	5.2/9.1[b]	23.7/32.5[c] 0.58 (0.32–1.05)
Caballero et al,[97] 2013	604	Retrospective 2-center	17 mo	AF, PCI-S ACS 75.8% Octogenarians 15.7%	OAC/no OAC at discharge	20.9/21.2	9.7/15.4	NR	22.2/44.4[c] 3.75 (0.97–14.53)	NR	2.2/19.4[d]	NR	NR	NR	8.9/18.9	28.9/58.3[d] 4.30 (1.26–14.56)
Dabrowska et al,[98] 2013	104	Prospective single-center	1 y	AF, PCI-S ACS NR	TT/DAPT	11.1/6.9	27.8/10.3	38.9/17.2	0/13.8	NR	3.4/11.1[e]	NR	0/0	NR	NR	NR
Dewilde et al,[32] 2013	573	RCT open-label multicenter	1 y	PCI-S AF 69% ACS NR	TT/OAC + Clopidogrel	5.6/3.2	NR	44.4/19.4[d] 0.36 (0.26–0.50)	6.3/2.5[d] 0.39 (0.16–0.93)	2.5/1.1	4.6/3.2	6.7/7.2	3.2/1.4	2.8/0.7[c] 0.25 (0.05–1.17)	NR	NR
Fosbol et al,[99] 2013	1648	Retrospective multicenter	1 y	AF, NSTEMI, PCI-S	TT/DAPT	15.5/12.8[c] 1.29 (0.96–1.74)	NR	NR	12.9/13.3	NR	6.3/6.8	NR	NR	1.6/2.2	NR	19.4/20.6
Gao et al,[100] 2010	622	Prospective single-center	1 y	AF, DES ACS 14.1%	TT/DAPT/ OAC + AT[f]	2.9/1.8/2.5	8.8/3.3/ 5.0[d]	11.8/5.1/ 7.4[d]	4.4/9.0/5.8	NR	2.9/5.4/ 5.8	3.7/4.5/ 4.1	0.7/0.9/1.7	0.7/3.6/0.8[c] NR	NR	8.8/20.1/ 14.9[d]
Gilard et al,[101] 2009	359	Prospective multicenter	1 y	PCI-S AF 69.1% ACS NR	TT/DAPT	5.6/2.1[d]	NR	18.4/16.0	8/5.6	4.0/2.6	5.0/4.3[e]	NR	1.6/1.7	0.8/3	0.8/0	NR
Ho et al,[76] 2013	602	Retrospective single-center	2 y	AF, PCI-S ACS NR	TT/DAPT	24.5/20.4	NR	NR	1.6/5.3 (CHADS$_2$ ≤2) 11.4/10.0 (CHADS$_2$ >2)	NR	NR	NR	NR	2.2/1.8	NR	NR
Kang et al,[102] 2015	367	Retrospective single-center	2 y	AF, DES	TT/DAPT	16.7/4.6[d] 3.54 (1.65–7.58)	NR	NR	8.7/1.8[d] 5.3 (1.8–16.0)	NR	NR	NR	NR	NR	NR	22.1/17.7
Karjalainen et al,[103] 2007	478	Retrospective multicenter	1 y	PCI-S AF 35.1% ACS 53.8%	TT/DAPT	8.2/2.6[d] 3.3 (1.3–8.6)	NR	NR	NR	NR	10.0/4.8[d] 2.2 (1.0–4.7)	11.0/7.5	4.1/1.3	3.2/2.2[c] 3.2 (0.8–12.1)	NR	21.9/11.0[d] 2.3 (1.3–3.8)

(continued on next page)

Study	n	Design	Follow-up	Population	Compared Regimens	Clinical Outcomes[a]										
						Major Bleeding	Minor Bleeding	Any Bleeding	Death	CV Death	MI	TVR	Stent Thrombosis	Stroke	SE	MAC(C)E Overall
Lamberts et al,[34] 2013	12,165	Retrospective nationwide	1 y	AF, PCI MI 77.2%	TT/DAPT/ OAC + ASA/ OAC + clopidogrel DAPT as a reference	14.3^d/6.9/ 9.7^d/10.9^d 2.08 (1.64– 2.65) 1.44 (1.14– 1.83) 1.63 (1.15– 2.30).	NR	NR	8.9^d/17.5/ 15.6^d/7.1^d 0.61 (0.47– 0.77) 0.54 (0.35– 0.76)	2.5^d/5.3/3.9/ 1.2 0.58 (0.36– 0.92)^{ig}	16.2^c/ 21.3/ 17.7^d/ 9.6^d 0.83 (0.68– 1.00)^h 0.78 (0.66– 0.91)^h 0.56 (0.40– 0.79)^h	NR	NR	4.1^d/6.3/ 5.6^d/ 2.8^d 0.67 (0.46– 0.98) 0.81 (0.61– 1.08) 0.51 (0.28– 0.95)	NR	NR
Lamberts et al,[29] 2014	8700	Retrospective nationwide	3.3 y	AF, stable CAD	TT/OAC + ASA/OAC + clopidogrel/ OAC/ DAPT/ clopidogrel + aspirin OAC as a reference	10.1^d/7.0^d/ 5.2^d/3.9/ 4.4/4.9/ 2.9 2.81 (1.82– 4.33) 1.84 (1.11– 3.06) 1.50 (1.23– 1.82)	NR	NR	12.5^d/10.3/ 7.1/8.5/ 16.1^d/15.0^d/ 13.5^d 1.89 (1.25– 2.65) 1.81 (1.52– 2.16) 1.61 (1.28– 2.01) 1.49 (1.32– 1.67)	NR	7.8^d/4.4/ 4.7/4.7/ 11.5 ^{d}/ 9.0^d/8.4^d 1.76 (1.05– 2.94)^h 2.24 (1.76– 2.84)^h 1.73 (1.27– 2.34)^h 1.73 (1.48– 2.02)^h	NR	NR	3.6/4.6/2.3/ 3.0/6.6^d/ 5.8^d/ 4.3^{b,d} 1.77 (1.32– 2.38) 1.73 (1.18– 2.53) 1.34 (1.13– 1.70)	NR	NR
Lopes et al,[104] 2016	1827	Retrospective multicenter	1 y	AF, PCI-S	TT/DAPT/ OAC + AT	5.68/5.06/ 5.85	NR	NR	4.14/9.34/ 5.41	2.76/5.54/ 2.71	NR	NR	NR	NR	NR	8.67/6.74/ 5.08
Mennuni et al,[105] 2015	859	Retrospective multicenter	1 y	AF, PCI-S MI 24%	TT/DAPT	11.5/6.4 1.8 (1.1–2.9)	NR	NR	NR	NR	NR	NR	NR	NR	NR	20.0/17.0
Mutuberria et al,[106] 2013	640	Prospective multicenter	1 y	AF, PCI-S ACS NR	TT/DAPT	5.3/0	NR	NR	8.4/1.3^d	8.4/0^d	NR	NR	NR	NR	1.1/1.3	13.7/9.3
Rossini et al,[107] 2008	204	Prospective Single-center	18 mo	PCI-S AF 66.6% ACS 78.9%	TT/DAPT	2.9/2	7.8/2.9	10.8/4.9	2.9/1.0	1/1	2/2	1/2.9	1/2	1/2	NR	5.8/4.9
Rubboli et al,[108] 2012	632	Prospective multicenter	1 y	PCI-S AF 58% ACS 63%	TT/DAPT/ OAC + ASA	5.0/2.0/2.6	NR	NR	9.9/8.5/10.2	NR	11.3/5.5/ 9.3^c	12.3/10.3/ 11.9	2.7/1.7/2.0	1.0/4.1/ 1.1^c	1.8/2.8/0^c	NR

Ruiz-Nodar et al,[109] 2008	426	Retrospective 2-center	594 d	AF, PCI-S ACS 83.9%	TT/DAPT	14.9/9.0	12.6/9.0	NR	17.8/27.8[d]	NR	6.5/10.4	7.1/8.4	1.2/1.3	NR	1.7/6.9[d]	26.5/38.7	4.9 (2.17–11.09)
Ruiz-Nodar et al,[110] 2012	420	Retrospective 2-center	1 y	AF, PCI-S ACS 86.4% HAS-BLED ≥3	OAC/no OAC at discharge	11.8/4.0[d] 3.03 (1.24–7.38)	NR	9.3/20.1[d] 0.45 (0.26–0.78)	NR	NR	NR	NR	NR	NR	NR	13.0/26.4[d]	0.48 (0.29–0.77)
Sambola et al,[111] 2009	405	Prospective multicenter	6 mo	PCI-S AF 67.6% ACS NR	TT/DAPT/ OAC + AT[f]	4.3/1.2/6.5[d]	11.2/2.5/6.5[d]	15.5/3.7/13[d] 6.8/1.2/10.9[c]	NR	4.3/0/8.7[d]	3.6/0/4.3	NR	0.3/1.2/2.2[b]	0.3/1.2/2.2[b]	NR	7.9/1.2/15.2[d]	
Sambola et al,[112] 2016	585	Prospective multicenter	1 y	AF, PCI-S ACS 73.2%	TT/DAPT	CHA$_2$DS$_2$-VASc = 1: 4.9/0[d]; ≥2: 8.4/3.1[d] 2.6 (1.03–6.5)	NR	CHA$_2$DS$_2$-VASc = 1: 19.5/6.9[d] 3.18 (1.16–8.69); ≥2: 21.8/15.6	CHA$_2$DS$_2$-VASc = 1: 7.4/5.5; ≥2: 9.2/10.6	NS CHA$_2$DS$_2$-VASc ≥2: NS	NR	NS CHA$_2$DS$_2$-VASc ≥2: NS		CHA$_2$DS$_2$-VASc = 1: 1.2/1.3; ≥2: 1.7/5.3[d] 3.23 (1.01–10.30)	CHA$_2$DS$_2$-VASc = 1: 0/0; ≥2: 1.77/5.5[d] 4.49 (1.48–13.6)	CHA$_2$DS$_2$-VASc = 1: 11.1/13.3; ≥2: 16.8/20.3	
Smith et al,[113] 2012	318	Retrospective Single-center	1 y	ACS, PCI-S AF 19.8%	TT/DAPT	13.4/3.8[d]	NR	4.5/2.5	NR	NR	NR	3.8/1.3[e]	NR	NR	1.9/1.9	0/0	NR
Uchida et al,[114] 2010	575	Prospective, single-center	459 d	DES AF 5% ACS 39.1%	TT/DAPT	20/2.7[d] 8.02 (3.34–19.15)	20/9.9[d]	40/12.8[d]	8/3.4	NR	0/0.2	14/7.4[c]	0/0	4/1.1	0/0	NR	22/12 1.74 (0.91–3.35)[c]

Abbreviations: ACS, acute coronary syndrome; AF, atrial fibrillation; AT, single antiplatelet therapy; CHADS$_2$, congestive heart failure, hypertension, age, diabetes, stroke; CV, cardiovascular; DAPT, dual antiplatelet therapy; DES, drug-eluting stent; MAC(C)E, major adverse cardiac (and cerebral) events; MI, myocardial infarction; NR, not reported; NS, not significant; NSTEMI, myocardial infarction without ST-segment elevation; OAC, oral anticoagulation; PCI(-S), percutaneous coronary intervention (with stenting); RCT, randomized controlled trial; SE, systemic embolism; TT, triple antithrombotic therapy; TVR, target vessel revascularization.

a Rate of events in groups, %; odds or hazard ratio (95% confidence interval) for significant associations when available.
b Stroke or systemic embolism.
c Trend toward between-groups difference.
d Significant difference in event rates.
e Acute coronary syndrome.
f More than 80% of patients in OAC plus single antiplatelet group were receiving clopidogrel.
g CORONARY death or fatal stroke.
h MI/coronary death.

Table 4
Meta-analyses and systematic reviews on efficacy and safety of triple antithrombotic therapy versus dual antiplatelet therapy in patients with AF undergoing PCI with stent implantation

Reference	Number of Studies Included	Clinical Outcomes, OR (95% CI)					
		All-Cause Death	MI	Stent Thrombosis	Ischemic Stroke	MACE[a]	Major Bleeding
Andrade et al,[115] 2013	18	NR	NR	NR	NR	NR	2.38 (1.05–5.38) at 1 mo 2.87 (1.47–5.62) at 6 mo
Bavishi et al,[116] 2016	17	0.81 (0.61–1.08)	0.74 (0.51–1.06)	0.67 (0.35–1.30)	0.59 (0.38–0.92)[b]	NR	1.20 (1.03–1.39)[b]
Gao et al,[117] 2011	9	1.20 (0.63–2.27)	0.84 (0.57–1.23)	0.54 (0.16–1.81)	0.29 (0.15–0.58)[b]	NR	2.00 (1.41–2.83)[b]
Gao et al,[118] 2015	16	0.98 (0.76–1.27)	1.01 (0.77–1.31)	0.91 (0.49–1.69)	0.57 (0.35–0.94)[b]	1.06 (0.82–1.39)	1.52 (1.11–2.10)[b]
Saheb et al,[119] 2013	10	NR	0.57 (0.22–1.50)	0.63 (0.32–1.22)	0.27 (0.13–0.57)[b]	0.76 (0.54–1.07)	1.47 (1.22–1.78)[b]
Singh et al,[120] 2011	6	NR	NR	NR	NR	0.72 (0.56–0.98)[b]	2.74 (1.08–6.98)[b]
Washam et al,[121] 2014	14	1.04 (0.59–1.83)	1.85 (1.13–3.02)[b]	NR	1.01 (0.38–2.67)	NR	1.46 (1.07–2.00)[b]
Zhao et al,[122] 2011	9	0.59 (0.39–0.90)[b]	NR	NR	0.38 (0.12–1.22)	0.60 (0.42–0.86)[b]	2.12 (1.05–4.29)[b]

Abbreviations: CI, confidence interval; MACE, major adverse cardiovascular events (composite of death, myocardial infarction/reinfarction, stent thrombosis, target vessel revascularization, stroke and bleeding); MI, myocardial infarction; NR, not reported; OR, odds ratio.
[a] Definitions vary across the studies.
[b] Significant increase (reduction) in risk.

Table 5 Antithrombotic therapy in patients with AF undergoing elective PCI				
Timing after PCI	**Elective PCI in Stable CAD**			
Stroke/SE risk CHA$_2$DS$_2$-VASc	Moderate 1 in males 2 in females		High ≥2 in males ≥3 in females	
Bleeding risk HAS-BLED	Low/Moderate 0–2	High ≥3	Low/Moderate 0–2	High ≥3
1 mo	Triple therapy of OAC + DAPT or OAC + SAPT[a] or DAPT	OAC + SAPT[a] or DAPT	Triple therapy of OAC + DAPT or OAC + SAPT[a]	Triple therapy of OAC + DAPT or OAC + SAPT[a] or DAPT
12 mo	OAC + SAPT[b] or DAPT		OAC + SAPT[b]	OAC + SAPT[b]
Life-long	OAC or OAC + SAPT[c]			

Abbreviations: INR, international normalized ratio; OAC, oral anticoagulation, either warfarin (INR 2.0–2.5) or non-VKA oral anticoagulant at the lower tested dose in AF (dabigatran 110 mg bid, rivaroxaban 15 mg every day, edoxaban 30 mg every day or apixaban 2.5 mg bid); PCI, percutaneous coronary intervention; SAPT, single antiplatelet therapy; SE, systemic embolism.

[a] Clopidogrel 75 mg every day.
[b] Either clopidogrel 75 mg every day or aspirin 75 to 100 mg every day.
[c] Selected cases, such as stenting of the left main, proximal bifurcation, recurrent MI.

Data from Lip GY, Windecker S, Huber K, et al. Management of antithrombotic therapy in atrial fibrillation patients presenting with acute coronary syndrome and/or undergoing percutaneous coronary or valve interventions: a joint consensus document of the European Society of Cardiology Working Group on Thrombosis, European Heart Rhythm Association (EHRA), European Association of Percutaneous Cardiovascular Interventions (EAPCI) and European Association of Acute Cardiac Care (ACCA) endorsed by the Heart Rhythm Society (HRS) and Asia-Pacific Heart Rhythm Society (APHRS). Eur Heart J 2014;35(45):3173.

Stenting, NCT00596570) registry there were no differences between triple therapy and combination of OAC and clopidogrel, with respect to any major adverse cardiovascular event, as well as bleeding events, but only fewer than 10% of patients received dual antithrombotic therapy.[35]

In summary, there potentially may be a place for combination of OAC and clopidogrel as a start of antithrombotic therapy and omitting aspirin in patients with AF after stent implantation, particularly in those with overall lower stroke risk and high bleeding risk.

Duration of Triple Antithrombotic Therapy

In the European consensus document, the recommended duration of triple therapy after elective PCI is at least 1 month, following which it can be replaced by OAC and clopidogrel, particularly in patients at high bleeding risk and moderate stroke risk (see Table 5).[5] After primary PCI for patients with ACS, the recommended duration of triple therapy is 6 months with an option to shorten to 1 month or replace with OAC plus clopidogrel if bleeding risk is particularly high (see Table 6).[5]

One assumption is that the shorter the duration of triple therapy, the lower the risk of bleeding complications, and a higher risk of ischemic events. In the ISAR-TRIPLE trial (Triple therapy in patients on oral anticoagulation after drug-eluting stent [DES] implantation, NCT00776633),[36] more than 600 patients receiving OAC and in whom DES implantation was performed, were randomized to either a 6-week or a 6-month clopidogrel therapy to investigate whether shortening clopidogrel therapy would be associated with better net clinical outcomes (combined endpoint of death, MI, definite stent thrombosis, stroke or thrombolysis in myocardial infarction [TIMI] major bleeding) at 9 months. There were no significant differences in rate of occurrence of primary combined endpoint between the 2 arms: 9.8% versus 8.8% in the 6-week and 6-month groups, respectively (HR 1.14, 95% CI 0.68–1.91).[36] Ischemic events, including cardiac death, MI, definite stent thrombosis, and ischemic stroke, were not significantly different: 4.0% versus 4.3% (HR 0.93, 95% CI 0.43–2.05), as was TIMI major bleeding (5.3% vs 4.0%, HR 1.35, 95% CI 0.64–2.84).[36]

Table 6
Antithrombotic therapy in patients with AF undergoing primary PCI

Timing after PCI			Primary PCI in ACS	
Stroke/SE risk CHA$_2$DS$_2$-VASc	Moderate 1 in males 2 in females		High ≥2 in males ≥3 in females	
Bleeding risk HAS-BLED	Low/Moderate 0–2	High ≥3	Low/Moderate 0–2	High ≥3
1 mo	Triple therapy of OAC + DAPT	Triple therapy of OAC + DAPT or OAC + SAPT[a]	Triple therapy of OAC + DAPT	Triple therapy of OAC + DAPT or OAC + SAPT[a]
6 mo		OAC + SAPT[b]		OAC + SAPT[b]
12 mo	OAC + SAPT[b]		OAC + SAPT[b]	
Life-long	OAC or OAC + SAPT[c]			

Abbreviations: ACS, acute coronary syndrome; AF, atrial fibrillation; INR, international normalized ratio; OAC, oral antico-agulation, either warfarin (INR 2.0–2.5) or non-VKA oral anticoagulant at the lower tested dose in AF (dabigatran 110 mg bid, rivaroxaban 15 mg every day, edoxaban 30 mg every day or apixaban 2.5 mg twice a day); PCI, percutaneous coro-nary intervention; SE, systemic embolism.
   [a] Clopidogrel 75 mg every day.
   [b] Either clopidogrel 75 mg every day or aspirin 75 to 100 mg every day.
   [c] Selected cases like as stenting of the left main, proximal bifurcation, recurrent MI.
   Data from Lip GY, Windecker S, Huber K, et al. Management of antithrombotic therapy in atrial fibrillation patients pre-senting with acute coronary syndrome and/or undergoing percutaneous coronary or valve interventions: a joint consensus document of the European Society of Cardiology Working Group on Thrombosis, European Heart Rhythm Association (EHRA), European Association of Percutaneous Cardiovascular Interventions (EAPCI) and European Association of Acute Cardiac Care (ACCA) endorsed by the Heart Rhythm Society (HRS) and Asia-Pacific Heart Rhythm Society (APHRS). Eur Heart J 2014;35(45):3173.

Is There a Place in Triple Therapy for Non–Vitamin K Oral Anticoagulants and New-Generation P2Y$_{12}$ Inhibitors?

The NOACs are increasingly used for stroke pre-vention in patients with AF. Pharmacologic char-acteristics and practical aspects of the NOACs were extensively reviewed,[37,38] as summarized in Tables 7 and 8. All the NOACs were noninfe-rior and often superior in prevention of stroke and SE, ischemic strokes, total and cardiovascu-lar mortality, major bleeding and intracranial hemorrhage compared with INR-adjusted warfarin in the phase 3 RCTs.[37–43]

The NOACs have several advantages over vitamin K antagonists (VKAs), which makes their periprocedural use in patients with CAD undergo-ing PCI also favorable.[44,45] First, NOACs offer a pre-dictable mode of anticoagulant action with fixed doses. Warfarin initiation, on the contrary, requires at least several days to reach target INR and further adjustment may be needed periodically during follow-up. Presence of particular genetic polymor-phisms (eg, CYP2C9, VKORC1) makes warfarin dose adjustment even more challenging.[46] A phar-macogenetic approach may improve the quality of anticoagulation with higher times in therapeutic range (TTR) achieved[47]; however, improvement in TTR was observed when compared with fixed VKA dosing algorithms but no difference was seen when compared with clinical algorithms. Also, a pharmacogenetic approach did not lead to reduction of composite of death, thromboembo-lism, and major bleeding.[48]

The onset of anticoagulant with the NOACs is fast, with peak concentration reached within 1 to 4 hours, as is the offset with half-life times of 8 to 17 hours (compared with 40 hours when warfarin is used). Renal clearance of the NOACs is high-est for dabigatran (80%) and lowest for apixaban (27%), whereas warfarin is not cleared through kidneys.[37,38] Despite much fewer drug interac-tions with the NOACs, one should be aware that they are transported with the P-glycopro-tein (P-gp) in the intestine; therefore, their con-centration is affected by potent P-gp inducers and inhibitors.[37,38]

Albeit regular laboratory monitoring is not required for NOACs, and this was suggested to reduce patient adherence to OAC, published real-world data show a higher rate of persistence of treatment while on the NOACs compared with warfarin.[49,50]

Absence of routinely accessible laboratory assays is also not a concern for most patients, as precise measurement of anticoagulant effect is not needed in most clinical scenarios. Whether a patient is under trough or peak anticoagulant effect can be anticipated based on knowledge of when the patient did take the last dosage as well as qualitatively assessed with some routine coagulation tests; for example, activated partial thromboplastin time for dabigatran or prothrombin time for factor Xa inhibitors.[51,52]

When life-threating major bleeding develops or urgent surgery cannot be postponed, the list of nonspecific reversal agents (prothrombin complex concentrate, activated prothrombin complex concentrate, activated factor VII) is now enhanced with idarucizumab as a specific antidote for dabigatran. Andexanet alpha, a specific antidote for factor Xa inhibitors is being considered in the accelerated approval pathway of the US Food and Drug Administration.[37,53]

Overall, there are no major issues to use one of the NOACs instead of warfarin as part of triple antithrombotic therapy, but such a recommendation assumes equal anticoagulation effect provided by therapeutic concentrations with standard dosing regimens of the NOACs and warfarin, because patients with either ACS or requiring DAPT were excluded from the stroke prevention trials. Similarly, patients with AF were excluded from the ACS trials performed with the NOACs in combination with DAPT.[4,5,45] In the ACS trials, dabigatran and apixaban showed no improvement with respect to ischemic outcomes but caused increased rate of major bleeds.[54,55] Only rivaroxaban 2.5 mg twice a day (ie, 4 times lower than the usual dose for stroke prevention in AF) added to DAPT resulted in reduction of combined endpoint of death from cardiovascular causes, MI, or stroke, as well as all-cause and cardiovascular mortality, but at cost of increased rate of major bleeding including intracranial hemorrhage when tested in the phase 3 ATLAS ACS 2–TIMI 51 trial (An Efficacy and Safety Study for Rivaroxaban in Patients With Acute Coronary Syndrome, NCT00809965).[56]

For patients who developed ACS or referred to elective PCI, the rapid onset of action of the NOACs makes bridging with parenteral anticoagulation unnecessary. In prespecified analyses of subgroups with concomitant use of aspirin or without it (aspirin was allowed by the NOACs phase 3 trials criteria with dose less than 100 mg in all trials, except ARISTOTLE with apixaban, in which a dose up to 165 mg was permitted) no impact on relative efficacy and safety outcomes was observed.

Despite all advantages of the NOACs, one should still remember that warfarin is a more versatile OAC that can be used in situations when the NOACs are contraindicated; for example, in patients with advanced kidney dysfunction (reduction of estimated glomerular filtration rate below 30 mL/min/1.73 m^2).[37,38] Also, when effectively managed in terms of INR control with high TTR reached, warfarin therapy is a safe and effective means of OAC. In the Swedish national quality registry for atrial fibrillation and anticoagulation (Auricula), for example, an average population TTR of 76.5% translated into rate of severe bleeding, intracranial hemorrhage, and thromboembolism to be as low as 2.24%, 0.37%, and 2.65%, respectively.[57] Given that TTR varies greatly across countries both within Europe and worldwide, the ESC guidelines give preference to the NOACs, whereas no such preference is stated in the AHA/ACC/HRS guidelines.[11,17]

Thus, if a patient is taking one of the NOACs, the patient should not be switched to warfarin, because this instead places patients at higher risk of thromboembolic events, and vice versa, warfarin-experienced with well-adjusted dose and high TTR could continue on warfarin.[5] In new-onset AF, the SAMe-TT$_2$R$_2$ score (see Table 1) may aid decision making to predict whether a patient will do well on VKA by achieving a good TTR.[58]

The newer third-generation P2Y$_{12}$ receptor inhibitors, prasugrel and ticagrelor, are increasingly the preferred component of DAPT in nonpatients with AF after ACS due to superior effectiveness compared with clopidogrel. Despite their potency to reduce ischemic events in patients with ACS, when used in combination with OAC for stroke prevention may result in unacceptably high risk of bleeding complications.[59] Hence, such a combination is not supported for routine use.[5,45]

How to Improve Safety of Triple Antithrombotic Therapy?

Apart from discouraging use of the third-generation P2Y$_{12}$ receptor inhibitors as part of combination therapy, reduction of hemorrhagic complications can be achieved through use of proton pump inhibitors, radial access, new-generation DESs, and discouraging bridging therapy periprocedurally.

Patients with the first-generation DES implanted were more prone to develop stent thrombosis because of delayed endothelialization and required longer minimal duration of

Table 7
Pharmacologic characteristics of the non–vitamin K oral anticoagulants

Parameter	Dabigatran	Rivaroxaban	Apixaban	Edoxaban
Mechanism of action	Direct thrombin inhibitor (free or bound), reversible	Factor Xa inhibitor (free or bound), reversible	Factor Xa inhibitor (free or bound), reversible	Factor Xa inhibitor (free or bound), reversible
Bioavailability, %	6.5	>80	>50	62
T_{max}, hour	1.0–3.0	2.5–4.0	1.0–3.0	1.0–2.0
$T_{1/2}$, hour	12–17	9–13	8–15	10–14
Renal excretion	80	35	27	50
Drug transporter	P-gp	P-gp, BCRP	P-gp, BCRP	P-gp
Drug-drug interactions[a]	Potent P-gp inhibitors and inducers	Potent CYP3A4 and P-gp inhibitors	Potent CYP3A4 and P-gp inhibitors	Potent P-gp inhibitors and inducers
Coagulation measurement	TT, dTT, aPTT, ECA	Anti-FXa is preferred method Changes in PT, aPTT, INR are highly variable	Anti-FXa is preferred method Changes in PT, aPTT, INR are highly variable	Anti-FXa is preferred method Changes in PT, aPTT, INR are highly variable
Reversal agents	Activated charcoal or hemodialysis (overdose); PCCs or recombinant FVII (uncontrolled bleeding)	Andexanet, aripazine (investigational) PCCs, recombinant FVIIa	Andexanet, aripazine (investigational) PCCs, recombinant FVIIa	Andexanet, aripazine (investigational) PCCs, recombinant FVIIa
Dosing for AF (European labeling)	150 mg bid 110 mg bid in high bleeding risk, concomitant verapamil, age ≥80 y	20 mg qd if CrCl >50 mL/min 15 mg qd if CrCl 15–50 mL/min	5 mg bid 2.5 mg bid if • CrCl 15–29 mL/min or • Any 2 of the following are present: age ≥80 y, body weight ≤60 kg, serum creatinine ≥133 µmol/L	60 mg qd in patients with CrCl of >50 to ≤95 mL/min 30 mg qd in patients with one or more • CrCl of 15–50 mL/min • Body weight ≤60 kg, • P-gp inhibitors (cyclosporine, dronedarone, erythromycin, ketoconazole)

Dosing for AF (US labeling)	150 mg bid 75 mg bid if CrCl 15–30 mL/min or CrCl 30–50 mL/min with concomitant dronedarone or ketoconazole	20 mg qd 15 mg qd if CrCl 15–50 mL/min	5 mg bid 2.5 mg bid if • Any 2 of the following are present: age ≥80 y, body weight ≤60 kg, serum creatinine ≥133 μmol/L • Currently on 5 mg bid and coadministered with strong dual inhibitors of CYP3A4 and P-gp (ketoconazole, itraconazole, ritonavir, clarithromycin)	60 mg qd in patients with CrCl of >50 to ≤95 mL/min 30 mg qd in patients with CrCl of 15–50 mL/min
Avoidance of concomitant use	US labeling P-gp inducers P-gp inhibitors if CrCl <30 mL/min	US labeling • Combined P-gp and moderate CYP3A4 inhibitors if CrCl 15–80 mL/min • Combined P-gp and strong CYP3A4 inducers and inhibitors European labeling • Strong dual P-gp and CYP3A4 inhibitors • Strong CYP3A4 inducers	US labeling • Strong dual CYP3A4 and P-gp inhibitors if current dose 2.5 mg bid • Strong dual CYP3A4 and P-gp inducers European labeling • Strong dual inhibitors of CYP3A4 and P-gp • Strong CYP3A4 and P-gp inducers (use cautiously)	US labeling P-gp inducer rifampin European labeling P-gp inducers (use cautiously)

Abbreviations: aPTT, activated partial thromboplastin time; BCRP, breast cancer resistance protein; bid, twice a day; CrCl, creatinine clearance; dTT, diluted thrombin time; ECT, ecarin clotting time; PCC, prothrombin complex concentrate; P-gp, P-glycoprotein; TT, triple antithrombotic therapy; qd, every day.

[a] Strong CYP3A4 and P-gp inducers include rifampicin, phenytoin, carbamazepine, phenobarbital or St. John's wort; strong dual inhibitors of CYP3A4 and P-gp include azole antimycotics (ketoconazole, itraconazole), and HIV protease inhibitors (lopinavir/ritonavir, ritonavir, indinavir, conivaptan).

Data from Refs.[37,123,124]

Table 8
Summary of the phase 3 stroke prevention in AF trials with the non–vitamin K oral anticoagulants

Clinical Trial	RE-LY[39,40,125]		ROCKET AF[41]	ARISTOTLE[42,126]	ENGAGE AF - TIMI 48[43,127]	
Non-VKA OAC examined	Dabigatran		Rivaroxaban	Apixaban	Edoxaban	
Trial design	PROBE		Double-blind, double-dummy	Double-blind, double-dummy	Double-blind, double-dummy	
Patients	18,113		14,264	18,201	21,105	
Age, y	71		73	70	72	
Mean CHADS$_2$ score	2.1		3.5	2.1	2.8	
Non-VKA OAC dosing arm	110 mg bid	150 mg bid	20 (15) mg qd	5 (2.5) mg bid	30 (15) mg qd	60 (30) mg qd
Prior stroke or transient ischemic attack, %	20 (including SE)		55	19 (including SE)	28.5	
Mean TTR, warfarin arm; %	64		55	62	68.4	
Hazard ratios (95% CI) for NOACs vs warfarin						
Stroke or systemic embolism	0.90 (0.74–1.10)	0.65 (0.52–0.81)	0.88 (0.75–1.03)	0.79 (0.66–0.96)	1.13 (0.96–1.34)	0.87 (0.73–1.04)
Ischemic stroke	1.11 (0.89–1.40)[a]	0.76 (0.60–0.98)[a]	0.94 (0.75–1.17)	0.92 (0.74–1.13)	1.41 (1.19–1.67)	1.00 (0.83–1.19)
Hemorrhagic stroke	0.31 (0.17–0.56)	0.26 (0.14–0.49)	0.59 (0.37–0.93)	0.51 (0.35–0.75)	0.33 (0.22–0.50)	0.54 (0.38–0.77)
Systemic embolism	1.26 (0.57—2.78)[b]	1.61 (0.76–3.42)[b]	0.23 (0.09–0.61)	0.87 (0.44–1.75)	1.24 (0.72–2.15)	0.65 (0.34–1.24)

All-cause mortality	0.91 (0.80–1.03)	0.88 (0.77–1.00)	0.85 (0.70–1.02)	0.89 (0.80–0.998)	0.87 (0.79–0.96)	0.92 (0.83–1.01)
Cardiovascular mortality	0.90 (0.77–1.06)	0.85 (0.72–0.99)	0.89 (0.73–1.10)	0.89 (0.76–1.04)	0.85 (0.76–0.96)	0.86 (0.77–0.97)
Myocardial infarction	1.29 (0.96–1.75)	1.27 (0.94–1.71)	0.81 (0.63–1.06)	0.88 (0.66–1.17)	1.19 (0.95–1.49)	0.94 (0.74–1.19)
Stroke and SE bleeding if antiplatelet agent concomitantly (yes/no)	0.93 (0.70–1.25)/ 0.87 (0.66–1.15)	0.8 (0.59–1.08)/ 0.52 (0.38–0.72)	0.87 (0.67–1.13)/ 0.88 (0.72–1.09)	0.58 (0.39–0.85)/ 0.84 (0.66–1.07)[c]	1.03 (0.76–1.39)/ 1.19 (0.99–1.43)	0.70 (0.50–0.98)/ 0.94 (0.77–1.15)
Major bleeding	0.80 (0.70–0.93)	0.93 (0.81–1.07)	1.04 (0.90–1.20)	0.69 (0.60–0.80)	0.47 (0.41–0.55)	0.80 (0.71–0.91)
Major or clinically relevant non major bleeding	NA	NA	1.03 (0.96–1.11)	0.68 (0.61–0.75)	0.62 (0.57–0.67)	0.86 (0.80–0.92)
Intracranial hemorrhage	0.30 (0.19–0.45)	0.41 (0.28–0.60)	0.67 (0.47–0.93)	0.42 (0.30–0.58)	0.30 (0.21–0.43)	0.47 (0.34–0.63)
Gastrointestinal bleeding	1.09 (0.85–1.39)	1.49 (1.19–1.88)	1.47 (1.20–1.81)	0.88 (0.67–1.14)	0.67 (0.53–0.83)	1.23 (1.02–1.50)
Major bleeding if antiplatelet agent concomitantly (yes/no)	0.82 (0.67–1.0)/ 0.79 (0.64–0.96)	0.93 (0.76–1.12)/ 0.94 (0.78–1.15)	0.78 (0.57–1.07)/ 0.79 (0.62–1.01)	0.77 (0.60–0.99)/ 0.65 (0.55–0.78)[c]	0.51 (0.39–0.66)/ 0.56 (0.46–0.67)	0.82 (0.65–1.04)/ 0.80 (0.68–0.95)

Abbreviations: ARISTOTLE, Apixaban for Reduction In STroke and Other ThromboemboLic Events in atrial fibrillation; bid, twice daily; CHADS$_2$, congestive heart failure, hypertension, age ≥75 years, diabetes mellitus, stroke or transient ischemic attack (2 points); CI, confidence interval; ENGAGE AF – TIMI 48, Effective aNticoaGulation with factor Xa next GEneration in Atrial Fibrillation–Thrombolysis In Myocardial Infarction 48; NA, data not available; OAC, oral anticoagulant; PROBE, prospective, randomized, open-label, blinded end point; qd, once daily; RE-LY, Randomized Evaluation of Long-term anticoagulation therapy; ROCKET AF, Rivaroxaban Once daily oral direct factor Xa inhibition Compared with vitamin K antagonism for prevention of stroke and Embolism Trial in Atrial Fibrillation; SE, systemic embolism; TTR, time in therapeutic range; VKA, vitamin K antagonist.

[a] Ischemic or uncertain stroke.

[b] Pulmonary embolism.

[c] Patients on aspirin ≥165 mg per day and those who required treatment with both aspirin and a P2Y$_{12}$ receptor antagonist at baseline were not eligible to be enrolled in the ARIS-TOTLE trial.

DAPT compared with bare-metal stenting (BMS). That is not the case with the new-generation DES, which is now recommended for all patients who require PCI with stent implantation.[3,5]

In one of the most recent studies, zotarolimus-eluting stents were implanted to stable patients with CAD and in the ACS setting if they were considered as uncertain DES candidates; for example, had high bleeding risk (including combination with OAC) and/or the presence of relative or absolute contraindications to long-term dual antiplatelet treatment, high thrombosis risk, and/or low restenosis risk based on angiographic findings (Zotarolimus-eluting Endeavor Sprint Stent in Uncertain DES Candidates [ZEUS] Study, NCT01385319).[60] Outcomes were compared with those in patients with BMS implantation. At 1-year follow-up, major adverse cardiovascular events (death, MI, or target vessel revascularization) were found in 17.5% of patients with DES and 22.1% with BMS (HR 0.76, 95% CI 0.61–0.95), and definite or probable stent thrombosis was significantly lower with DES as well (2.0% vs 4.1%).[60] In a sub-group analysis of patients with at least one high bleeding risk criterion, there were worse outcomes, but benefits of DES remained (22.6% vs 29%, HR 0.75, 95% CI 0.57–0.98).[61] Everolimus-eluting stents also showed superiority to BMS in various clinical scenarios.[62,63] In 2644 patients at high risk for bleeding undergoing PCI-S, the LEADERS FREE trial found that a polymer-free umirolimus-coated stent was superior to a BMS for safety and efficacy endpoints, even when used with a 1-month course of DAPT.[64,65]

No excess of major adverse cardiovascular and cerebrovascular events with DES compared with BMS have been confirmed by other observational data in patients with AF undergoing PCI.[66]

Overall, heparin bridging in patients undergoing PCI with stent implantation remains common practice, despite resulting in worse outcomes; however, uninterrupted OAC is increasingly used.[67–71]

In the AFCAS registry, those patients with AF who were discharged on low molecular weight heparin as part of triple therapy had a twofold increase in both BARC (Bleeding Academic Research Consortium) major bleeding as well as MACCE compared with triple therapy, including VKA; that is, 11.5% versus 6.0% and 11.5% versus 5.0%, respectively.[69]

In the ORBIT-AF registry (Outcomes Registry for Better Informed Treatment of Atrial Fibrillation), bleeding events were again more common in bridged than nonbridged patients (5.0% vs 1.3%, OR 3.84, 95% CI 2.07–7.14), as was the composite endpoint of MI, stroke or SE, major bleeding, hospitalization, or death within 30 days (13% vs 6.3%, OR 1.94, 95% CI 1.38–2.71).[70] In the substudy of the Randomized Evaluation of Long-term anticoagulation therapy (RE-LY) trial, bridging before elective surgery or procedure was used in interruption in 27.5% of patients on warfarin and 15.4% on dabigatran. Significantly more major bleeds developed in bridged patients both in dabigatran and warfarin arms (6.5% vs 1.8%, and 6.8% vs 1.6%, respectively), with no difference in rate of stroke and SE.[68] In the WOEST trial, MACCE and major bleeding rates were similar in patients with uninterrupted OAC and those bridged periprocedurally.[71]

Currently it is recommended to perform PCI if INR is above 2 while on warfarin, but NOACs are advised to be discontinued 24 to 48 hours before the procedure.[5] In the X-PLORER trial (Exploring the efficacy and safety of rivaroxaban to support elective percutaneous coronary intervention, NCT01442792), patients with stable CAD referred for elective PCI had lower levels of thrombin-antithrombin complex at 2 hours after procedure with rivaroxaban taken 2 to 4 hours before the procedure (with or without unfractionated heparin) when compared with unfractionated heparin alone.[72] Thus, effective suppression of coagulation was seen, but whether this biomarker effect will translate into clinical benefits is less certain.

Radial artery access compared with femoral artery access for PCI is known to be safe and effective, particularly in terms of fewer bleeding complications.[73] A meta-analysis of 15 RCTs and 17 cohort studies involving more than 44,000 patients with ACS found reductions in major bleeding (OR 0.45, 95% CI 0.33–0.61), access-related complications (OR 0.27, 95% CI 0.18–0.39), mortality (OR 0.64, 95% CI 0.54–0.75), and major adverse cardiac events (MACE) (OR 0.70, 95% CI 0.57–0.85).[74] In another meta-analysis of 9 studies with more than 220,000 patients with ACS without persistent ST elevation, radial access was associated with significant reduction in major bleeding (OR 0.52, 95% CI 0.36–0.73), access-site bleeding (OR 0.41, 95% CI 0.22–0.78), need for blood transfusions (OR 0.61, 95% CI 0.41–0.91), and 1-year mortality (OR 0.72, 95% CI 0.55–0.95).[75]

Triple antithrombotic therapy in patients with AF is associated with a fivefold increase in gastrointestinal bleeding compared with DAPT.[76] Therefore, proton pump inhibitors are a compulsory component among strategies to reduce risk of bleeding complications.[73]

Also, where OAC is combined with antiplatelet agents, a lower intensity of anticoagulation should be maintained with INR for VKA ranging from 2.0 to 2.5. If an NOAC is used, the lower tested dose for stroke prevention should be used in combination therapy with antiplatelet therapy; for example, dabigatran 110 mg twice a day, apixaban 2.5 mg twice a day, rivaroxaban 15 mg every day, or edoxaban 30 mg every day.[5]

ONGOING TRIALS

Current gaps in evidence will be bridged by several ongoing trials, which are recruiting patients with AF undergoing PCI with stent implantation. In the REDUAL-PCI trial (Evaluation of dual therapy with dabigatran vs triple therapy with warfarin in patients with AF that undergo a PCI with stenting, NCT02164864) a dual antithrombotic therapy regimen of dabigatran 110 mg twice a day plus clopidogrel or ticagrelor and dabigatran 150 mg twice a day plus clopidogrel or ticagrelor are compared with a triple antithrombotic therapy of warfarin plus clopidogrel or ticagrelor plus aspirin once daily in patients with AF who undergo elective PCI with stenting or due to an ACS.[77]

In the PIONEER AF–PCI (a study exploring 2 strategies of rivaroxaban and one of oral vitamin K antagonist in patients with atrial fibrillation who undergo percutaneous coronary intervention, NCT01830543), there are 3 arms: rivaroxaban 2.5 mg twice a day in combination with aspirin 75 to 100 mg every day and clopidogrel 75 mg every day (or prasugrel 10 mg every day, or ticagrelor 90 mg twice a day) followed by rivaroxaban 15 mg every day (or 10 mg every day for individuals with moderate renal impairment) in combination with low-dose aspirin 75 to 100 mg every day; the same antithrombotic regimen, but with dose-adjusted VKA instead of rivaroxaban (target INR 2.0–3.0 or 2.0–2.5 at the investigator discretion); and rivaroxaban 15 mg every day (or 10 mg every day for subjects with moderate renal impairment) plus clopidogrel 75 mg every day (or prasugrel 10 mg every day or ticagrelor 90 mg every day) for 12 months. Randomization is stratified by the intended duration of DAPT of 1, 6, or 12 months.[78]

The AUGUSTUS (Study of apixaban in patients with atrial fibrillation, not caused by a heart valve problem, who are at risk for thrombosis due to having had a recent coronary event, such as a heart attack or a procedure to open the vessels of the heart, NCT02415400) aims to determine whether apixaban is safer than warfarin when combined with clopidogrel with or without aspirin. Outcomes will be assessed after 6 months of treatment.[79]

In the recently announced ENTRUST AF–PCI trial, edoxaban 60 mg every day (or 30 mg every day in patients with creatinine clearance $\leq$50 mL/min or body weight $\leq$60 kg, or concomitant use of P-gp inhibitors except amiodarone) plus P2Y$_{12}$ inhibitor (clopidogrel 75 mg every day preferably, or ticagrelor 90 mg twice a day, or prasugrel 10 mg every day) will be compared with warfarin plus clopidogrel 75 mg every day (or prasugrel 10 mg every day, or ticagrelor 90 mg twice a day) plus low-dose aspirin.[80]

The observational WOEST 2 registry (What is the optimal antiplatelet and anticoagulant therapy in patients with oral anticoagulation undergoing revascularization 2, NCT02635230) will involve unselected patients receiving combination of chronic OAC (either VKA or NOAC) and a P2Y$_{12}$ inhibitor (clopidogrel, prasugrel, or ticagrelor) with or without aspirin.[81]

SUMMARY

Managing antithrombotic therapy in patients with AF who also require DAPT in the setting of a presentation with an ACS or where PCI is undertaken represents a challenging area. Risks of stroke/SE, stent thrombosis, and bleeding should be balanced when choosing between regimens of antithrombotic therapy. Thus far, no large RCT has been completed to show which strategy offered the most beneficial profile of safety and efficacy. Newer antiplatelet agents, oral anticoagulants, DES, and so forth, all continuously change the landscape of management of such patients. Ongoing RCTs will help to understand how various antithrombotic regimens translate into efficacy and safety outcomes, and that allow the highest net clinical benefit.

REFERENCES

1. Dzeshka MS, Lip GY. Antithrombotic and anticoagulant therapy for atrial fibrillation. Cardiol Clin 2014;32(4):585–99.
2. Dzeshka MS, Brown RA, Lip GY. Patients with atrial fibrillation undergoing percutaneous coronary intervention. Current concepts and concerns: part I. Pol Arch Med Wewn 2015;125(1–2):73–81.
3. Authors/Task Force members, Windecker S, Kolh P, et al. 2014 ESC/EACTS Guidelines on myocardial revascularization: The Task Force on

Myocardial Revascularization of the European Society of Cardiology (ESC) and the European Association for Cardio-Thoracic Surgery (EACTS) Developed with the special contribution of the European Association of Percutaneous Cardiovascular Interventions (EAPCI). Eur Heart J 2014; 35(37):2541–619.

4. De Caterina R, Husted S, Wallentin L, et al. Oral anticoagulants in coronary heart disease (Section IV). Position paper of the ESC Working Group on Thrombosis - Task Force on Anticoagulants in Heart Disease. Thromb Haemost 2016;115(4): 685–711.

5. Lip GY, Windecker S, Huber K, et al. Management of antithrombotic therapy in atrial fibrillation patients presenting with acute coronary syndrome and/or undergoing percutaneous coronary or valve interventions: a joint consensus document of the European Society of Cardiology Working Group on Thrombosis, European Heart Rhythm Association (EHRA), European Association of Percutaneous Cardiovascular Interventions (EAPCI) and European Association of Acute Cardiac Care (ACCA) endorsed by the Heart Rhythm Society (HRS) and Asia-Pacific Heart Rhythm Society (APHRS). Eur Heart J 2014;35(45):3155–79.

6. Dzeshka MS, Lane DA, Lip GY. Stroke and bleeding risk in atrial fibrillation: navigating the alphabet soup of risk-score acronyms (CHADS2, CHA2 DS2 -VASc, R2 CHADS2, HAS-BLED, ATRIA, and more). Clin Cardiol 2014;37(10):634–44.

7. Dzeshka MS, Lip GY. Stroke and bleeding risk assessment: where are we now? J Atr Fibrillation 2014;6(6):49–57.

8. Overvad TF, Bronnum Nielsen P, Larsen TB, et al. Left atrial size and risk of stroke in patients in sinus rhythm. A systematic review. Thromb Haemost 2016;116(2):206–19.

9. Dzeshka MS, Lip GY, Snezhitskiy V, et al. Cardiac fibrosis in patients with atrial fibrillation: mechanisms and clinical implications. J Am Coll Cardiol 2015;66(8):943–59.

10. Szymanski FM, Lip GY, Filipiak KJ, et al. Stroke risk factors beyond the CHA2DS2-VASc Score: can we improve our identification of "high stroke risk" patients with atrial fibrillation? Am J Cardiol 2015; 116(11):1781–8.

11. Camm AJ, Lip GY, De Caterina R, et al. 2012 focused update of the ESC Guidelines for the management of atrial fibrillation: an update of the 2010 ESC Guidelines for the management of atrial fibrillation. Developed with the special contribution of the European Heart Rhythm Association. Eur Heart J 2012;33(21):2719–47.

12. Nielsen PB, Chao TF. The risks of risk scores for stroke risk assessment in atrial fibrillation. Thromb Haemost 2015;113(6):1170–3.

13. Olesen JB, Torp-Pedersen C. Stroke risk in atrial fibrillation: Do we anticoagulate CHADS2 or CHA2DS2-VASc >/=1, or higher? Thromb Haemost 2015;113(6):1165–9.

14. Lip GY, Skjoth F, Rasmussen LH, et al. Oral anticoagulation, aspirin, or no therapy in patients with nonvalvular AF with 0 or 1 stroke risk factor based on the CHA2DS2-VASc score. J Am Coll Cardiol 2015;65(14):1385–94.

15. Lip GY, Nielsen PB, Skjoth F, et al. Atrial fibrillation patients categorized as "not for anticoagulation" according to the 2014 Canadian Cardiovascular Society algorithm are not "low risk". Can J Cardiol 2015;31(1):24–8.

16. Lip GY, Skjoth F, Nielsen PB, et al. Non-valvular atrial fibrillation patients with none or one additional risk factor of the CHA2DS2-VASc score. A comprehensive net clinical benefit analysis for warfarin, aspirin, or no therapy. Thromb Haemost 2015;114(4):826–34.

17. January CT, Wann LS, Alpert JS, et al. 2014 AHA/ACC/HRS guideline for the management of patients with atrial fibrillation: a report of the American College of Cardiology/American Heart Association Task Force on Practice Guidelines and the Heart Rhythm Society. J Am Coll Cardiol 2014;64(21):e1–76.

18. Huisman MV, Rothman KJ, Paquette M, et al. Antithrombotic treatment patterns in patients with newly diagnosed nonvalvular atrial fibrillation: the GLORIA-AF registry, Phase II. Am J Med 2015;128(12):1306–13.e1.

19. Lip GY, Laroche C, Dan GA, et al. A prospective survey in European Society of Cardiology member countries of atrial fibrillation management: baseline results of EURObservational Research Programme Atrial Fibrillation (EORP-AF) Pilot General Registry. Europace 2014;16(3):308–19.

20. Golwala H, Jackson LR 2nd, Simon DN, et al. Racial/ethnic differences in atrial fibrillation symptoms, treatment patterns, and outcomes: Insights from Outcomes Registry for Better Informed Treatment for Atrial Fibrillation Registry. Am Heart J 2016;174:29–36.

21. Kakkar AK, Mueller I, Bassand J-P, et al. Risk profiles and antithrombotic treatment of patients newly diagnosed with atrial fibrillation at risk of stroke: perspectives from the international, observational, prospective GARFIELD registry. PLoS One 2013;8(5):e63479.

22. Lubitz SA, Yin X, Rienstra M, et al. Long-term outcomes of secondary atrial fibrillation in the community: the Framingham Heart Study. Circulation 2015;131(19):1648–55.

23. Podolecki T, Lenarczyk R, Kowalczyk J, et al. Stroke and death prediction with CHA2DS2-vasc score after myocardial infarction in patients

without atrial fibrillation. J Cardiovasc Med 2015; 16(7):497–502.

24. Almendro-Delia M, Valle-Caballero MJ, Garcia-Rubira JC, et al. Prognostic impact of atrial fibrillation in acute coronary syndromes: results from the ARIAM registry. Eur Heart J Acute Cardiovasc Care 2014;3(2):141–8.

25. Lopes RD, Pieper KS, Horton JR, et al. Short- and long-term outcomes following atrial fibrillation in patients with acute coronary syndromes with or without ST-segment elevation. Heart 2008;94(7): 867–73.

26. Bengtson LG, Lutsey PL, Loehr LR, et al. Impact of atrial fibrillation on healthcare utilization in the community: the Atherosclerosis Risk in Communities study. J Am Heart Assoc 2014;3(6):e001006.

27. Simsekyilmaz S, Liehn EA, Militaru C, et al. Progress in interventional cardiology: challenges for the future. Thromb Haemost 2015;113(3):464–72.

28. Undas A. Fibrin clot properties and their modulation in thrombotic disorders. Thromb Haemost 2014;112(1):32–42.

29. Lamberts M, Gislason GH, Lip GY, et al. Antiplatelet therapy for stable coronary artery disease in atrial fibrillation patients taking an oral anticoagulant: a nationwide cohort study. Circulation 2014; 129(15):1577–85.

30. Lip GY, Laroche C, Popescu MI, et al. Improved outcomes with European Society of Cardiology guideline-adherent antithrombotic treatment in high-risk patients with atrial fibrillation: a report from the EORP-AF General Pilot Registry. Europace 2015;17(12):1777–86.

31. Ancedy Y, Lecoq C, Saint Etienne C, et al. Antithrombotic management in patients with atrial fibrillation undergoing coronary stent implantation: What is the impact of guideline adherence? Int J Cardiol 2016;203:987–94.

32. Dewilde WJM, Oirbans T, Verheugt FWA, et al. Use of clopidogrel with or without aspirin in patients taking oral anticoagulant therapy and undergoing percutaneous coronary intervention: an open-label, randomised, controlled trial. Lancet 2013;381(9872):1107–15.

33. Lamberts M, Olesen JB, Ruwald MH, et al. Bleeding after initiation of multiple antithrombotic drugs, including triple therapy, in atrial fibrillation patients following myocardial infarction and coronary intervention: a nationwide cohort study. Circulation 2012;126(10):1185–93.

34. Lamberts M, Gislason GH, Olesen JB, et al. Oral anticoagulation and antiplatelets in atrial fibrillation patients after myocardial infarction and coronary intervention. J Am Coll Cardiol 2013;62(11): 981–9.

35. Rubboli A, Schlitt A, Kiviniemi T, et al. One-year outcome of patients with atrial fibrillation

undergoing coronary artery stenting: an analysis of the AFCAS registry. Clin Cardiol 2014;37(6): 357–64.

36. Fiedler KA, Maeng M, Mehilli J, et al. Duration of triple therapy in patients requiring oral anticoagulation after drug-eluting stent implantation: the ISAR-TRIPLE trial. J Am Coll Cardiol 2015;65(16): 1619–29.

37. Heidbuchel H, Verhamme P, Alings M, et al. Updated European Heart Rhythm Association Practical Guide on the use of non-vitamin K antagonist anticoagulants in patients with non-valvular atrial fibrillation. Europace 2015;17(10):1467–507.

38. Dzeshka MS, Lip GY. Non-vitamin K oral anticoagulants in atrial fibrillation: Where are we now? Trends Cardiovasc Med 2015;25(4):315–36.

39. Connolly SJ, Ezekowitz MD, Yusuf S, et al. Dabigatran versus warfarin in patients with atrial fibrillation. N Engl J Med 2009;361(12):1139–51.

40. Connolly SJ, Ezekowitz MD, Yusuf S, et al. Randomized evaluation of long-term anticoagulation therapy I. Newly identified events in the RE-LY trial. N Engl J Med 2010;363(19):1875–6.

41. Patel MR, Mahaffey KW, Garg J, et al. Rivaroxaban versus warfarin in nonvalvular atrial fibrillation. N Engl J Med 2011;365(10):883–91.

42. Granger CB, Alexander JH, McMurray JJ, et al. Apixaban versus warfarin in patients with atrial fibrillation. N Engl J Med 2011;365(11):981–92.

43. Giugliano RP, Ruff CT, Braunwald E, et al. Edoxaban versus warfarin in patients with atrial fibrillation. N Engl J Med 2013;369(22):2093–104.

44. Htun NM, Peter K. Non-vitamin K antagonist oral anticoagulants (NOACs) in the cardiac catherisation laboratory: friends or foes? Thromb Haemost 2015;114(2):214–6.

45. Dzeshka MS, Brown RA, Lip GY. Patients with atrial fibrillation undergoing percutaneous coronary intervention: current concepts and concerns: part II. Pol Arch Med Wewn 2015;125(3):172–80.

46. Shahabi P, Scheinfeldt LB, Lynch DE, et al. An expanded pharmacogenomics warfarin dosing table with utility in generalised dosing guidance. Thromb Haemost 2016;116(2):337–48.

47. Cerezo-Manchado JJ, Roldan V, Corral J, et al. Genotype-guided therapy improves initial acenocoumarol dosing. Results from a prospective randomised study. Thromb Haemost 2016;115(1): 117–25.

48. Belley-Cote EP, Hanif H, D'Aragon F, et al. Genotype-guided versus standard vitamin K antagonist dosing algorithms in patients initiating anticoagulation. A systematic review and meta-analysis. Thromb Haemost 2015;114(4):768–77.

49. Hecker J, Marten S, Keller L, et al. Effectiveness and safety of rivaroxaban therapy in daily-care patients with atrial fibrillation. Results from the

Dresden NOAC Registry. Thromb Haemost 2016; 115(5):939–49.

50. Martinez C, Katholing A, Wallenhorst C, et al. Therapy persistence in newly diagnosed non-valvular atrial fibrillation treated with warfarin or NOAC. A cohort study. Thromb Haemost 2016; 115(1):31–9.

51. Van Blerk M, Bailleul E, Chatelain B, et al. Influence of dabigatran and rivaroxaban on routine coagulation assays. A nationwide Belgian survey. Thromb Haemost 2015;113(1):154–64.

52. Douxfils J, Chatelain B, Chatelain C, et al. Edoxaban: Impact on routine and specific coagulation assays. A practical laboratory guide. Thromb Haemost 2015;115(2):368–81.

53. Greinacher A, Thiele T, Selleng K. Reversal of anticoagulants: an overview of current developments. Thromb Haemost 2015;113(5):931–42.

54. Oldgren J, Budaj A, Granger CB, et al. Dabigatran vs. placebo in patients with acute coronary syndromes on dual antiplatelet therapy: a randomized, double-blind, phase II trial. Eur Heart J 2011;32(22):2781–9.

55. Alexander JH, Lopes RD, James S, et al. Apixaban with antiplatelet therapy after acute coronary syndrome. N Engl J Med 2011;365(8):699–708.

56. Mega JL, Braunwald E, Wiviott SD, et al. Rivaroxaban in patients with a recent acute coronary syndrome. N Engl J Med 2012;366(1):9–19.

57. Sjogren V, Grzymala-Lubanski B, Renlund H, et al. Safety and efficacy of well managed warfarin. A report from the Swedish quality register Auricula. Thromb Haemost 2015;113(6):1370–7.

58. Ruiz-Ortiz M, Bertomeu V, Cequier A, et al. Validation of the SAMe-TT2R2 score in a nationwide population of nonvalvular atrial fibrillation patients on vitamin K antagonists. Thromb Haemost 2015;114(4):695–701.

59. Sarafoff N, Martischnig A, Wealer J, et al. Triple therapy with aspirin, prasugrel, and vitamin K antagonists in patients with drug-eluting stent implantation and an indication for oral anticoagulation. J Am Coll Cardiol 2013;61(20): 2060–6.

60. Valgimigli M, Patialiakas A, Thury A, et al. Zotarolimus-eluting versus bare-metal stents in uncertain drug-eluting stent candidates. J Am Coll Cardiol 2015;65(8):805–15.

61. Ariotti S, Adamo M, Costa F, et al. Is bare-metal stent implantation still justifiable in high bleeding risk patients undergoing percutaneous coronary intervention? A pre-specified analysis from the ZEUS trial. JACC Cardiovasc Interv 2016;9(5):426–36.

62. Siontis GC, Stefanini GG, Mavridis D, et al. Percutaneous coronary interventional strategies for treatment of in-stent restenosis: a network meta-analysis. Lancet 2015;386(9994):655–64.

63. Sabate M, Brugaletta S, Cequier A, et al. Clinical outcomes in patients with ST-segment elevation myocardial infarction treated with everolimus-eluting stents versus bare-metal stents (EXAMI-NATION): 5-year results of a randomised trial. Lancet 2016;387(10016):357–66.

64. Urban P, Meredith IT, Abizaid A, et al. Polymer-free drug-coated coronary stents in patients at high bleeding risk. N Engl J Med 2015;373(21): 2038–47.

65. Naber CK, Urban P, Ong PJ, et al. Biolimus-A9 polymer-free coated stent in high bleeding risk patients with acute coronary syndrome: a Leaders Free ACS sub-study. Eur Heart J 2016 [pii: ehw203].

66. Kiviniemi T, Puurunen M, Schlitt A, et al. Bare-metal vs. drug-eluting stents in patients with atrial fibrillation undergoing percutaneous coronary intervention. Circ J 2014;78(11):2674–81.

67. Capodanno D, Musumeci G, Lettieri C, et al. Impact of bridging with perioperative low-molecular-weight heparin on cardiac and bleeding outcomes of stented patients undergoing non-cardiac surgery. Thromb Haemost 2015; 114(2):423–31.

68. Douketis JD, Healey JS, Brueckmann M, et al. Perioperative bridging anticoagulation during dabigatran or warfarin interruption among patients who had an elective surgery or procedure. Substudy of the RE-LY trial. Thromb Haemost 2015;113(3):625–32.

69. Kiviniemi T, Airaksinen KE, Rubboli A, et al. Bridging therapy with low molecular weight heparin in patients with atrial fibrillation undergoing percutaneous coronary intervention with stent implantation: the AFCAS study. Int J Cardiol 2015; 183:105–10.

70. Steinberg BA, Peterson ED, Kim S, et al. Use and outcomes associated with bridging during anticoagulation interruptions in patients with atrial fibrillation: findings from the Outcomes Registry for Better Informed Treatment of Atrial Fibrillation (ORBIT-AF). Circulation 2015;131(5):488–94.

71. Dewilde WJ, Janssen PW, Kelder JC, et al. Uninterrupted oral anticoagulation versus bridging in patients with long-term oral anticoagulation during percutaneous coronary intervention: subgroup analysis from the WOEST trial. EuroIntervention 2015;11(4):381–90.

72. Vranckx P, Leebeek FW, Tijssen JG, et al. Peri-procedural use of rivaroxaban in elective percutaneous coronary intervention to treat stable coronary artery disease. The X-PLORER trial. Thromb Haemost 2015;114(2):258–67.

73. Vries MJ, van der Meijden PE, Henskens YM, et al. Assessment of bleeding risk in patients with coronary artery disease on dual antiplatelet

therapy. A systematic review. Thromb Haemost 2016;115(1):7–24.

74. Ruiz-Rodriguez E, Asfour A, Lolay G, et al. Systematic review and meta-analysis of major cardiovascular outcomes for radial versus femoral access in patients with acute coronary syndrome. South Med J 2016;109(1):61–76.

75. Bavishi C, Panwar SR, Dangas GD, et al. Meta-analysis of radial versus femoral access for percutaneous coronary interventions in non-ST-segment elevation acute coronary syndrome. Am J Cardiol 2016;117(2):172–8.

76. Ho KW, Ivanov J, Freixa X, et al. Antithrombotic therapy after coronary stenting in patients with nonvalvular atrial fibrillation. Can J Cardiol 2013; 29(2):213–8.

77. Kim MH, Bell KF, Makenbaeva D, et al. Health care burden of dyspepsia among nonvalvular atrial fibrillation patients. J Manag Care Spec Pharm 2014;20(4):391–9.

78. Gibson CM, Mehran R, Bode C, et al. An open-label, randomized, controlled, multicenter study exploring two treatment strategies of rivaroxaban and a dose-adjusted oral vitamin K antagonist treatment strategy in subjects with atrial fibrillation who undergo percutaneous coronary intervention (PIONEER AF-PCI). Am Heart J 2015; 169(4):472–8.e5.

79. Min T, Benjamin S, Cozma L. Thromboembolic complications of thyroid storm. Endocrinol Diabetes Metab Case Rep 2014;2014:130060.

80. Capodanno D, Lip GY, Windecker S, et al. Triple antithrombotic therapy in atrial fibrillation patients with acute coronary syndromes or undergoing percutaneous coronary intervention or transcatheter aortic valve replacement. EuroIntervention 2015;10(9):1015–21.

81. Kuroki K, Tada H, Kunugida F, et al. Hybrid epicardial and endocardial ablation of a persistent atrial tachycardia arising from the marshall bundle: the importance of a detailed analysis of the local potentials. Heart Vessels 2015;30(3): 416–9.

82. Lip GY, Nieuwlaat R, Pisters R, et al. Refining clinical risk stratification for predicting stroke and thromboembolism in atrial fibrillation using a novel risk factor-based approach: the Euro Heart Survey on atrial fibrillation. Chest 2010;137(2): 263–72.

83. Pisters R, Lane DA, Nieuwlaat R, et al. A novel user-friendly score (HAS-BLED) to assess 1-year risk of major bleeding in patients with atrial fibrillation: the Euro Heart Survey. Chest 2010;138(5): 1093–100.

84. Apostolakis S, Sullivan RM, Olshansky B, et al. Factors affecting quality of anticoagulation control among patients with atrial fibrillation on warfarin:

the SAMe-TT(2)R(2) score. Chest 2013;144(5): 1555–63.

85. Chan W, Ajani AE, Clark DJ, et al. Impact of periprocedural atrial fibrillation on short-term clinical outcomes following percutaneous coronary intervention. Am J Cardiol 2012;109(4):471–7.

86. Gizurarson S, Stahlman M, Jeppsson A, et al. Atrial fibrillation in patients admitted to coronary care units in western Sweden—focus on obesity and lipotoxicity. J Electrocardiol 2015;48(5): 853–60.

87. Jabre P, Jouven X, Adnet F, et al. Atrial fibrillation and death after myocardial infarction: a community study. Circulation 2011;123(19):2094–100.

88. Lau DH, Huynh LT, Chew DP, et al. Prognostic impact of types of atrial fibrillation in acute coronary syndromes. Am J Cardiol 2009;104(10): 1317–23.

89. Lopes RD, Elliott LE, White HD, et al. Antithrombotic therapy and outcomes of patients with atrial fibrillation following primary percutaneous coronary intervention: results from the APEX-AMI trial. Eur Heart J 2009;30(16):2019–28.

90. Lopes RD, Li L, Granger CB, et al. Atrial fibrillation and acute myocardial infarction: antithrombotic therapy and outcomes. Am J Med 2012;125(9): 897–905.

91. Meyer ML, Jaensch A, Mons U, et al. Atrial fibrillation and long-term prognosis of patients with stable coronary heart disease: relevance of routine electrocardiogram. Int J Cardiol 2016; 203:1014–5.

92. Pilgrim T, Kalesan B, Zanchin T, et al. Impact of atrial fibrillation on clinical outcomes among patients with coronary artery disease undergoing revascularisation with drug-eluting stents. EuroIntervention 2013;8(9):1061–71.

93. Rene AG, Genereux P, Ezekowitz M, et al. Impact of atrial fibrillation in patients with ST-elevation myocardial infarction treated with percutaneous coronary intervention (from the HORIZONS-AMI [Harmonizing Outcomes With Revascularization and Stents in Acute Myocardial Infarction] trial). Am J Cardiol 2014;113(2):236–42.

94. Rohla M, Vennekate CK, Tentzeris I, et al. Long-term mortality of patients with atrial fibrillation undergoing percutaneous coronary intervention with stent implantation for acute and stable coronary artery disease. Int J Cardiol 2015;184:108–14.

95. Ruff CT, Bhatt DL, Steg PG, et al. Long-term cardiovascular outcomes in patients with atrial fibrillation and atherothrombosis in the REACH Registry. Int J Cardiol 2014;170(3):413–8.

96. Bernard A, Fauchier L, Pellegrin C, et al. Anticoagulation in patients with atrial fibrillation undergoing coronary stent implantation. Thromb Haemost 2013;110(3):560–8.

97. Caballero L, Ruiz-Nodar JM, Marin F, et al. Oral anticoagulation improves the prognosis of octogenarian patients with atrial fibrillation undergoing percutaneous coronary intervention and stenting. Age Ageing 2013;42(1):70–5.

98. Dabrowska M, Ochala A, Cybulski W, et al. Balancing between bleeding and thromboembolism after percutaneous coronary intervention in patients with atrial fibrillation. Could triple anticoagulant therapy be a solution? Postepy Kardiol Interwencyjnej 2013;9(3):234–40.

99. Fosbol EL, Wang TY, Li S, et al. Warfarin use among older atrial fibrillation patients with non-ST-segment elevation myocardial infarction managed with coronary stenting and dual antiplatelet therapy. Am Heart J 2013;166(5):864–70.

100. Gao F, Zhou YJ, Wang ZJ, et al. Comparison of different antithrombotic regimens for patients with atrial fibrillation undergoing drug-eluting stent implantation. Circ J 2010;74(4):701–8.

101. Gilard M, Blanchard D, Helft G, et al. Antiplatelet therapy in patients with anticoagulants undergoing percutaneous coronary stenting (from STENTing and oral antiCOagulants [STENTICO]). Am J Cardiol 2009;104(3):338–42.

102. Kang DO, Yu CW, Kim HD, et al. Triple antithrombotic therapy versus dual antiplatelet therapy in patients with atrial fibrillation undergoing drug-eluting stent implantation. Coron Artery Dis 2015;26(5):372–80.

103. Karjalainen PP, Porela P, Ylitalo A, et al. Safety and efficacy of combined antiplatelet-warfarin therapy after coronary stenting. Eur Heart J 2007;28(6):726–32.

104. Lopes RD, Rao M, Simon DN, et al. Triple vs dual antithrombotic therapy in patients with atrial fibrillation and coronary artery disease. Am J Med 2016;129(6):592–9.e1.

105. Mennuni MG, Halperin JL, Bansilal S, et al. Balancing the Risk of Bleeding and Stroke in Patients With Atrial Fibrillation After Percutaneous Coronary Intervention (from the AVIATOR Registry). Am J Cardiol 2015;116(1):37–42.

106. Mutuberria Urdaniz M, Sambola A, Bosch E, et al. Outcomes in patients with atrial fibrillation undergoing coronary artery stenting with a low-moderate CHA2DS2VASc score: do they need anticoagulation? Eur Heart J 2013;34(Suppl 1):P4093.

107. Rossini R, Musumeci G, Lettieri C, et al. Long-term outcomes in patients undergoing coronary stenting on dual oral antiplatelet treatment requiring oral anticoagulant therapy. Am J Cardiol 2008;102(12):1618–23.

108. Rubboli A, Magnavacchi P, Guastaroba P, et al. Antithrombotic management and 1-year outcome of patients on oral anticoagulation undergoing coronary stent implantation (from the Registro Regionale Angioplastiche Emilia-Romagna Registry). Am J Cardiol 2012;109(10):1411–7.

109. Ruiz-Nodar JM, Marin F, Hurtado JA, et al. Anticoagulant and antiplatelet therapy use in 426 patients with atrial fibrillation undergoing percutaneous coronary intervention and stent implantation implications for bleeding risk and prognosis. J Am Coll Cardiol 2008;51(8):818–25.

110. Ruiz-Nodar JM, Marin F, Roldan V, et al. Should we recommend oral anticoagulation therapy in patients with atrial fibrillation undergoing coronary artery stenting with a high HAS-BLED bleeding risk score? Circ Cardiovasc Interv 2012;5(4):459–66.

111. Sambola A, Ferreira-Gonzalez I, Angel J, et al. Therapeutic strategies after coronary stenting in chronically anticoagulated patients: the MUSICA study. Heart 2009;95(18):1483–8.

112. Sambola A, Mutuberria M, Garcia Del Blanco B, et al. Effects of triple therapy in patients with non-valvular atrial fibrillation undergoing percutaneous coronary intervention regarding thromboembolic risk stratification. Circ J 2016;80(2):354–62.

113. Smith JG, Wieloch M, Koul S, et al. Triple antithrombotic therapy following an acute coronary syndrome: prevalence, outcomes and prognostic utility of the HAS-BLED score. EuroIntervention 2012;8(6):672–8.

114. Uchida Y, Mori F, Ogawa H, et al. Impact of anticoagulant therapy with dual antiplatelet therapy on prognosis after treatment with drug-eluting coronary stents. J Cardiol 2010;55(3):362–9.

115. Andrade JG, Deyell MW, Khoo C, et al. Risk of bleeding on triple antithrombotic therapy after percutaneous coronary intervention/stenting: a systematic review and meta-analysis. Can J Cardiol 2013;29(2):204–12.

116. Bavishi C, Koulova A, Bangalore S, et al. Evaluation of the efficacy and safety of dual antiplatelet therapy with or without warfarin in patients with a clinical indication for DAPT and chronic anticoagulation: a meta-analysis of observational studies. Catheter Cardiovasc Interv 2016;88(1):E12–22.

117. Gao F, Zhou YJ, Wang ZJ, et al. Meta-analysis of the combination of warfarin and dual antiplatelet therapy after coronary stenting in patients with indications for chronic oral anticoagulation. Int J Cardiol 2011;148(1):96–101.

118. Gao XF, Chen Y, Fan ZG, et al. Antithrombotic regimens for patients taking oral anticoagulation after coronary intervention: a meta-analysis of 16 clinical trials and 9,185 patients. Clin Cardiol 2015;38(8):499–509.

119. Saheb KJ, Deng BQ, Hu QS, et al. Triple antithrombotic therapy versus double antiplatelet

therapy after percutaneous coronary intervention with stent implantation in patients requiring chronic oral anticoagulation: a meta-analysis. Chin Med J 2013;126(13):2536–42.

120. Singh PP, Singh M, Bedi U, et al. Safety and efficacy of triple antithrombotic therapy after percutaneous coronary intervention in patients needing long-term anticoagulation. Ther Adv Cardiovasc Dis 2011;5(1):23–31.

121. Washam JB, Dolor RJ, Jones WS, et al. Dual antiplatelet therapy with or without oral anticoagulation in the postdischarge management of acute coronary syndrome patients with an indication for long term anticoagulation: a systematic review. J Thromb Thrombolysis 2014;38(3): 285–98.

122. Zhao HJ, Zheng ZT, Wang ZH, et al. "Triple therapy" rather than "triple threat": a meta-analysis of the two antithrombotic regimens after stent implantation in patients receiving long-term oral anticoagulant treatment. Chest 2011;139(2): 260–70.

123. Dzeshka MS, Lip GY. Warfarin versus dabigatran etexilate: an assessment of efficacy and safety in patients with atrial fibrillation. Expert Opin Drug Saf 2015;14(1):45–62.

124. Dzeshka MS, Lip GY. Edoxaban for reducing the risk of stroke and systemic embolism in patients with non-valvular atrial fibrillation. Expert Opin Pharmacother 2015;16(17):2661–78.

125. Dans AL, Connolly SJ, Wallentin L, et al. Concomitant use of antiplatelet therapy with dabigatran or warfarin in the Randomized Evaluation of Long-Term Anticoagulation Therapy (RE-LY) trial. Circulation 2013;127(5):634–40.

126. Alexander JH, Lopes RD, Thomas L, et al. Apixaban vs. warfarin with concomitant aspirin in patients with atrial fibrillation: insights from the ARISTOTLE trial. Eur Heart J 2014;35(4):224–32.

127. Xu H, Ruff CT, Giugliano RP, et al. Concomitant use of single antiplatelet therapy with edoxaban or warfarin in patients with atrial fibrillation: analysis from the ENGAGE AF-TIMI48 Trial. J Am Heart Assoc 2016;5(2):e002587.

Antiplatelet Therapy for Secondary Prevention After Acute Myocardial Infarction

Ilaria Cavallari, MD, Marc P. Bonaca, MD, MPH*

KEYWORDS

- Antiplatelet therapy • Myocardial infarction • Secondary prevention

---

KEY POINTS

- Patients with prior myocardial infarction (MI) are at heightened risk for recurrent ischemic complications over the long term.
- Prolonged intensive antiplatelet therapy reduces cardiovascular and all-cause death in patients with history of MI at the cost of an increase in nonfatal bleeding events.
- Risk scores are useful tools to identify patients who would derive a net benefit from long-term intensive antiplatelet therapy.

Antiplatelet therapy represents the cornerstone of short- and long-term prevention of atherothrombosis. In the setting of acute coronary syndrome (ACS), especially in patients with myocardial infarction (MI), randomized studies have shown a reduction in ischemic risk with dual antiplatelet therapy (DAPT) with aspirin and the $P2Y_{12}$ receptor inhibitor clopidogrel versus aspirin alone for a year after the acute event. Subsequent studies have shown even greater benefit with the more potent agents, prasugrel and ticagrelor, as compared with clopidogrel.[1–4] As a result, practice guidelines in the United States and Europe currently recommend treatment with a $P2Y_{12}$ inhibitor, in addition to aspirin, for up to 1 year after MI, regardless of medical or invasive management[5–7] with a preference for more potent agents where appropriate (Fig. 1). However, patients who suffer an MI remain at heightened risk for ischemic complications beyond 1 year[8–10]

with 1 in 5 subjects experiencing an event during a mean follow-up of 2.5 years[10] (Fig. 2). Recent trials have demonstrated that extension of intensive long-term antiplatelet therapy as long-term secondary prevention reduces this ischemic risk and increased bleeding.[11–13]

In light of available data, a recent consensus document by the American College of Cardiology/American Heart Association assigned a class IIb recommendation for continuation of DAPT beyond 12 months; this strategy may be considered for patients at higher ischemic risk with lower bleeding risk (see Fig. 1).[7] Since these guidelines have been published, emerging data have begun to characterize key subgroups that derive robust absolute benefit from intensive strategies. In addition, risk scores have attempted to integrate markers of ischemic and bleeding risk to improve patient selection.

The aim of this review is to describe the residual risk of patients with prior MI, summarize

---

Disclosures: I. Cavallari has nothing to disclose. M.P. Bonaca is a consultant for Bayer, AstraZeneca, and Merck. TRA2P-TIMI 50 was funded by a grant from Merck to Brigham and Women's Hospital. PEGASUS-TIMI 54 was funded by a grant from AstraZeneca to Brigham and Women's Hospital.
TIMI Study Group, Division of Cardiovascular Medicine, Brigham and Women's Hospital, Harvard Medical School, 350 Longwood Avenue, Boston, MA 02115, USA
* Corresponding author. TIMI Study Group, 350 Longwood Avenue, 1st Floor Offices, Boston, MA 02115.
E-mail address: mbonaca@partners.org

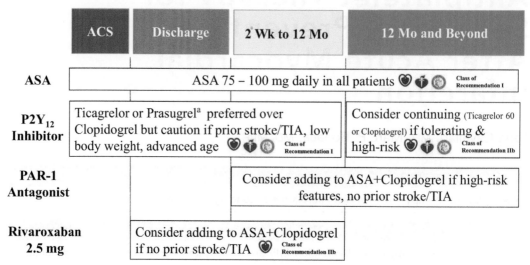

Fig. 1. Algorithm for the use of antithrombotic therapy in patients with ACS. [a] Prasugrel only for patients treated with PCI. ASA, aspirin.

current evidence on prolonged intensive antiplatelet therapy for the secondary prevention of recurrent ischemic events, and introduce the concept of tailored duration of intensive antiplatelet therapy.

RESIDUAL RISK AFTER MYOCARDIAL INFARCTION

Several observational studies have characterized long-term ischemic risk in patients with prior atherothrombosis (see Fig. 2). An analysis of 64,977 stable outpatients enrolled in the REACH (REduction of Atherothrombosis for Continued Health) registry evaluated the risk of cardiovascular (CV)

death, MI, and stroke based on a clinical history of either CV risk factors only, known atherosclerosis but no prior ischemic event, or a prior ischemic event.[8] Patients with a prior ischemic event had the highest risk of CV death, MI, or stroke at 4 years (18.3%) compared with patients with stable atherosclerosis (12.2%) or risk factors only (9.1%). This observation appears biologically plausible; those with prior spontaneous MI, mediated by plaque rupture, may be at greater risk for future plaque rupture events than those without prior MI. Multiple factors have been hypothesized to explain this risk, including a long-term heightened inflammatory state, persisting platelet activation, and higher vulnerable plaque burden

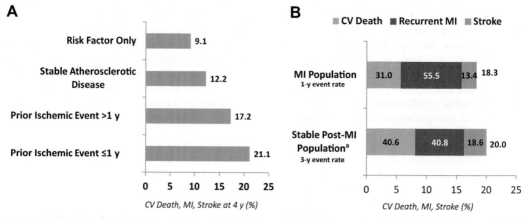

Fig. 2. Residual risk after MI. [a] Alive patients who did not experience MI or stroke during the first 365 days after MI. (Data from Bhatt DL, Eagle KA, Ohman EM, et al. Comparative determinants of 4-year cardiovascular event rates in stable outpatients at risk of or with atherothrombosis. JAMA 2010;304:1350–7; and Jernberg T, Hasvold P, Henriksson M, et al. Cardiovascular risk in post-myocardial infarction patients: nationwide real world data demonstrate the importance of a long-term perspective. Eur Heart J 2015;36:1163–70.)

prone to rupture.[14] Of note, the risk of recurrent events is largely driven by de novo events with stent-related complications rare in the stable phase. In fact, for patients discharged after MI, the risk of recurrent spontaneous events remains relatively constant, whereas the risk of stent-related complications decreases over time (Fig. 3).[15] In addition, data from the REACH registry indicate that the risk of long-term ischemic complications is highest for patients within 1 year of the acute event (21.1%) but remains heightened over the long term even for those who have survived beyond a year from their most recent event (17.2%).

In the same line of evidence, another retrospective cohort study including 108,315 patients admitted to hospital with a primary MI in Sweden showed that within the first year, the rate of recurrent MI, stroke, or CV death was 18.3%, with most of these events being recurrent MI (56%), followed by CV death (31.0%), and ischemic stroke (13.4%).[10] For those patients who survived 1 year after their MI without a recurrent event, the rate of subsequent CV death, MI, or stroke was 20% over 3 years. Although recurrent MI was the most frequent event (40.8%), the relative proportion of CV death (40.6%) and stroke (18.6%) was higher than that seen within the first year.[10] Similarly, other national registries have estimated comparable rates of subsequent recurrent MI, stroke, or mortality, ranging from 16.7% to 21.3% at 3 years in patients who had survived 1 year from MI.[16] Taken together, these data indicate the need for close monitoring and more aggressive treatment strategies to reduce long-term ischemic risk in the post-MI population.

CURRENT EVIDENCE ON PROLONGED INTENSIVE ANTIPLATELET THERAPY IN PATIENTS WITH PRIOR MYOCARDIAL INFARCTION

Aspirin has been studied for ischemic risk reduction in multiple randomized trials and analyzed in a meta-analysis conducted by the Antithrombotic Trialists' Collaborative.[17] In the secondary prevention population including 17,000 individuals, aspirin was shown to reduce any serious vascular event by 19% (hazard ratio [HR] 0.81, 95% confidence interval [CI] 0.75–0.87) with an ARR of 1.49% per year versus placebo.[17] There

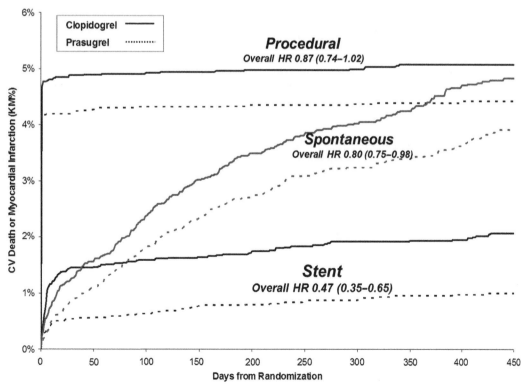

Fig. 3. Ischemic events after ACS. (*From* Scirica B, Morrow D, Antman E, et al. Timing and clinical setting of cardiovascular death or myocardial infarction following PCI for ACS—observations from the TRITON-TIMI 38 trial. J Am Coll Cardiol 2012;59(13s1):E340; with permission.)

were consistent reductions in coronary mortality, MI, and ischemic stroke.[17] However, aspirin increased the risk of major extracranial bleeding, primarily gastrointestinal (ARI of 0.4% per year), and hemorrhagic stroke (ARI of 0.01% per year).[17,18] In the setting of ACS, the addition of clopidogrel to aspirin reduced the rate of recurrence of major CV events in the first 30 days and through 12 months by 20%, depending on the endpoint and whether the population was non-ST-elevation or ST-elevation ACS.[1,2] Although the treatment duration was 3 to 12 months after non-ST-elevation ACS, the survival curves demonstrated continued separation over the course of follow-up, suggesting continued benefit over time.[19] Subsequently, post hoc landmark analyses from other studies enrolling ACS patients have shown a variable degree of protection from recurrent CV events with the use of longer duration of more intensive antiplatelet therapy but at the price of higher risk of major but not fatal bleeding complications.[4,19–22]

CHARISMA (Clopidogrel for High Atherothrombotic Risk and Ischemic Stabilization, Management, and Avoidance) was the first dedicated trial designed with the aim to investigate the efficacy and safety of long-term clopidogrel added to aspirin in a broad population of 15,603 patients with established CV disease or multiple risk factors.[23] After a median follow-up of 28 months, the addition of clopidogrel resulted in a nonsignificant 7.1% relative risk (RR) reduction in the primary efficacy endpoint of CV death, MI, or stroke (95% CI, −4.5%–17.5%; P = .22) at the cost of an increase in the occurrence of global use of strategies to open occluded arteries (GUSTO) moderate bleeding (2.1% vs 1.3%, HR 1.63, 95% CI 1.27–2.09; P<.001).[24] However, a subsequent post hoc analysis suggested that patients with symptomatic vascular disease defined as prior MI, ischemic stroke, or symptomatic peripheral artery disease in the clopidogrel arm derived a benefit for the primary efficacy endpoint compared with placebo (7.3% vs 8.8%, HR 0.83, 95% CI 0.72–0.96; P = .01), whereas patients without symptomatic disease had no benefit and a trend toward harm.[25] A further evaluation showed that those patients with prior MI appeared to derive the greatest magnitude of benefit with a 23% RR reduction of major adverse CV events (HR 0.77, 95% CI 0.61–0.98, P = .031).[25] Long-term clopidogrel increased GUSTO moderate or severe bleeding driven by an increase in moderate bleeding.[24]

The protease activated receptor 1 (PAR-1), which is the primary receptor for thrombin on human platelets, has also been tested as a target for secondary prevention.[26] The Thrombin Receptor Antagonist in Secondary Prevention of Atherothrombotic Ischemic Events (TRA2P)–Thrombolysis in Myocardial Infarction (TIMI) 50 trial randomized a broad population of patients with atherosclerotic vascular disease to receive vorapaxar, an oral competitive antagonist of PAR-1, 2.5 mg daily, or a matching placebo.[27] Background antithrombotic therapy in the trial was at the discretion of the treating physicians and included antiplatelet monotherapy as well as DAPT with aspirin and clopidogrel. At 3 years, vorapaxar significantly reduced the primary endpoint of CV death, MI, or stroke (HR 0.87, 95% CI 0.80–0.94, P<.001), while increasing the rate of GUSTO moderate or severe bleeding (HR 1.66, 95% CI 1.43–1.93, P<.001) and intracranial hemorrhage (HR 1.94, 95% CI 1.39–2.70, P<.001).[27] Of note, the risk of intracranial hemorrhage with vorapaxar was highest in those with a history of stroke (absolute risk increase [ARI] 1.5%, 2.4% with vorapaxar vs 0.9% with placebo, P<.001) relative to those without a history of stroke (ARI 0.2%, 0.6% with vorapaxar group vs 0.4% with placebo, P = .049).[28] This finding is consistent with others showing increased risk of intracranial bleeding with long-term potent antiplatelet strategies in patients with prior stroke.[3,29–31] As a result, vorapaxar was approved for clinical use based on the overall efficacy; however, it is contraindicated in patients with prior stroke or transient ischemic attack (TIA) due to the increased risk of intracranial hemorrhage in that population.[11]

In the subgroup of 17,779 patients with prior MI (including those with prior stroke/TIA), vorapaxar reduced the primary endpoint of CV death, MI, or stroke by 20%, translating into an absolute risk reduction (ARR) of 1.6% at 3 years (0.53% per year) when added to aspirin monotherapy (98%) or DAPT with aspirin and clopidogrel (78%).[21] GUSTO moderate or severe bleeding was increased with vorapaxar with an ARI of 1.3% at 3 years (0.43% per year, HR 1.61, 95% CI 1.31–1.97, P<.001). Similarly to previous trials, the rates of intracranial hemorrhage (0.6% vs 0.4%, HR 1.54, 95% CI 0.96–2.48, P = .076) and fatal bleeding (0.2% vs 0.1%, HR 1.56, 95% CI 0.67–3.60, P = .30) were similar between the randomization treatment groups.[21] Overall, in the post-MI population, the net outcome of all-cause mortality, MI, stroke, or GUSTO severe bleeding at 3 years was significantly reduced with vorapaxar (ARR 1.3%, HR 0.86, 95% CI 0.78–0.95, P = .003).[21]

The addition of vorapaxar to standard therapy in patients with prior MI appeared to be particularly beneficial in subgroups at high risk of recurrent ischemic events, such as those with diabetes.[32] Although the relative effect of vorapaxar on the primary endpoint was similar in patients with and without diabetes (P for interaction = 0.51), by nature of their greater absolute risk, patients with diabetes had a robust ARR (2.9% at 3 years, 1.0% per year) with a resulting number needed to treat (NNT) of 29, as compared with patients without diabetes (ARR 1.3% at 3 years, NNT = 74).[32] This benefit translated into a significant reduction in the net outcome of all-cause mortality, MI, stroke, or GUSTO severe bleeding (HR 0.77, 95% CI 0.65–0.93, P = .006) in the diabetic population.[32] In addition, vorapaxar had consistent efficacy in reducing CV death, MI, or stroke in patients planned for aspirin monotherapy (HR 0.75, 95% CI 0.60–0.94, P = .011) and in those planned for DAPT with aspirin and clopidogrel (HR 0.80, 95% CI 0.70–0.91, P<.001) with similar safety profiles (P for interaction 0.37).[33]

Addressing a related but distinct question, the DAPT (Dual Antiplatelet Therapy) trial enrolled 9961 patients treated with aspirin and a thienopyridine after coronary stenting.[13] Those who were adherent to therapy and had not had a major adverse CV or cerebrovascular event, repeat revascularization, or moderate or severe bleeding at 12 months were randomized to continued thienopyridine or placebo for an additional 18 months. Continuation of clopidogrel or prasugrel on a background of aspirin for more than 12 months was associated with a significant reduction in nonfatal ischemic events.[13] This ischemic risk reduction was accompanied by a significant increase in GUSTO moderate or severe bleeding with prolonged DAPT (2.5% vs 1.6%, P = .001) and potentially a higher risk of death from non-CV causes (2.0% vs 1.5%; HR 1.36, 95% CI 1.00–1.85, P = .05).[13] Of note and similar to the CHARISMA trial, the reduction of major adverse CV and cerebrovascular events for continued thienopyridine was greater for patients with MI (3.9% vs 6.8%; P<.001) compared with those presenting without MI (4.4% vs 5.3%; P = .08; P for interaction = 0.03).[34] Moreover, in both groups there was a significant decrease in the occurrence of de novo MI events as well as stent thrombosis.[34] The increase in non-CV mortality appeared in the non-MI patients (1.0% vs 0.5%) with no apparent excess in patients with prior MI (0.6% vs 0.5%).

The PEGASUS-TIMI 54 (Prevention of Cardiovascular Events in Patients with Prior Heart Attack Using Ticagrelor Compared to Placebo on a Background of Aspirin–Thrombolysis in Myocardial Infarction 54) trial prospectively tested the hypothesis that long-term therapy with ticagrelor (90 mg or 60 mg twice daily) added to low-dose aspirin would reduce the risk of major adverse CV events in stable patients with a history of MI 1 to 3 years before randomization.[12] In contrast to DAPT, patients could be randomized as a "continue on DAPT" strategy from their index MI or could be reinitiated on P2Y$_{12}$ inhibitor therapy from aspirin monotherapy. A total of 21,162 patients were randomized, and after a median follow-up of 33 months, both doses of ticagrelor resulted in an approximately 15% relative reduction in the risk of CV death, MI and stroke, as compared with placebo (HR for 90 mg of ticagrelor vs placebo, 0.85, 95% CI 0.75–0.96; P = .008; HR for 60 mg of ticagrelor vs placebo, 0.84, 95% CI 0.74–0.95; P = .004).[12] Rates of TIMI major bleeding, but not intracranial hemorrhage or fatal bleeding, were higher with ticagrelor (2.60% with 90 mg and 2.30% with 60 mg) than with placebo (1.06%) (P<.001 for each dose vs placebo). There was no heterogeneity in the efficacy or safety of ticagrelor among major clinical subgroups. Overall, the 60-mg dose appeared to have similar efficacy but better tolerability than the 90-mg twice-daily dose.[35] These findings resulted in ticagrelor 60-mg dose twice daily being recently approved by the US Food and Drug Administration for the treatment of patients with a history of MI beyond the first year.

Udell and colleagues[36] subsequently performed a study-level meta-analysis to evaluate the efficacy and safety of long-term P2Y$_{12}$ inhibition in patients with prior MI. The meta-analysis included greater than 33,000 patients with previous MI to better understand the CV benefits and risks of this strategy (Fig. 4).[36] This meta-analysis demonstrated that extended DAPT decreases the risk of each individual component of major adverse CV events compared with aspirin alone (6.4% vs 7.5%; RR 0.78, 95% CI 0.67–0.90; P = .001), including CV death (2.3% vs 2.6%; RR 0.85, 95% CI 0.74–0.98; P = .03).[36] This benefit was paralleled by an increased risk of major bleeding (1.85% vs 1.09%; RR 1.73, 95% CI 1.19–2.50; P = .004) but not fatal bleeding (0.14 vs 0.17%; RR 0.91, 95% CI 0.53–1.58; P = .75), with no difference in the occurrence of non-CV death (RR 1.03, 95% CI 0.86–1.23; P = .76).[33] These results remained unchanged when the analysis was restricted to include only studies that randomized patients to prolonged DAPT after 1 year from the acute event and had a minimum of 2 years follow-up.[37] In the latter

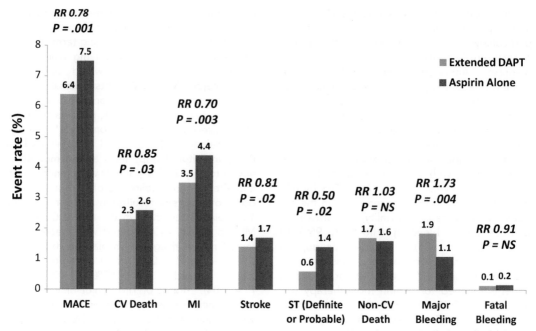

Fig. 4. Efficacy and safety of extended DAPT in patients with prior MI. NS, not significant. (*Data from* Bohula EA, Aylward PE, Bonaca MP, et al. Efficacy and safety of vorapaxar with and without a thienopyridine for secondary prevention in patients with previous myocardial infarction and no history of Stroke or transient ischemic attack: results from TRA 2°P-TIMI 50. Circulation 2015;132:1871–9.)

meta-analysis, extended DAPT was shown to prevent 6 major CV events/1000 patients/y and 2 CV deaths/1000 patients/y, with an excess of 0.6 major bleeding/1000 patients/y with use of clopidogrel as second antiplatelet drug and of 1.9 major bleeding/1000 patients/y with use of prasugrel or ticagrelor.[37]

CONTINUING ON AT 1 YEAR AFTER MYOCARDIAL INFARCTION VERSUS RESTARTING IN ALL PATIENTS WITH HISTORY OF MYOCARDIAL INFARCTION

A prespecified analysis from PEGASUS-TIMI 54 evaluated the efficacy and safety of long-term ticagrelor by time from last dose of a $P2Y_{12}$ inhibitor before randomization. The greatest reduction in ischemic events with prolonged DAPT was observed for patients in whom $P2Y_{12}$ inhibition was continued or restarted only after a brief interruption ($\leq$30 days) (HR 0.73; 95% CI 0.61–0.87 for ticagrelor pooled doses, ARR 2.2% at 3 years), whereas the benefit was uncertain in the group who was started on therapy after having remained event free on aspirin monotherapy for a prolonged period (>1 year) (HR 1.01; 95% CI 0.80–1.27 for ticagrelor pooled doses, ARR 0.3% at 3 years).[38] In addition, tolerability was better and drug discontinuation rates were much lower in

patients who had taken and tolerated ticagrelor therapy for 1 year (adverse events leading to discontinuation: 13%–16% in the first year vs 6.0%–6.5% over the subsequent 2 years).[35] These data confirm that the most natural translation of the PEGASUS-TIMI 54 and DAPT trials data would be to continue $P2Y_{12}$ inhibition in patients with MI who have tolerated and adhered to therapy without significant bleeding in the first year after MI. Although selected high-risk individuals may benefit from restarting therapy after a prolonged interruption (eg, >1 year), the data suggest that routine application of this practice to patients who have been event free may only provide a modest absolute benefit.

CLINICAL FACTORS GUIDING PATIENT SELECTION

Although some clinicians may consider the tradeoff of efficacy and safety in the PEGASUS-TIMI 54 cohort that continued on $P2Y_{12}$ inhibition and the DAPT subgroup with history of MI compelling enough to routinely apply in clinical practice, others may wish to consider additional factors to further select patients who are most likely to accrue a robust efficacy benefit relative to bleeding risk. Several post hoc analyses showed greater absolute benefits of prolonged

Table 1
Efficacy and safety of prolonged intensive antiplatelet therapy with the addition of vorapaxar in high-risk subgroups of patients

Subgroup	TRA2P-TIMI 50 MACE	
	3-y Event Rate in Placebo (%)	3-y ARR/ARI with Vorapaxar (%)
Diabetes	14.3	−2.9
No diabetes	7.6	−1.3
Prior CABG	13.7	−3.7
No prior CABG	7.8	—
	Major Bleeding	
Diabetes	2.6	+1.7
No diabetes	1.9	+1.0
Prior CABG	4.1	+2.2
No prior CABG	—	—

intensive antiplatelet therapy in selected high-risk subgroups of patients, such as those with diabetes, renal dysfunction, peripheral artery disease, multivessel coronary artery disease, and previous coronary artery bypass grafting, including significant net benefit and reductions in CV and all-cause mortality in some subgroups (Tables 1 and 2).[32,39–44] Subgroup analyses should be interpreted with caution because they are generally not powered to show significant differences on their own. In addition, individual subgroups may enrich for several factors. For example, patients with diabetes mellitus are also more likely to have multivessel coronary disease and peripheral artery disease relative to those without diabetes. Therefore, although subgroups may be attractive because they are easy to apply in clinical practice, they may oversimplify patient selection.

A more complex method of individualizing the application of clinical trial is through the use of clinical risk scores and decision tools. One such tool derived from the DAPT trial to select patients most likely to benefit and least likely to be harmed from prolonged DAPT after percutaneous coronary intervention (PCI) is called the DAPT score (Table 3).[45] The DAPT score, with values ranging from −2 to 10, assigns points to the following variables: age, vein graft PCI, cigarette smoking, diabetes, MI at presentation, stent diameter, history of congestive heart failure or left ventricular ejection fraction less than 30%, prior PCI or prior MI, and paclitaxel-eluting stents. Among patients with DAPT scores ≥2, continued thienopyridine was associated with reductions in MI and stent

Table 2
Efficacy and safety of prolonged intensive antiplatelet therapy with the addition of ticagrelor doses pooled in high-risk subgroups of patients

Subgroup	PEGASUS-TIMI 54 MACE	
	3-y Event Rate in Placebo (%)	3-y ARR/ARI with Ticagrelor (%)
Diabetes	11.6	−1.5
No diabetes	7.8	−1.1
Renal disease (eGFR <60 mL/min)	13.99	−2.7
No renal disease	7.43	−0.6
PAD	19.3	−4.1
No PAD	8.4	−1.0
	Major Bleeding	
Diabetes	0.98	+1.6
No diabetes	1.09	+1.3
Renal disease (eGFR <60 mL/min)	1.34	+1.19
No renal disease	0.99	+1.42
PAD	1.56	+0.1
No PAD	1.03	—

Table 3
Tailored extended intensive antiplatelet therapy: the Dual Antiplatelet Therapy, Thrombolysis in Myocardial Infarction, and Patterns of Nonadherence to Antiplatelet Regimen in Stented Patients Risk Scores

DAPT Score Variable	Points	TIMI Risk Score Variable	Points	PARIS Thrombotic Risk Score Variable	Points	PARIS Bleeding Risk Score Variable	Points
Age		Age ≥75	1	Non-insulin-dependent diabetes mellitus (DM)	1	Age	
≥75	-2					50-59	1
65 to <75	-1			Insulin-dependent DM	3	60-69	2
<65	0					70-79	3
						≥80	4
Diabetes	1	CHF	1	Tn-negative ACS	1	BMI	
				Tn-positive ACS	2	<25 or ≥35 kg/m²	2
Cigarette smoking	1	Current smoking	1	Current smoking	1	Current smoking	2
Prior PCI or prior MI	1	Diabetes	1	CrCl <60 mL/min	1	Anemia	3
Congestive heart failure (CHF) or left ventricular ejection fraction <30%	2	Hypertension	2	Prior PCI	2	CrCl <60 mL/min	2
MI at presentation	1	Prior stroke	1	Prior CABG	2	Triple therapy at discharge	2
Paclitaxel-eluting stent	1	Peripheral artery disease	1				
Vein graft stent	2	Family history of coronary artery disease	2				
Stent diameter <3 mm	1	Prior coronary artery bypass graft (CABG)	1				
		Renal dysfunction (estimated glomerular filtration rate [eGFR] <60 mL/min/1.73 m²)	1				

DAPT Score	NNT with Thieno	TIMI Risk Score	PARIS Thrombotic Risk Score	NNT with Vorapaxar	PARIS Bleeding Risk Score
Low (<2)	153	Low (0–1)	Low (0–2)	145	Low (0–3)
High (≥2)	34	Intermediate (2–3)	Intermediate (3–4)	41	Intermediate (4–7)
		High (≥4)	High (≥5)	28	High (≥8)

(Data from Refs. [45–48])

thrombosis regardless of MI status at presentation (2.7% vs 6.0%, P<.001 any MI; 2.6% vs 5.2%, P = .002 no MI, P for interaction = 0.68).[46] Rates of GUSTO moderate or severe bleeding were 1.5% versus 1.1% for continued thienopyridine versus placebo among those with any MI (P = .24) and 2.2% versus 2.0% for those with no MI (P = .68; P for interaction = 0.59). Among patients with DAPT scores less than 2, in both groups, continued thienopyridine was associated with increased bleeding (3.2% vs 1.2%, P = .01; 2.9% vs 1.6%, P = .004, respectively, P for interaction = 0.38), and MI and stent thrombosis rates of 2.1% versus 3.2% (P = .17) and 1.5% versus 2.0% (P = .21), respectively (P for interaction = 0.76). The DAPT score represents an important step toward a decision tool for post-PCI patients. Some limitations include that it is not applicable to patients with prior MI managed medically, paclitaxel-eluting stents are not used commonly, and angiographic factors (eg, stent diameter, vein graft intervention) may not be easily knowable to clinicians in the outpatient setting more than a year after the procedure. In addition, the DAPT score must be validated in other prospective trials of long-term secondary prevention.

A second score that was derived primarily to predict ischemic risk in patients with prior MI is the TIMI Risk Score for Stable Ischemic Heart Disease. The score was derived in a population of 8200 placebo-treated stable patients a history of MI enrolled in TRA2P-TIMI 50 trial to predict CV death, recurrent MI, and ischemic stroke[47] (see Table 3). This score uses clinical variables such as age, congestive heart failure, smoking, diabetes, hypertension, prior stroke, peripheral arterial disease, family history of coronary artery disease, prior coronary artery bypass grafting, and renal function as estimated by glomerular filtration rate. In both the derivation and validation cohorts, the TIMI Risk Score showed a strong graded relationship with the rate of CV death, recurrent MI, and ischemic stroke. In patients eligible for clinical use, the addition of vorapaxar in those at intermediate (score 2–3) and high (score ≥4) risk resulted in a 2.4% and 3.6% ARR of CV death, recurrent MI, and ischemic stroke, translating into a NNT of 41 and 28 in the intermediate- and high-risk groups.[47] In addition and similar to the DAPT score, the greatest bleeding excess with vorapaxar appeared confined to lower ischemic risk patients resulting in an increasingly favorable net outcome with vorapaxar with increasing TIMI Risk Scores. Similarly, Baber and colleagues[48] developed and validated separate models to predict risks for out-of-hospital

thrombotic and bleeding events after PCI with DES using data from the PARIS registry (Patterns of Non-Adherence to Antiplatelet Regimen in Stented Patients) registry (see Table 3). Independent predictors of thrombotic events at 2 years included ACS, prior revascularization, diabetes, renal dysfunction and current smoking. On the other hand, older age, extremely high or low body mass index, prescribed anticoagulant therapy in addition to DAPT (triple therapy) at discharge, anemia, current smoking, and renal dysfunction were found to be associated with major bleeding.

SUMMARY

Several observational and randomized trial data sets have clearly demonstrated that a history of MI indicates an ongoing disease state characterized by long-term risk of spontaneous atherothrombotic events. This risk is for de novo spontaneous MI, ischemic stroke, and CV death; although in the era of better stent technology, very late stent complications are increasingly rare. Long-term intensive antiplatelet strategies reduce this ischemic risk at a cost of bleeding. Patient selection for application of intensive antiplatelet therapies requires thoughtful assessment of benefit and risk as well as consideration of patient preference. Long-term intensive antiplatelet therapy may be a reasonable therapeutic approach for patients who have not experienced adverse events during the first year of treatment after MI and are not at heightened risk of complication (eg, prior stroke/TIA). Emerging subgroup analyses continue to identify patient groups at further heightened ischemic risk that derive greater absolute benefit. Ultimately, risk tools such as the DAPT and TIMI Risk Scores may be the optimal mechanism to guide the physician to appropriately select patients who derive a net benefit from prolonged intensive antiplatelet therapy.

REFERENCES

1. Yusuf S, Zhao F, Mehta SR, et al. Effects of clopidogrel in addition to aspirin in patients with acute coronary syndromes without ST-segment elevation. N Engl J Med 2001;345:494–502.
2. Sabatine MS, Cannon CP, Gibson CM, et al. Addition of clopidogrel to aspirin and fibrinolytic therapy for myocardial infarction with ST-segment elevation. N Engl J Med 2005;352:1179–89.
3. Wiviott SD, Braunwald E, McCabe CH, et al. Prasugrel versus clopidogrel in patients with acute coronary syndromes. N Engl J Med 2007;357:2001–15.

4. Wallentin L, Becker RC, Budaj A, et al. Ticagrelor versus clopidogrel in patients with acute coronary syndromes. N Engl J Med 2009;361:1045–57.

5. Roffi M, Patrono C, Collet JP, et al. 2015 ESC guidelines for the management of acute coronary syndromes in patients presenting without persistent ST-segment elevation: task force for the management of acute coronary syndromes in patients presenting without persistent ST-segment elevation of the European Society of Cardiology (ESC). Eur Heart J 2016;37:267–315.

6. Steg PG, James SK, Atar D, et al. ESC guidelines for the management of acute myocardial infarction in patients presenting with ST-segment elevation. Eur Heart J 2012;33:2569–619.

7. Levine GN, Bates ER, Bittl JA, et al. 2016 ACC/AHA Guideline focused update on duration of dual antiplatelet therapy in patients with coronary artery disease: a report of the American College of Cardiology/American Heart Association task force on clinical practice guidelines. J Am Coll Cardiol 2016. [Epub ahead of print].

8. Bhatt DL, Eagle KA, Ohman EM, et al. Comparative determinants of 4-year cardiovascular event rates in stable outpatients at risk of or with atherothrombosis. JAMA 2010;304:1350–7.

9. Fox KA, Carruthers KF, Dunbar DR, et al. Underestimated and under-recognized: the late consequences of acute coronary syndrome (GRACE UK-Belgian study). Eur Heart J 2010;31:2755–64.

10. Jernberg T, Hasvold P, Henriksson M, et al. Cardiovascular risk in post-myocardial infarction patients: nationwide real world data demonstrate the importance of a long-term perspective. Eur Heart J 2015; 36:1163–70.

11. Magnani G, Bonaca MP, Braunwald E, et al. Efficacy and safety of vorapaxar as approved for clinical use in the United States. J Am Heart Assoc 2015;4: e001505.

12. Bonaca MP, Bhatt DL, Cohen M, et al. Long-term use of ticagrelor in patients with prior myocardial infarction. N Engl J Med 2015;372:1791–800.

13. Mauri L, Kereiakes DJ, Yeh RW, et al. Twelve or 30 months of dual antiplatelet therapy after drug-eluting stents. N Engl J Med 2014;371:2155–66.

14. Ault KA, Cannon CP, Mitchell J, et al. Platelet activation in patients after an acute coronary syndrome: results from the TIMI-12 trial. Thrombolysis in myocardial infarction. J Am Coll Cardiol 1999;33:634–9.

15. Scirica B, Morrow D, Antman E, et al. Timing and clinical setting of cardiovascular death or myocardial infarction following PCI for ACS—Observations from the TRITON-TIMI 38 trial. J Am Coll Cardiol 2012;59(13s1):E340.

16. Rapsomaniki E, Shah A, Perel P, et al. Prognostic models for stable coronary artery disease based on electronic health record cohort of 102 023 patients. Eur Heart J 2014;35:844–52.

17. Antithrombotic Trialists' (ATT) Collaboration, Baigent C, Blackwell L, Collins R, et al. Aspirin in the primary and secondary prevention of vascular disease: collaborative meta-analysis of individual participant data from randomised trials. Lancet 2009;373:1849–60.

18. Derry S, Loke YK. Risk of gastrointestinal haemorrhage with long term use of aspirin: meta-analysis. BMJ 2000;321:1183–7.

19. Yusuf S, Mehta SR, Zhao F, et al. Early and late effects of clopidogrel in patients with acute coronary syndromes. Circulation 2003;107:966–72.

20. Antman EM, Wiviott SD, Murphy SA, et al. Early and late benefits of prasugrel in patients with acute coronary syndromes undergoing percutaneous coronary intervention: a TRITON-TIMI 38 (trial to assess improvement in therapeutic outcomes by optimizing platelet inhibition with prasugrel-thrombolysis in myocardial infarction) analysis. J Am Coll Cardiol 2008;51:2028–33.

21. Scirica BM, Bonaca MP, Braunwald E, et al. Vorapaxar for secondary prevention of thrombotic events for patients with previous myocardial infarction: a prespecified subgroup analysis of the TRA 2 degrees P-TIMI 50 trial. Lancet 2012;380:1317–24.

22. Wiviott SD, White HD, Ohman EM, et al. Prasugrel versus clopidogrel for patients with unstable angina or non-ST-segment elevation myocardial infarction with or without angiography: a secondary, prespecified analysis of the TRILOGY ACS trial. Lancet 2013;382:605–13.

23. Bhatt DL, Fox KA, Hacke W, et al. Clopidogrel and aspirin versus aspirin alone for the prevention of atherothrombotic events. N Engl J Med 2006;354: 1706–17.

24. Berger PB, Bhatt DL, Fuster V, et al. Bleeding complications with dual antiplatelet therapy among patients with stable vascular disease or risk factors for vascular disease: results from the Clopidogrel for High Atherothrombotic Risk and Ischemic Stabilization, Management, and Avoidance (CHARISMA) trial. Circulation 2010;121:2575–83.

25. Bhatt DL, Flather MD, Hacke W, et al. Patients with prior myocardial infarction, stroke, or symptomatic peripheral arterial disease in the charisma trial. J Am Coll Cardiol 2007;49:1982–8.

26. Bonaca MP, Morrow DA. SCH 530348: a novel oral thrombin receptor antagonist. Future Cardiol 2009; 5:435–42.

27. Morrow DA, Braunwald E, Bonaca MP, et al. Vorapaxar in the secondary prevention of atherothrombotic events. N Engl J Med 2012;366:1404–13.

28. Morrow DA, Alberts MJ, Mohr JP, et al. Efficacy and safety of vorapaxar in patients with prior ischemic stroke. Stroke 2013;44:691–8.

29. Diener HC, Bogousslavsky J, Brass LM, et al. Aspirin and clopidogrel compared with clopidogrel alone after recent ischaemic stroke or transient ischaemic attack in high-risk patients (MATCH): randomised, double-blind, placebo-controlled trial. Lancet 2004;364:331–7.

30. Sacco RL, Diener HC, Yusuf S, et al. Aspirin and extended-release dipyridamole versus clopidogrel for recurrent stroke. N Engl J Med 2008;359:1238–51.

31. Benavente OR, Hart RG, McClure LA, et al. Effects of clopidogrel added to aspirin in patients with recent lacunar stroke. N Engl J Med 2012;367: 817–25.

32. Cavender MA, Scirica BM, Bonaca MP, et al. Vorapaxar in patients with diabetes mellitus and previous myocardial infarction: findings from the thrombin receptor antagonist in secondary prevention of atherothrombotic ischemic events-TIMI 50 trial. Circulation 2015;131:1047–53.

33. Bohula EA, Aylward PE, Bonaca MP, et al. Efficacy and safety of vorapaxar with and without a thienopyridine for secondary prevention in patients with previous myocardial infarction and no history of stroke or transient ischemic attack: results from TRA 2°P-TIMI 50. Circulation 2015;132:1871–9.

34. Yeh RW, Kereiakes DJ, Steg PG, et al. Benefits and risks of extended duration dual antiplatelet therapy after PCI in patients with and without acute myocardial infarction. J Am Coll Cardiol 2015;65:2211–21.

35. Bonaca MP, Bhatt DL, Ophuis TO, et al. Long-term tolerability of treatment with ticagrelor for the secondary prevention of major adverse cardiovascular events: a secondary analysis of the PEGASUS-TIMI 54 trial. JAMA Cardiol 2016;1:425–32.

36. Udell JA, Bonaca MP, Collet JP, et al. Long-term dual antiplatelet therapy for secondary prevention of cardiovascular events in the subgroup of patients with previous myocardial infarction: a collaborative meta-analysis of randomized trials. Eur Heart J 2016;37:390–9.

37. Patti G, Cavallari I. Extended duration dual antiplatelet therapy in patients with myocardial infarction: a study-level meta-analysis of controlled randomized trials. Am Heart J 2016;176:36–43.

38. Bonaca MP, Bhatt DL, Steg PG, et al. Ischaemic risk and efficacy of ticagrelor in relation to time from $P2Y_{12}$ inhibitor withdrawal in patients with prior myocardial infarction: Insights from PEGASUS-TIMI 54. Eur Heart J 2016;37:1133–42.

39. Bhatt DL, Bonaca MP, Bansilal S, et al. Reduction in ischemic events with ticagrelor in diabetic patients: from the PEGASUS-TIMI 54 trial. J Am Coll Cardiol 2016;67:2732–40.

40. Magnani G, Storey RF, Steg G, et al. Efficacy and safety of ticagrelor for long-term secondary prevention of atherothrombotic events in relation to renal function: insights from the PEGASUS-TIMI 54 trial. Eur Heart J 2016;37:400–8.

41. Bonaca MP, Gutierrez JA, Creager MA, et al. Acute limb ischemia and outcomes with vorapaxar in patients with peripheral artery disease: results from the trial to assess the effects of vorapaxar in preventing heart attack and stroke in patients with atherosclerosis-thrombolysis in myocardial infarction 50 (TRA2°P-TIMI 50). Circulation 2016; 133:997–1005.

42. Bonaca MP, Bhatt DL, Storey RF, et al. Efficacy and safety of ticagrelor as long-term secondary prevention in patients with peripheral artery disease and prior myocardial infarction. J Am Coll Cardiol 2016. http://dx.doi.org/10.1016/j.jacc.2016.03.524.

43. Bansilal S, Bonaca M, Cornel JH, et al. Efficacy and safety of ticagrelor for long-term secondary prevention of atherothrombotic events in patients with prior MI and multivessel coronary disease: insights for the PEGASUS-TIMI 54 trial. J Am Coll Cardiol 2016;67(13_S):2146.

44. Kosova EC, Bonaca MP, Dellborg M, et al. Vorapaxar in patients with coronary artery bypass grafting: findings from the TRA 2°P-TIMI 50 trial. Eur Heart J Acute Cardiovasc Care 2016. [Epub ahead of print].

45. Yeh RW, Secemsky EA, Kereiakes DJ, et al. Development and validation of a prediction rule for benefit and harm of dual antiplatelet therapy beyond 1 year after percutaneous coronary intervention. JAMA 2016;315:1735–49.

46. Kereiakes DJ, Yeh RW, Massaro JM, et al. DAPT score utility for risk prediction in patients with or without previous myocardial infarction. J Am Coll Cardiol 2016;67:2492–502.

47. Bohula EA, Bonaca MP, Aylward PE, et al. Development of a TIMI risk score for stable ischemic heart disease. Circulation 2015;132:A17338.

48. Baber U, Mehran R, Giustino G, et al. Coronary thrombosis and major bleeding after PCI with drug-eluting stents: risk scores from Paris. J Am Coll Cardiol 2016;67:2224–34.

Antithrombotic Therapy to Reduce Ischemic Events in Acute Coronary Syndromes Patients Undergoing Percutaneous Coronary Intervention

Freek W.A. Verheugt, MD, FESC

KEYWORDS

- Percutaneous coronary intervention • Acute coronary syndromes • Oral anticoagulation
- Parenteral anticoagulation • Oral antiplatelet therapy • Parenteral antiplatelet therapy

---

KEY POINTS

- Because coronary thrombosis plays a pivotal role in the pathogenesis in most patients with acute coronary syndromes (ACS), antithrombotic therapy is essential in the management of ACS in the short and long term.
- Antiplatelet therapy should be started almost immediately after diagnosis and continued for at least 1 year after invasive therapy.
- Parenteral anticoagulation is indicated during coronary intervention for ACS.
- Possibly at discharge, oral anticoagulation may have a role in secondary prevention.
- There are major trials running that are studying the long-term antithrombotic protection of patients who have undergone percutaneous coronary intervention for ACS.

Blood coagulation is pivotal in the pathogenesis of acute vascular disease as shown in a large number of clinical trials on the effectiveness of antiplatelet drugs in vascular disease.[1] Because recently formed thrombi are mainly composed of fibrin and aggregated platelets, vasoactive mediators such as thromboxane A_2 released from platelets may occlude arteries. It has therefore been suggested that antiplatelet drugs like aspirin may be active in the prevention of vascular disease. Indeed, in a retrospective study in patients treated with high-dose aspirin for rheumatoid arthritis, the drug seemed to reduce the incidence of myocardial infarction, angina pectoris, sudden death, and cerebral infarction.[2] In patients presenting with acute coronary syndromes (ACS), revascularization is recommended in most cases,[3–6] of which percutaneous coronary intervention (PCI) by far is the most common. The most frequent complication of PCI is myocardial infarction, which has prognostic consequences.[7] It can be effectively prevented by aspirin.[8] Further reductions can be achieved by the use of platelet P2Y12 blockers.[8,9] The combination of aspirin and platelet P2Y12 blockers, dual antiplatelet therapy (DAPT), has become crucial after stenting had been introduced in the PCI practice. Clopidogrel, prasugrel, and ticagrelor are the available P2Y12 blockers for PCI in ACS.[3–6] The strongest platelet inhibition can be applied by platelet glycoprotein (GP) IIb/IIIa receptor antagonists,[10–14] but their role seems to diminish since the introduction of DAPT.

Conflict of Interest: The author has received educational and research grants from Bayer HealthCare as well as honoraria for consultancies/presentations from The Medicines Company, Bayer HealthCare, AstraZeneca, and Eli Lilly.
Division of Cardiology, Onze Lieve Vrouwe Gasthuis (OLVG), Oosterpark 9, Amsterdam 1091 AC, Netherlands
E-mail address: f.w.a.verheugt@olvg.nl

In addition to antiplatelet therapy parenteral anticoagulation is important in the fight against thrombotic complications during PCI (Fig. 1, Tables 1–4). Unfractionated heparin is the most often used agent. Less common are low-molecular-weight heparin[15] and the recombinant thrombin blocker bivalirudin.[16,17]

NON-ST ELEVATION ACUTE CORONARY SYNDROME

In non-ST-elevation ACS (NSTE-ACS), coronary plaque rupture followed by thrombotic phenomena usually is the pathophysiologic basis. Therefore, NSTE-ACS patients are at increased risk for ongoing thrombosis and ischemia. To prevent these complications, antiplatelet and anticoagulation therapies are recommended for all patients with NSTE-ACS.[5,6]

As said, the most common complication is myocardial infarction, which can now be better detected by the high-sensitive troponin assays.[7] Embolization of atheromatous and/or thrombotic material in the area of the dilated lesion(s) is thought to be responsible for the infarction. Currently, stenting of the dilated vessels is standard practice, which introduces a second thrombotic risk: acute, subacute, or late stent thrombosis.[18]

Preprocedural Antithrombotic Therapy

With regard to antiplatelet therapy, treatment usually is started at first medical contact irrespective of a decision for an invasive strategy. When the latter is adopted, current guidelines recommend aspirin 200 mg chewed followed by 80 to 100 mg daily and possibly ticagrelor with loading dose of 180 mg followed by 90 mg twice a day (Box 1). There is no consensus as to whether DAPT should be started before coronary angiography.[5,6] Only for high-risk patients, GP IIb/IIIa blockers may be added to this regimen (see Box 1). Diabetes mellitus and ongoing ischemia are features of a high risk. The experience of the combination ticagrelor with GP IIb/IIIa blockers, however, is limited.

In patients in whom coronary surgery is anticipated, P2Y12 blockers may be withheld until coronary angiography. After PCI, prasugrel can then be used instead of ticagrelor.[5,6] A loading dose of 60 mg of prasugrel is necessary followed by 10 mg daily in patients less than the age of

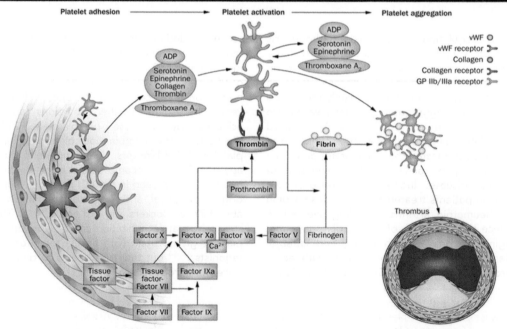

Fig. 1. Mechanisms of coronary thrombosis. ADP, adenosine 5′-diphosphate; vWF, von Willebrand factor. (*From* Franchi F, Angiolillo DJ. Novel antiplatelet agents in acute coronary syndrome. Nat Rev Cardiol 2015;12(1):30–47; with permission.)

| Table 1 |
| Recommendations for antiplatelet therapy with percutaneous coronary intervention in non-ST-elevation–acute coronary syndromes from European Society of Cardiology (A) and American College of Cardiology/American Heart Association (B) |

A

Recommendations	COR	LOE
Aspirin is recommended for all patients without contraindications at an initial oral loading dose[d] of 150–300 mg (in aspirin-naive patients) and a maintenance dose of 75–100 mg/d long term regardless of treatment strategy.	I	A
A P2Y$_{12}$ inhibitor is recommended, in addition to aspirin, for 12 mo unless there are contraindications such as excessive risk of bleeds.	I	A
Ticagrelor (180-mg loading dose, 90 mg twice daily) is recommended, in the absence of contraindications, for all patients at moderate to high risk of ischemic events (eg, elevated cardiac troponins). Regardless of initial treatment strategy and including those pretreated with clopidogrel (which should be discontinued when ticagrelor is started).	I	B
Prasugrel (60-mg loading dose, 10-mg daily dose) is recommended in patients who are proceeding to PCI if no contraindication.	I	B
Clopidogrel (300–600-mg loading dose, 75-mg daily dose) is recommended for patients who cannot receive ticagrelor or prasugrel or who require oral anticoagulation.	I	B
P2Y$_{12}$ inhibitor administration for a shorter duration of 3–6 mo after drug-eluting stent (DES) implantation may be considered in patients deemed at high bleeding risk.	IIb	A

B

Recommendations	Dosing and Special Considerations	COR	LOE
Aspirin			
Nonenteric-coated aspirin to *all* patients promptly after presentation	162 mg–325 mg	I	A
Aspirin maintenance dose continued indefinitely	81 mg/d–325 mg/d	I	A
P2Y$_{12}$ inhibitors			
Clopidogrel loading dose followed by daily maintenance 75-mg dose in patients unable to take aspirin	75 mg	I	B
P2Y$_{12}$ inhibitor, in addition to aspirin, for up to 12 mo for patients treated initially with either an early invasive or initial ischemia-guided strategy:	300-mg or 600-mg loading dose, then 75 mg/d	I	B
Clopidogrel			
Ticagrelor	180-mg loading dose, then 90 mg bid		
P2Y$_{12}$ inhibitor therapy (clopidogrel, prasugrel, or ticagrelor) continued for at least 12 mo in post-PCI patients treated with coronary stents	N/A	I	B
Ticagrelor in preference to clopidogrel for patients treated with an early invasive or ischemia-guided strategy	N/A	IIa	B
GP IIb/IIIa inhibitors			
GP IIb/IIIa inhibitor in patients treated with an early invasive strategy and DAPT with intermediate-/high-risk features (eg, positive troponin)	Preferred options are eptifibatide or tirofiban	IIb	B

Abbreviations: COR, class of recommendation; LOE, level of evidence.

Table 2
Recommendations for anticoagulant therapy with percutaneous coronary intervention in non-ST-elevation–acute coronary syndromes from European Society of Cardiology (A) and American College of Cardiology/American Heart Association (B)

A Recommendations		COR	LOE
Parenteral anticoagulation is recommended at the time of diagnosis according to both ischemic and bleeding risks.		I	B
Fondaparinux (2.5 mg SC daily) is recommended as having the most favorable efficacy-safety profile regardless of the management strategy.		I	B
Bivalirudin (0.75 mg/kg IV bolus, followed by 1.75 mg/kg/h for up to 4 h after the procedure) is recommended as an alternative to unfractionated heparin (UFH) plus GP IIb/IIIa inhibitors during PCI.		I	A
UFH 70–100 IU/kg IV (50–70 IU/kg if concomitant with GP IIb/IIIa inhibitors) is recommended in patients undergoing PCI who did not receive any anticoagulant.		I	B
In patients on fondaparinux (2.5 mg SC daily) undergoing PCI, a single IV bolus of UFH (70–85 IU/kg, or 50–60 IU/kg in the case of concomitant use of GP IIb/IIIa inhibitors) is recommended during the procedure.		I	B
Enoxaparin (1 mg/kg SC twice daily) or UFH is recommended when fondaparinux is not available.		I	B

B Recommendations	Dosing and Special Considerations	COR	LOE
SC enoxaparin for duration of hospitalization or until PCI is performed	• 1 mg/kg SC every 12 h (reduce dose to 1 mg/kg/d SC in patients with CrCl <30 mL/min) • Initial 30 mg IV loading dose in selected patents	I	A
Bivalirudin until diagnostic angiography or PCI is performed in patients with early invasive strategy only	• Loading dose 0.10 mg/kg loading dose followed by 0.25 mg/kg/h • Only provisional use of GP IIb/IIa inhibitor in patients also treated with DAPT	I	B
SC fondaparinux for the duration of hospitalization or until PCI is performed	2.5 mg SC daily	I	B
Administer additional anticoagulant with anti-IIa activity if PCI is performed while patient is on fondaparinux	N/A	I	B
IV UFH for 48 h or until PCI is performed	• Initial loading dose 60 II/kg (maximum 4000 IU) with initial infusion 12 IU/kg/h (maximum 1000 IU/h) • Adjusted to therapeutic activated partial thromboplastin time range	I	B
IV fibrinolytic treatment not recommended in patients with NSTE-ACS	N/A	III: Harm	A

Abbreviations: COR, class of recommendation; LOE, level of evidence.

75 years and 5 mg for the elderly. Also, here treatment for at least 1 year after NSTE-ACS is recommended.

Procedural Antithrombotic Therapy
Recently, the intravenous (IV) platelet P2Y12 blocker cangrelor has been approved in PCI patients. The drug has a very rapid onset and offset of action, which is preferable in ACS both in the acute phase and in case of urgent surgery or major bleeding. It has been shown to reduce early myocardial infarction in NSTE-ACS,[19] where it may be used in P2Y12 blocker-naive patients.[5]

Table 3
Recommendations for antiplatelet therapy with percutaneous coronary intervention in ST-elevation myocardial infarction from European Society of Cardiology (A) and American College of Cardiology/American Heart Association (B)

A	COR	LOE
Aspirin oral or IV (if unable to swallow) is recommended	I	B
An ADP-receptor blocker is recommended in addition to aspirin. Options are:	I	A
Prasugrel in clopidogrel-naive patients, if no history of prior stroke/transient ischemic attack (TIA), age <75 y	I	B
Ticagrelor	I	B
Clopidogrel, preferably when prasugrel or ticagrelor are either not available or contraindicated	I	C
GP IIb/IIIa inhibitors should be considered for bailout therapy if there is angiographic evidence of massive thrombus, slow or no-reflow, or a thrombotic complication.	IIa	C
Routine use of a GP IIb/IIIa inhibitor as an adjunct to primary PCI performed with unfractionated heparin may be considered in patients without contraindications.	IIb	B
Upstream use of a GP IIb/IIIa inhibitor (vs in-lab use) may be considered in high-risk patients undergoing transfer for primary PCI.	IIb	B
Options for GP IIb/IIIa inhibitors are (with LoE for each agent):		
Abciximab		A
Eptifibatide (with double bolus)		B
Tirofiban (with a high bolus dose)		B

B	COR	LOE
Aspirin		
162- to 325-mg load before procedure	I	B
81- to 325-mg daily maintenance dose (indefinite)	I	A
81 mg daily is the preferred maintenance dose	IIa	B
P2Y$_{12}$ inhibitors		
Loading doses		
Clopidogrel: 600 mg as early as possible or at time of PCI	I	B
Prasugrel: 60 mg as early as possible or at time of PCI	I	B
Ticagrelor: 180 mg as early as possible or at time of PCI	I	B
Maintenance doses and duration of therapy		
DES placed: Continue therapy for 1 y with:		
Clopidogrel: 75 mg daily	I	B
Prasugrel: 10 mg daily	I	B
Ticagrelor: 90 mg twice a day	I	B
BMS placed: Continue therapy for 1 y with:		
Clopidogrel: 75 mg daily	I	B
Prasugrel: 10 mg daily	I	B
Ticagrelor: 90 mg twice a day	I	B
DES placed:		
Clopidogrel, prasugrel, or ticagrelor continued beyond 1 y	IIb	C
Patients withSTEMI with prior stroke or TIA: prasugrel	III: Harm	B

(continued on next page)

B	COR	LOE
IV GP IIb/IIIa receptor antagonists In conjunction with UFH or bivalirudin in selected patients		
Abciximab: 0.25-mg/kg IV bolus, then 0.125 µg/kg/min (maximum 10 µg/min)	IIa	A
Tirofiban: (high-bolus dose): 25-µg/kg IV bolus, then 0.15 µg/kg/min	IIa	B
In patients with CrCl <30 mL/min, reduce infusion by 50%		
Eptifibatide: (double bolus): 180-µg/kg IV bolus, then 2 µg/kg/min; a second 180-µg/kg bolus is administered 10 min after the first bolus	IIa	B
In patients with CrCl <50 mL/min, reduce infusion by 50%		
Avoid in patients on hemodialysis		
Precatheterization laboratory administration of IV GP IIb/IIIa receptor antagonist	IIb	B
Intracoronary abciximab 0.25-mg/kg bolus	IIb	B

Abbreviations: COR, class of recommendation; LOE, level of evidence.

For anticoagulation, unfractionated heparin is given as an IV bolus either under activated clotting time (ACT) guidance in the range of 250 to 350 seconds (see Box 1) or 200 to 250 seconds if a GP IIb/IIIa inhibitor is given or in a weight-adjusted manner (usually 70–100 IU/kg, or 50–70 IU/kg in combination with a GP IIb/IIIa inhibitor). Heparin should be stopped after PCI unless

| Table 4 |
| Recommendations for anticoagulant therapy with percutaneous coronary intervention in ST-elevation myocardial infarction from European Society of Cardiology (A) and American College of Cardiology/American Heart Association (B) |

A	COR	LOE
An injectable anticoagulant must be used in primary PCL	I	C
Bivalirudin (with use of GP IIb/IIIa blocker restricted to bailout) is recommended over unfractionated heparin and a GP IIb/IIIa blocker	I	B
Enoxaparin (with or without routine GP IIb/IIIa blocker) may be preferred over unfractionated heparin	IIb	B
Unfractionated heparin with or without routine GP IIb/IIIa blocker must be used in patients not receiving bivalirudin or enoxaparin.	I	C
Fondaparinux is not recommended for primary PCI.	III	B
The use of fibrinolysis before planned primary PCI is not recommended.	III	A

B	COR	LOE
UFH:	I	C
With GP IIb/IIIa receptor antagonist planned: 50- to 70-U/kg IV bolus to achieve therapeutic ACT		
With no GP IIb/IIIa receptor antagonist planned: 70- to 100-U/kg bolus to achieve therapeutic ACT	I	C
Bivalirudin: 0.75-mg/kg IV bolus, then 1.75-mg/kg/h infusion with or without prior treatment with UFH. An additional bolus of 0.3 mg/kg can be given if needed.	I	B
Reduce infusion to 1 mg/kg/h with estimated CrCl <30 mL/min		
Preferred over UFH with GP IIb/IIIa receptor antagonist in patients at high risk of bleeding	IIa	B

Abbreviations: COR, class of recommendation; LOE, level of evidence.

> **Box 1**
> **Most common antithrombotic therapy around and after percutaneous coronary intervention for non-ST-elevation–acute coronary syndromes**
>
> *Anticoagulation*
> - Unfractionated heparin IV bolus 5000 U followed by infusion with a target ACT of 300 to 350 seconds
>
> *Antiplatelet therapy*
> - Aspirin 200 mg chewed followed by 80 to 100 mg daily lifelong
> - Ticagrelor 180 mg loading dose followed by 90 mg twice a day for 1 year
> - In post-PCI patients not pretreated with P2Y12 blockers: prasugrel 60-mg loading dose followed by 10 mg daily (5 mg in patients >75 years) for 1 year)
> - In high-risk patients or bailout: abciximab bolus 250 µg/kg loading dose followed by 0.125 µg/kg/min for 12 to 24 hours with a maximum of 10 µg/min. Reduce heparin dose to ACT 250 to 300 seconds
> - Or tirofiban bolus 25 µg/kg loading dose followed by 0.15 µg/kg/min for 12 to 24 hours. Reduce heparin dose to ACT 250 to 300 seconds
> - Or eptifibatide bolus 180 µg/kg followed by 2 µg/kg/min for 12 to 24 hours. Reduce heparin dose to ACT 250 to 300 seconds

there is an established indication related to the procedure or to the patient's condition. Alternatively, 3 anticoagulation schedules may be considered. First, the low-molecular-weight heparin enoxaparin 1 mg/kg twice a day can be continued subcutaneously as an anticoagulant in patients undergoing PCI. If the last dose was administered less than 8 hours before PCI, no additional anticoagulation is needed, whereas an additional 0.3 mg/kg IV bolus is recommended if the last enoxaparin dose was administered 8 hours or more before PCI. Second, if fondaparinux 2.5 mg every day is used as an anticoagulant in patients undergoing PCI, a single IV bolus of unfractionated heparin (70–85 IU/kg, or 50–60 IU/kg in the case of concomitant use of GP IIb/IIIa inhibitors) must be given in the catheterization laboratory.[5,6] Finally, in high-risk patients, the IV direct thrombin blocker bivalirudin may be administered in a dose of 0.75 mg/kg bolus, followed by 1.75 mg/kg/h for up to 4 hours after the procedure as an alternative to unfractionated heparin plus GP IIa/IIIa blockers.[5,6]

ST-ELEVATION ACUTE CORONARY SYNDROME

ACS with ST-elevation on the presenting electrocardiogram (ECG) usually is caused by an acute thrombotic occlusion of a major epicardial coronary artery resulting in myocardial infarction: ST-elevation myocardial infarction (STEMI). Most important is the establishment of timely reperfusion of the occluded artery for optimal salvage of the myocardium at risk. Either fibrinolytic

therapy, primary PCI with stenting, or both are suitable options and should be accompanied and followed by vigorous antithrombotic therapy. Given the urge of time, antithrombotic therapy must be started ahead of the reperfusion procedure.[20]

Preprocedural Antithrombotic Therapy
An aspirin loading dose together with a bolus of unfractionated heparin is given at first medical contact when the ECG shows ST-segment elevation (ambulance or emergency department). Whether P2Y12 blockade should be started then is still unclear.[21] The advantage is that an effective DAPT is initiated at the first possible moment; the disadvantage is the risk of excess bleeding when early coronary surgery is needed. Nevertheless, in randomized trials this risk seems acceptable.[22,23] Preprocedural administration of GP inhibitors is feasible, but is with the co-administration of heparin complex. It has not shown convincing clinical benefit.[24] The same holds true for the use of preprocedural alternative anticoagulation with bivalirudin[25] as well as for facilitation of primary PCI with fibrinolytic therapy.[26]

Procedural Antithrombotic Therapy
During PCI, aspirin must be given, if it has not been started before (Box 2). Because the oral P2Y12 blockers prasugrel and ticagrelor have a slow onset of action in STEMI,[27,28] cangrelor on top of aspirin is an attractive form of P2Y12 blockade,[19] because it has a very rapid onset of action as well as a rapid offset, which may be of use if urgent cardiac surgery is mandated.

Box 2
Most common antithrombotic therapy around and after percutaneous coronary intervention for ST-elevation myocardial infarction

Anticoagulation

- Unfractionated heparin IV bolus followed by infusion with a target ACT of 250 to 350 seconds

Antiplatelet therapy

- Aspirin 200 mg chewed followed by 80 to 100 mg daily lifelong
- A P2Y12 blocker (clopidogrel loading dose 300–600 mg followed by 75 mg for 1 year, or prasugrel 180 mg followed by 90 mg twice a day for 1 year, or prasugrel loading dose 60 mg followed by 10 mg or 5 mg in patients over 75 years) for 1 year
- In high-risk patients or bailout: abciximab bolus 250 µg/kg loading dose followed by infusion of 10 µg/kg/min with a maximum of 10 µg/min for 12 to 24 hours. Reduce heparin dose to ACT 250 to 300 seconds
- Or tirofiban bolus 25 µg/kg loading dose followed by 0.15 µg/kg/min for 12 to 24 hours. Reduce heparin dose to ACT 250 to 300 seconds
- Or eptifibatide bolus 180 µg/kg followed by 2 µg/kg/min for 12 to 24 hours. Reduce heparin dose to ACT to 250 to 300 seconds

---

Alternatively, GP IIb/IIIa inhibitors may be applied because of their faster onset of action,[29] but they have a slow offset of action, need prolonged infusion, and increase the bleeding risk considerably. They may be used though as a bailout in case of residual thrombus load.

Anticoagulation with unfractionated heparin should be administered at a target ACT of 250 to 350 seconds, or in the case of GP IIb/IIIa inhibitor use, a target ACT of 250 to 300 seconds must be applied. Heparin should be stopped after PCI unless there is an established indication related to the procedure or to the patient's condition.

ANTITHROMBOTIC THERAPY AFTER THE ACUTE PHASE OF ACUTE CORONARY SYNDROMES

Aspirin is the antiplatelet agent that must be given lifelong, whereas P2Y12 blockers are restricted for use of 1 year after ACS.[4] This regimen holds true for clopidogrel, prasugrel, and ticagrelor. There are data that DAPT prolongation beyond 1 year after ACS may be beneficial in terms of reinfarction and stroke,[30,31] but not mortality. Major bleeding is clearly increased with DAPT prolongation, and there is a signal to increased mortality.[32]

Oral anticoagulants should be considered only in patients with a clear indication like atrial fibrillation and/or mechanical heart valves. In many parts of the world, low-dose rivaroxaban in a dose of 2.5 mg has been approved for secondary prevention after ACS on top of DAPT with clopidogrel. It has been shown to reduce death[33] and stent thrombosis[34] when started at a mean of 4 days after ACS in stabilized patients.

FUTURE PERSPECTIVES

The medical and invasive management of ACS has significantly improved in the last decades.

Table 5
Trials of antiplatelet therapy in patients with acute coronary syndromes with or without aspirin

Trial	n	Experimental Arm	Control Arm	clinicaltrials.gov	Primary Endpoint
GlobalLeaders[36,a]	16,000	Ticagrelor	Ticagrelor Aspirin	01813435	Death or Q-wave MI
TWILIGHT[37]	9,000	Ticagrelor[b]	Ticagrelor Aspirin	02270242	Bleeding
GEMINI-ACS[38]	3,000	P2Y12 Rivaroxaban	P2Y12 Aspirin	02293395	Bleeding

[a] Also includes elective PCI where clopidogrel/aspirin is the control arm.
[b] With aspirin for the first 3 mo.

However, both the introduction of more potent antithrombotic therapy and the broad acceptance of an invasive strategy have increased the risk of major bleeding. Therefore, safer methods have been developed like radial access for PCI, and antithrombotic approaches like bivalirudin instead of heparin plus GP IIb/IIIa inhibitors. Alternatively, omitting older antiplatelet agents like aspirin in the antithrombotic cocktail seems attractive in the reduction of major bleeding after the first randomized trial in patients with atrial fibrillation undergoing PCI was published.[35] Currently, 3 large trials on long-term protection are evaluating such a strategy in ACS patients (Table 5).[36–38]

SUMMARY

Because coronary thrombosis plays a pivotal role in the pathogenesis in most ACS patients, antithrombotic therapy is essential in the management of ACS in the short and long term. Antiplatelet therapy should be started almost immediately after diagnosis and continued for at least 1 year after invasive therapy. In addition, parenteral anticoagulation is indicated during coronary intervention for ACS. Possibly, at discharge oral anticoagulation may have a role in secondary prevention. Finally, there are major trials running that are studying the long-term antithrombotic protection of patients who have undergone PCI for ACS.

REFERENCES

1. Antithrombotic Trialists' Collaboration. Collaborative meta-analysis of randomised trials of antiplatelet therapy for prevention of death, myocardial infarction, and stroke in high risk patients. BMJ 2002;324:71–86.
2. Linos A, Worthington JW, O'Fallon W, et al. Effect of aspirin on prevention of coronary and cerebrovascular disease in patients with rheumatoid arthritis. Mayo Clin Proc 1978;53:581–6.
3. Steg PG, James SK, Atar D, et al. ESC guidelines for the management of acute myocardial infarction in patients presenting with ST-segment elevation. Eur Heart J 2012;33:2569–619.
4. O'Gara PT, Kushner FD, Ascheim DD, et al. Guidelines for the management of ST-elevation myocardial infarction. Circulation 2013;127:e362–425.
5. Roffi M, Patrono C, Collet JP, et al. 2015 ESC guidelines for the management of acute coronary syndromes in patients presenting without persistent ST-segment elevation: task force for the management of acute coronary syndromes in patients presenting without persistent ST-segment elevation of the European Society of Cardiology (ESC). Eur Heart J 2016;37:267–315.
6. Amsterdam EA, Wenger NK, Brindis RG, et al. AHA/ACC guideline for the management of patients with non-ST elevation acute coronary syndromes: executive summary. Circulation 2014;130:2354–94.
7. Reichlin T, Schindler C, Drexler B, et al. One-hour rule-out and rule-in of acute myocardial infarction using high-sensitivity cardiac troponin T. Arch Intern Med 2012;172:1211–8.
8. Schwartz L, Bourassa MG, Lespérance J, et al. Aspirin and dipyridamole in the prevention of restenosis after percutaneous transluminal coronary angioplasty. N Engl J Med 1988;318:1714–9.
9. Bertrand ME, Legrand V, Boland J, et al. Randomized multicenter comparison of conventional anticoagulation versus antiplatelet therapy in unplanned and elective coronary stenting: the full anticoagulation versus aspirin and ticlopidine (FANTASTIC) study. Circulation 1998;98:1597–603.
10. Steinhubl SR, Berger PB, Mann JT, et al. Early and sustained dual oral antiplatelet therapy following percutaneous coronary intervention: a randomized controlled study. JAMA 2002;288:2411–20.
11. Use of a monoclonal antibody directed against the platelet glycoprotein IIb/IIIa receptor in high-risk coronary angioplasty. EPIC Investigation. N Engl J Med 1994;330:956–61.
12. RESTORE Investigators. The effects of platelet glycoprotein IIb/IIIa receptor blockade with tirofiban on adverse cardiac events in patients with stable angina or acute myocardial infarction undergoing coronary angioplasty. Circulation 1997;96:1445–53.
13. ESPRIT Investigators. Novel dosing regimen of eptifibatide in planned coronary stent implantation (ESPRIT): a randomised, placebo-controlled trial. Lancet 2000;356:2037–44.
14. Kastrati A, Mehilli J, Schühlen H, et al. A clinical trial of abciximab in elective percutaneous coronary intervention after pretreatment with clopidogrel. N Engl J Med 2004;350:232–8.
15. SYNERGY Trial Investigators. Enoxaparin versus unfractionated heparin in high-risk patients with non-ST-segment elevation acute coronary syndrome managed with an intended early invasive strategy. JAMA 2004;292:45–54.
16. Lincoff AM, Bittl JA, Harrington A, et al. Bivalirudin and provisional glycoprotein IIb/IIIa blockade compared with heparin and planned glycoprotein IIb/IIIa blockade during percutaneous coronary intervention: REPLACE-2 randomized trial. JAMA 2003;289:853–63.
17. Stone GW, McLaurin BT, Cox DA, et al. Bivalirudin for patients with acute coronary syndromes. N Engl J Med 2006;355:2203–16.

18. van Werkum JW, Heestermans AA, Zomer AC, et al. Predictors of coronary stent thrombosis: the Dutch Stent Thrombosis Registry. J Am Coll Cardiol 2009;53:1399–409.

19. Steg PG, Bhatt DL, Hamm CW, et al. Effect of cangrelor on periprocedural outcomes in percutaneous coronary interventions: a pooled analysis of patient-level data. Lancet 2013;382:1981–92.

20. Verheugt FW. Reperfusion therapy starts in the ambulance. Circulation 2006;113:2377–9.

21. Montalescot G, van 't Hof AW, Lapostolle F, et al. Prehospital ticagrelor in ST-segment elevation myocardial infarction. N Engl J Med 2014;371:1016–27.

22. Fox KA, Mehta SR, Peters RJG, et al. Benefits and risks of the combination of clopidogrel and aspirin in patients undergoing surgical revascularization for non-ST elevation acute coronary syndrome: the CURE trial. Circulation 2004;110:1202–8.

23. Held C, Asenblad N, Bassand JP, et al. Ticagrelor versus clopidogrel in patients with acute coronary syndromes undergoing coronary artery bypass surgery: results from the PLATO (platelet inhibition and patient outcomes) trial. J Am Coll Cardiol 2011;57:672–84.

24. Montalescot G, Borentain M, Payot L, et al. Early vs late administration of glycoprotein IIb/IIIa inhibitors in primary percutaneous coronary intervention of acute ST-segment elevation myocardial infarction: a meta-analysis. JAMA 2004;292:362–6.

25. Steg PG, van 't Hof A, Hamm CW, et al. Bivalirudin started during emergency transport for primary PCI. N Engl J Med 2013;369:2207–17.

26. Armstrong PW, Gershlick AH, Goldstein P, et al. Fibrinolysis or primary PCI in ST-segment elevation myocardial infarction. N Engl J Med 2013;368:1379–87.

27. Parodi G, Valenti R, Bellandi B, et al. Comparison of prasugrel and ticagrelor loading doses in ST-segment elevation myocardial infarction patients: RAPID (rapid activity of platelet inhibitor drugs) primary PCI study. J Am Coll Cardiol 2013;61:1601–6.

28. Alexopoulos D, Xanthopoulou I, Gkizas V, et al. Randomized assessment of ticagrelor versus prasugrel antiplatelet effects in patients with ST-segment-elevation myocardial infarction. Circ Cardiovasc Interv 2012;5:797–804.

29. Valgimigli M, Tebaldi M, Campo G, et al. Prasugrel versus tirofiban bolus with or without short post-bolus infusion with or without concomitant prasugrel administration in patients with myocardial infarction undergoing coronary stenting: the FABOLUS PRO (Facilitation through Aggrastat By drOpping or shortening Infusion Line in patients with ST-segment elevation myocardial infarction compared to or on top of PRasugrel given at loading dOse) trial. JACC Cardiovasc Interv 2012;5:268–77.

30. Mauri L, Kereiakes DJ, Yeh RW, et al. Twelve or 30 months of dual antiplatelet therapy after drug-eluting stents. N Engl J Med 2014;371:2155–66.

31. Bonaca MP, Bhatt DL, Cohen M, et al. Long-term use of ticagrelor in patients with prior myocardial infarction. N Engl J Med 2015;372:1791–800.

32. Navarese EP, Andreotti F, Schulze V, et al. Optimal duration of dual antiplatelet therapy after percutaneous coronary intervention with drug eluting stents: meta-analysis of randomised controlled trials. BMJ 2015;350:h1618.

33. Mega JL, Braunwald E, Wiviott SD, et al. Rivaroxaban in patients with a recent coronary syndrome. N Engl J Med 2012;366:9–19.

34. Verheugt FW. Combined antiplatelet and novel anticoagulant therapy after acute coronary syndrome: is three a crowd? Eur Heart J 2013;34:1618–20.

35. Dewilde WJ, Oirbans T, Verheugt FWA, et al. Use of clopidogrel with or without aspirin in patients taking oral anticoagulant therapy and undergoing percutaneous coronary intervention: an open-label, randomised controlled trial. Lancet 2013;381:1107–15.

36. Available at: www.clinicaltrials.gov/ct2/results?term=01813435&Search=Search. Accessed April 27, 2016.

37. Available at: www.clinicaltrials.gov/ct2/results?term=02270242&Search=Search. Accessed April 27, 2016.

38. Available at: www.clinicaltrials.gov/ct2/show/NCT02293395?term=gemini+rivaroxaban&rank=1. Accessed April 27, 2016.

Genetic Determinants of P2Y$_{12}$ Inhibitors and Clinical Implications

Larisa H. Cavallari, PharmD[a],[*],
Aniwaa Owusu Obeng, PharmD[b],[c]

KEYWORDS

- Clopidogrel • Prasugrel • Ticagrelor • Genotype • CYP2C19 • Pharmacogenomics

KEY POINTS

- There is significant interpatient variability in clopidogrel effectiveness in patients with an acute coronary syndrome and percutaneous coronary intervention (PCI).
- Clopidogrel is a prodrug that requires bioactivation, and cytochrome P450 (CYP) 2C19 is involved in both steps of the bioactivation process.
- Data consistently demonstrate reduced clopidogrel effectiveness after PCI in patients with the CYPC19 loss-of-function genotype.
- Neither prasugrel nor ticagrelor are affected by CYP2C19 genotype, and guidelines recommend consideration of one of these agents for PCI patients with the CYP2C19 LOF genotype.
- A number of institutions have implemented CYP2C19 genotyping for patients undergoing PCI to assist with antiplatelet selection.

INTRODUCTION

Clopidogrel is commonly prescribed in combination with aspirin for the prevention of ischemic events in patients with an acute coronary syndrome (ACS), whether managed medically or with percutaneous coronary intervention (PCI).[1,2] However, there is substantial interpatient response variability with clopidogrel. Contributions to this variability have been well-studied and include both clinical factors and genotype.[3–5] Prasugrel and ticagrelor are alternative agents shown to be superior to clopidogrel in clinical trials, but are associated with increased bleeding risk.[6,7] This review describes genetic contributions to variable response to platelet P2Y$_{12}$ inhibitors, guidelines for selecting antiplatelet therapy based on genotype, and examples of clinical implementation of genotype-guided antiplatelet therapy after PCI.

PHARMACOLOGY OF ADENOSINE DIPHOSPHATE ANTAGONISTS/P2Y$_{12}$ RECEPTOR INHIBITORS

Clopidogrel and prasugrel are thienopyridines that irreversibly bind to platelet P2Y$_{12}$ receptors, thereby inhibiting adenosine diphosphate (ADP)-mediated platelet activation and aggregation.

Disclosure Statement: The authors have nothing to disclose.
Funding Sources: Work by L.H. Cavallari is supported by NIH/NHGRI (U01 HG 007269). A.O. Obeng is supported in part by NIH/NHGRI (U01HG006380). The content is solely the responsibility of the authors and does not necessarily represent the official views of the NIH.
[a] Department of Pharmacotherapy and Translational Research, Center for Pharmacogenomics, University of Florida, 1333 Center Drive, PO Box 100486, Gainesville, FL 32610, USA; [b] Division of General Internal Medicine, Department of Medicine, The Charles Bronfman Institute for Personalized Medicine, Icahn School of Medicine at Mount Sinai, One Gustave L. Levy Place, New York, NY, USA; [c] Department of Pharmacy, The Mount Sinai Hospital, New York, NY, USA
* Corresponding author.
E-mail address: lcavallari@cop.ufl.edu

Both are administered as prodrugs that require hepatic bioactivation to their active moieties.[8] As shown in Fig. 1, a number of cytochrome P450 (CYP) enzymes are involved in the 2-step biotransformation of clopidogrel to its active compound (R1309641).[8,9] Notably, only 15% of ingested clopidogrel is converted into the active compound, and the remainder is inactivated by carboxyl esterases.[8,10]

A lack of uniformity in platelet inhibition after clopidogrel treatment has been observed, and patients with high on-treatment platelet reactivity tend to respond poorly to the drug, with an increased risk for major adverse cardiovascular events (MACE), including stent thrombosis.[11–14] Clopidogrel response variability has been attributed to factors such as age, body mass index, comedications, diabetes, renal failure, cardiac failure and most importantly loss-of-function (LOF) polymorphisms in the Cytochrome P450 2C19 (*CYP2C19*) gene.[3–5]

Prasugrel also undergoes hepatic bioactivation mediated by multiple enzymes, as shown in Fig. 2.[8] It has a more rapid onset of action and exhibits greater platelet inhibition than clopidogrel, with much less variability in response.[15] However, prasugrel is associated with an increased risk of major bleeding compared with clopidogrel, which has led to reduced dose (5 mg/d) recommendations for patients weighing 60 kg or less and those 75 years of age or older, who have excess formation of active metabolites.[15,16] Like clopidogrel, high on-treatment platelet reactivity has been reported with prasugrel, which confers

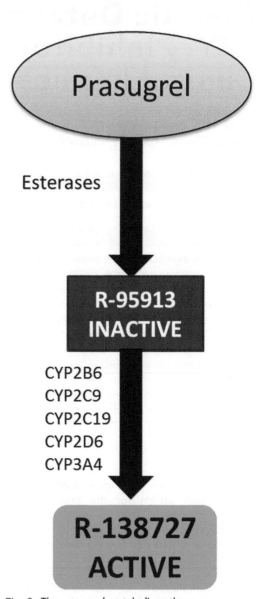

Fig. 2. The prasugrel metabolic pathway.

a greater risk of MACE after PCI.[17] Prasugrel is contraindicated in patients with pathologic bleeding or a history of transient ischemic attack or stroke.

Ticagrelor is a nonthienopyridine that reversibly binds the P2Y$_{12}$ receptor and does not require bioactivation. It has a quicker onset and offset of antiplatelet activity compared with clopidogrel, and this results in greater efficacy in terms of reduction in the risk for MACE in ACS patients.[7,18] Although risk for major bleeding is similar between ticagrelor and clopidogrel, ticagrelor is associated with an increased risk of noncoronary artery bypass graft related bleeding. Other adverse

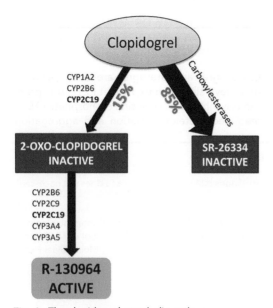

Fig. 1. The clopidogrel metabolic pathway.

events with ticagrelor include dyspnea, bradyarrhythmia, and minor spikes in serum creatinine and serum uric acid levels.[7,19,20] Ticagrelor is contraindicated in patients a history of intracranial hemorrhage, active bleeding, moderate to severe hepatic impairment, and any hypersensitivity reactions to ticagrelor.[20]

GENETIC DETERMINANTS OF CLOPIDOGREL RESPONSE
CYP2C19 Genotype

Polymorphisms in the CYP2C19 gene (specifically LOF variants) have been implicated consistently in clopidogrel response heterogeneity in both candidate gene and genome-wide association studies.[21–26] CYP2C19 or cytochrome P450, family 2, subfamily C, polypeptide 19, is located on chromosome 10 among a cluster of CYP genes including CYP2C18, CYP2C9, and CYP2C8.[27] Like many other cytochrome P450 genes, CYP2C19 possesses genetic polymorphisms that lead to variable hepatic expression, which in turn alters the function of the resultant protein (ie, CYP2C19 enzyme).

More than 30 CYP2C19 alleles have been identified (available from: http://www.cypalleles.ki.se/). The CYP2C19*1 allele represents a fully functional or normal activity allele. The most common LOF allele is the *2 allele (c.681 G > A; rs4244285), which occurs secondary to an aberrant splice site in exon 5 leading to a truncated protein.[27] The less common CYP2C19*3 (c.636 G > A; rs4986893) variation results in loss of enzyme activity secondary to premature termination of the amino acid sequence. CYP2C19*4 through *8 are LOF alleles observed in less than 1% of the general population.[27,28] Approximately 60% to 70% of

East Asians carry a LOF allele; the rate is lower (about 30%) in an ethnically and racially diverse population.[28,29] The CYP2C19*17 allele (c. -806C > T) occurs in the gene promoter region and results in enhanced enzymatic activity and is thus called a gain-of-function allele. Although several groups have observed greater clopidogrel-induced platelet inhibition and high bleeding risk in patients with a *17 allele compared with noncarriers, data are inconsistent.[22,30–32]

As shown in Table 1, CYP2C19 genotype confers 5 phenotypes:

- Normal (or extensive) metabolizers;
- Poor metabolizers (PMs);
- Intermediate metabolizers (IMs);
- Rapid metabolizers; and
- Ultra-rapid metabolizers.

The prevalence of CYP2C19 phenotypes by race is shown in Table 2. Consistent with having a higher frequency of LOF alleles, Asians have the highest prevalence of the PM and IM phenotypes.

CYP2C19 Genotype and Clopidogrel Pharmacokinetics and Pharmacodynamics

Carriers of a CYP2C19 LOF allele (ie, PMs and IMs) have diminished capacity to bioactive clopidogrel. A relative reduction of 32% in plasma concentrations of the active metabolite was reported in LOF carriers after clopidogrel exposure.[33] Consistent with this, LOF genotype is associated with high on-treatment platelet reactivity after PCI, which is an independent risk factor for MACE.[34] Therefore, it would follow that clopidogrel-treated LOF allele carriers may be at greater risk for MACE after PCI compared with noncarriers.

Table 1
CYP2C19 phenotypes derived from the CYP2C19 genotype

Genotype	Phenotype
*1/*1	Normal metabolizer
*2/*2, *2/*3, or other combination of 2 loss-of-function alleles	Poor metabolizer
*1/*2, *1/*3, *2/*17[a] or other genotypes with a single loss-of-function allele	Intermediate metabolizer
*1/*17	Rapid metabolizer
*17/*17	Ultrarapid metabolizer

[a] The IM phenotype assignment for genotypes with 1 loss-of-function and 1 gain-of-function allele (eg, *2/*17) is based on evidence of increased platelet aggregation among clopidogrel-treated patients with this genotype compared with the *1/*1 genotype, indicating that that the *17 allele is unable to completely compensate for reduced activity with the *2 allele.[29] However, the data are not completely consistent, and thus the intermediate metabolizer phenotype assignment is considered provisional.

Table 2 Prevalence of CYP2C19 phenotypes by race			
Race	Phenotype (%)		
	PMs	IMs	RMs or UMs
White	2	25	40
Black	4	30	45
Asian	14	50	<5

Abbreviations: IMs, intermediate metabolizers; PMs, poor metabolizers; RMs, rapid metabolizers; UMs, ultrarapid metabolizers.

CYP2C19 Genotype and Clinical Outcomes with Clopidogrel

In an early study of nearly 800 PCI patients, a 3-fold increase in the incidence of death and myocardial infarction at 1 year was observed in CYP2C19*2 allele carriers compared with the noncarriers.[21] This association was replicated in a number of subsequent studies.[22–25] In a meta-analysis including 9 studies and more than 9600 patients (54% with ACS and 91% with PCI), carriers of a LOF allele had an increased risk for MACE compared with noncarriers (hazard ratio, 1.57; 95% confidence interval [CI], 1.13–2.16).[35] The risk for stent thrombosis was even more marked, with a hazard ratio of 2.67 (95% CI, 1.69–4.22) in IMs and 3.97 (95% CI, 1.75–9.02) in PMs compared with non-LOF allele carriers.

The association between CYP2C19 genotype and adverse outcomes has not been demonstrated with all indications of clopidogrel. Specifically, among lower risk patients, such as those receiving clopidogrel for stable coronary disease, atrial fibrillation, or with ACS managed medically, no difference in clinical outcomes has been reported by genotype.[32,36] Similarly, a metaanalysis including studies of lower risk patients found only a modest association between genotype and clinical outcomes, which was abrogated when smaller studies were excluded.[37]

A more recent metaanalysis specifically aimed to assess outcomes among patients with and without PCI.[38] In non-PCI patients, no increased risk of cardiovascular events was apparent (relative risk, 0.99; 95% CI, 0.84–1.17). However, among those who underwent PCI, there were significantly more events among LOF allele carriers compared with non-carriers (relative risk, 1.20; 95% CI, 1.10–1.31). Overall, the data strongly and consistently support reduced clopidogrel effectiveness in carriers of a CYP2C19 LOF allele after ACS and PCI, but not in those at lower risk for adverse cardiovascular events.

Other Genes Associated with Clopidogrel Response

Other genes involved in the metabolic and pharmacodynamic pathways of clopidogrel have also been examined for their association with clopidogrel effectiveness. These include the ABCB1, CES1, CYP2B6, CYP2C9, CYP3A4, PON1, and P2Y12 genes.[22,39–43] However, none of these have been shown to contribute consistently to clopidogrel response heterogeneity. In a genome-wide association study conducted in healthy Amish volunteers given clopidogrel, only a cluster of polymorphisms on chromosome 10q24 in linkage disequilibrium with CYP2C19*2 reached genome-wide significance for its association with platelet aggregation, suggesting that no other gene has major contributions to clopidogrel response.[23]

THERAPEUTIC APPROACHES BASED ON CYP2C19 GENOTYPE

Clopidogrel Dose Escalation

Clopidogrel dose escalation as a means of compensating for reduced clopidogrel activation in the presence of a CYP2C19 LOF allele has been the subject of several studies. In healthy volunteers, a clopidogrel maintenance dose of 150 mg in IMs and 300 mg in PMs resulted in similar inhibition of ADP-induced platelet aggregation as a 75-mg dose in normal metabolizers.[44] However, among patients with coronary heart disease, a 300-mg dose failed to reduce platelet reactivity in PMs to a level achieved with a 75-mg dose in normal metabolizers.[45] In IMs, a dose of 225 mg in nondiabetics and 300 mg in diabetics resulted in desired on-treatment platelet reactivity.[46] Taken together, these data suggest that although adequate antiplatelet activity may be attained with tripling or quadrupling the dose in IMs, such an approach may not be effective in PMs. Use of alternative agents whose effects are not influenced by CYP2C19 genotype is a more viable option in IMs and PMs.

Alternative Antiplatelet Therapy

Unlike clopidogrel, the CYP2C19 genotype does not affect prasugrel pharmacokinetics or pharmacodynamics, despite being involved in prasugrel bioactivation.[22] This is likely because CYP2C19 has a minor role in the bioactivation of prasugrel compared with other enzymes involved.[47] Because ticagrelor does not require bioactivation, CYP450 enzymes do not influence the amount of drug initially entering the body.

Genetic substudies of large randomized controlled trials that compared the efficacy of clopidogrel with prasugrel or ticagrelor have been conducted.[48,49] In carriers of a *CYP2C19* LOF allele, both prasugrel and ticagrelor were shown to significantly reduce ischemic events compared with clopidogrel. However, prasugrel and clopidogrel were similarly effective in patients without a LOF allele.[49] Ticagrelor tended to remain superior to clopidogrel in the absence of the LOF genotype ($P = .06$).[48] The test for interaction between genotype and treatment group was not significant, leading the authors to conclude that ticagrelor is superior in reducing ischemic events compared with clopidogrel, regardless of genotype.

GUIDELINES FOR *CYP2C19* GENOTYPING WITH CLOPIDOGREL

In March 2010, the US Food and Drug Administration approved a revision to the clopidogrel labeling to add a boxed warning stating that[50]:

- The efficacy of clopidogrel is reduced in PMs with ACS or undergoing PCI;
- Tests are available to determine genotype for clinical purposes; and
- Alternative treatment strategies should be considered for PMs.

This followed 2 previous revisions to the label, the first of which added initial information about reduced clopidogrel response in PMs, and the second of which advised avoidance of clopidogrel in patients with decreased CYP2C19 enzyme activity secondary to LOF genotype or concomitant use of CYP2C19 inhibitors.

After the clopidogrel label revision, the American College of Cardiology Foundation and the American Heart Association issued guidance on the use of genetic testing to guide antiplatelet selection after PCI.[50] They state that the evidence base is insufficient to recommend routine genetic testing, citing a lack of data that routine testing improves outcomes. However, genetic testing may be considered before starting clopidogrel in patients at moderate to high risk for poor outcomes, such as those undergoing high-risk PCI procedures. For patients found to be PMs, then alternative therapy is recommended in the absence of contraindications.

The Clinical Pharmacogenetics Implementation Consortium (CPIC) also provides guidelines for clopidogrel use based on *CYP2C19* genotype.[29] The guidelines do not provide recommendations on whether or not to order a genetic test, but rather on how to interpret genetic test results and use them to optimize drug therapy. The clopidogrel guidelines were the second of 17 CPIC gene–drug pair guidelines available as of mid 2016, indicating the high level of evidence supporting *CYP2C19*-guided clopidogrel use relevant to genotype-guided therapy for other drugs. The recommendations are outlined in **Fig. 3**, with prasugrel or ticagrelor recommended after ACS and PCI in patients with a LOF allele.[29] The recommendations are graded as strong for PMs, meaning that the desirable effects clearly outweigh the undesirable effects, and moderate for IMs, meaning that there is close or uncertain balance between desirable and undesirable effects.

CLINICAL IMPLEMENTATION OF *CYP2C19* GENOTYPING
Examples of Clinical Implementation
A number of institutions have established a process for providing *CYP2C19* genotyping to help direct antiplatelet prescribing for patients undergoing PCI. Approaches vary from preemptive

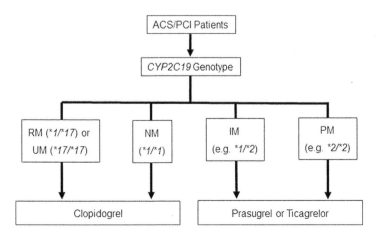

Fig. 3. Recommendations by the Clinical Pharmacogenetics Implementation Consortium (CPIC) for *CYP2C19*-guided antiplatelet therapy. ACS, acute coronary syndrome; IM, intermediate metabolizer; PCI, percutaneous coronary intervention; PM, poor metabolizer; RM, rapid metabolizer; UM, ultra-rapid metabolizer.

genetic testing in advance of patients needing dual antiplatelet therapy to reactive testing at the time of PCI when dual antiplatelet therapy is deemed necessary. For example, Vanderbilt University and the University of Maryland implemented CYP2C19 testing for patients scheduled to undergo left heart catheterization so that results would be available in the event that the patient proceeded to PCI.[51,52] At the University of Florida, the approach is more reactive, with the genotype test order defaulted on the post-PCI order set so that patients are automatically genotyped unless the physician chooses to unselect the order.[53]

Patient selection for genotyping also varies by site, with some sites broadly genotyping all patients undergoing left heart catheterization or PCI, as described. Other sites focus on high-risk patients. This is the approach at the University of North Carolina, where testing is recommended in PCI patients with high-risk anatomic findings.[54] Rather than being a defaulted order, genetic testing is actively ordered after angiography-guided risk stratification by the interventional cardiologist.

In the United States, genotyping must be performed in a Clinical Laboratory Improvement Amendments (CLIA)-certified laboratory for results to be entered into the electronic health record and used for clinical purposes. Recommendations for alternative antiplatelet therapy for patients with an LOF genotype may be provided to physicians via electronic decision support tools or through other forms of communication (eg, telephone call, secure email).[51–53] For example, at the University of Florida, an alert will pop up in the electronic health record in response to an order for clopidogrel for a patient with a LOF genotype, warning the clinician of potential reduced clopidogrel effectiveness and advising consideration of prasugrel or ticagrelor. Dosing information and contraindications for alternative agents are included in the alert to assist with the prescribing decision, and the physician may place the order for alternative therapy directly from the alert. Ultimately, the choice of antiplatelet therapy is left to the discretion of the physician. Recent preliminary data suggest that patients with an LOF allele who are switched to alternative therapy have a significant reduction in risk for MACE compared with LOF allele carriers continued on clopidogrel.[55]

Barriers to Clinical Implementation

Implementation of CYP2C19 testing requires overcoming a number of barriers. These barriers include establishing a process for genetic testing and the need to obtain genotype results before or soon after PCI. Ideally, a point-of-care platform would be available in the cardiac catheterization laboratory to rapidly provide genotype results. Although such a platform is available, placing it in the cardiac catheterization laboratory is inconsistent with quality standards in the United States, which requires that testing be done in a CLIA-licensed laboratory. Thus, a process must be established to transport samples efficiently to a CLIA-licensed laboratory for testing and efficient return of genotype results.

Another major barrier is the lack of data from large randomized clinical trials showing improved outcomes with genotype-guided clopidogrel use. Obviously, many sites feel that the available data linking CYP2C19 genotype to poor outcomes with clopidogrel are sufficient to support clinical implementation. However, others argue that implementation is premature in the absence of prospective clinical trial data. Although a clinical trial is currently underway, it is not expected to be completed until 2019 (ClinicalTrials.gov identifier: NCT01742117). In the meantime, it is anticipated that clinical outcome data will emerge from sites implementing genetic testing clinically, which may influence the landscape of clopidogrel pharmacogenetics.

The need for clinician preparedness to use genetic testing results is an additional barrier. Equipping clinicians with tools to translate genetic results into prescribing decisions at the time of care may be addressed through electronic decision support, as described at the University of Florida,[52] consultation with pharmacogenetic experts, or other means. Recognizing the knowledge and awareness barrier for pharmacogenetic testing, the National Institutes of Health and other stakeholders have also taken steps to better educate the clinician workforce on genomic medicine (Genetics/Genomics Competency Center [available from: http://g-2-c-2.org//]).

PHARMACOGENETICS OF PRASUGREL AND TICAGRELOR

Several investigators have examined associations between CYP450 genotypes and prasugrel response. One study reported overrepresentation of the CYP2C9*2 variant among individuals with a lower level of platelet inhibition with prasugrel,[56] whereas others have found no significant effect of CYP2C9, CYP2C19, CYP2B6, CYP3A4, or CYP1A2 genotypes on either prasugrel metabolite concentrations or antiplatelet effects.[22,41]

A genome-wide association study was conducted to identify associations with ticagrelor pharmacokinetics and clinical response.[57] A variant in the CYP3A4 gene was found to be associated with ticagrelor concentrations. Two additional polymorphisms, one in the SLCO1B1 gene, encoding for the organic anion transporter polypeptide, and another in UGT2B7, encoding for UDP-glucuronosyltransferase 2B7, were associated with concentrations of the major active metabolite of ticagrelor. However, effects were modest, and none of the polymorphisms were associated with reductions in ischemic events or risk for bleeding or dyspnea with ticagrelor.

SUMMARY

Data clearly and consistently demonstrate reduced clopidogrel effectiveness in preventing ischemic events after PCI in patients with a CYP2C19 LOF allele. Given the high prevalence of the LOF genotype, a substantial portion of the population is at risk for inadequate antiplatelet response to clopidogrel. The data have accumulated to the extent that an increasing number of institutions are beginning to offer CYP2C19 genotyping for patients undergoing PCI to assist with antiplatelet selection. Randomized controlled trial data, considered the gold standard evidence needed to broadly influence practice patterns, are forthcoming on the efficacy of genotype-guided antiplatelet therapy. In the meantime, efforts to implement CYP2C19 testing into practice to predict clopidogrel response will help to establish procedures for overcoming implementation barriers and may also provide useful "real-world" data on outcomes with pharmacogenetics testing to complement clinical trial findings.

REFERENCES

1. Sabatine MS, Cannon CP, Gibson CM, et al, Clopidogrel as Adjunctive Reperfusion Therapy -Thrombolysis in Myocardial Infarction I. Effect of clopidogrel pretreatment before percutaneous coronary intervention in patients with ST-elevation myocardial infarction treated with fibrinolytics: the PCI-CLARITY study. JAMA 2005;294:1224–32.

2. Mehta SR, Yusuf S, Peters RJ, et al, Clopidogrel in Unstable angina to prevent Recurrent Events trial I. Effects of pretreatment with clopidogrel and aspirin followed by long-term therapy in patients undergoing percutaneous coronary intervention: the PCI-CURE study. Lancet 2001;358: 527–33.

3. Khalil BM, Shahin MH, Solayman M, et al. Genetic and nongenetic factors affecting clopidogrel response in the Egyptian population. Clin Transl Sci 2016;9:23–8.

4. Cuisset T, Quilici J, Grosdidier C, et al. Comparison of platelet reactivity and clopidogrel response in patients </= 75 Years Versus > 75 years undergoing percutaneous coronary intervention for non-ST-segment elevation acute coronary syndrome. Am J Cardiol 2011;108:1411–6.

5. Hochholzer W, Trenk D, Fromm MF, et al. Impact of cytochrome P450 2C19 loss-of-function polymorphism and of major demographic characteristics on residual platelet function after loading and maintenance treatment with clopidogrel in patients undergoing elective coronary stent placement. J Am Coll Cardiol 2010;55:2427–34.

6. Wiviott SD, Braunwald E, McCabe CH, et al. Prasugrel versus clopidogrel in patients with acute coronary syndromes. N Engl J Med 2007;357:2001–15.

7. Wallentin L, Becker RC, Budaj A, et al. Ticagrelor versus clopidogrel in patients with acute coronary syndromes. N Engl J Med 2009;361:1045–57.

8. Laine M, Paganelli F, Bonello L. P2Y12-ADP receptor antagonists: days of future and past. World J Cardiol 2016;8:327–32.

9. Kazui M, Nishiya Y, Ishizuka T, et al. Identification of the human cytochrome P450 enzymes involved in the two oxidative steps in the bioactivation of clopidogrel to its pharmacologically active metabolite. Drug Metab Dispos 2010;38:92–9.

10. Karazniewicz-Lada M, Danielak D, Burchardt P, et al. Clinical pharmacokinetics of clopidogrel and its metabolites in patients with cardiovascular diseases. Clin Pharmacokinet 2014;53:155–64.

11. Gurbel PA, Bliden KP, Hiatt BL, et al. Clopidogrel for coronary stenting: response variability, drug resistance, and the effect of pretreatment platelet reactivity. Circulation 2003;107:2908–13.

12. Jaremo P, Lindahl TL, Fransson SG, et al. Individual variations of platelet inhibition after loading doses of clopidogrel. J Intern Med 2002;252:233–8.

13. Stone GW, Witzenbichler B, Weisz G, et al, ADAPT-DES Investigators. Platelet reactivity and clinical outcomes after coronary artery implantation of drug-eluting stents (ADAPT-DES): a prospective multicentre registry study. Lancet 2013;382:614–23.

14. Angiolillo DJ, Bernardo E, Sabate M, et al. Impact of platelet reactivity on cardiovascular outcomes in patients with type 2 diabetes mellitus and coronary artery disease. J Am Coll Cardiol 2007;50: 1541–7.

15. Wiviott SD, Trenk D, Frelinger AL, et al, PRINCIPLE-TIMI 44 Investigators. Prasugrel compared with high loading- and maintenance-dose clopidogrel in patients with planned percutaneous coronary intervention: the Prasugrel in comparison to

Clopidogrel for inhibition of platelet activation and aggregation-thrombolysis in myocardial infarction 44 trial. Circulation 2007;116:2923–32.

16. Roe MT, Goodman SG, Ohman EM, et al. Elderly patients with acute coronary syndromes managed without revascularization: insights into the safety of long-term dual antiplatelet therapy with reduced-dose prasugrel versus standard-dose clopidogrel. Circulation 2013;128:823–33.

17. Bonello L, Pansieri M, Mancini J, et al. High on-treatment platelet reactivity after prasugrel loading dose and cardiovascular events after percutaneous coronary intervention in acute coronary syndromes. J Am Coll Cardiol 2011;58:467–73.

18. Gurbel PA, Bliden KP, Butler K, et al. Randomized double-blind assessment of the ONSET and OFFSET of the antiplatelet effects of ticagrelor versus clopidogrel in patients with stable coronary artery disease: the ONSET/OFFSET study. Circulation 2009;120:2577–85.

19. Yousuf O, Bhatt DL. The evolution of antiplatelet therapy in cardiovascular disease. Nat Rev Cardiol 2011;8:547–59.

20. Htun WW, Steinhubl SR. Ticagrelor: the first novel reversible P2Y(12) inhibitor. Expert Opin Pharmacother 2013;14:237–45.

21. Trenk D, Hochholzer W, Fromm MF, et al. Cytochrome P450 2C19 681G>A polymorphism and high on-clopidogrel platelet reactivity associated with adverse 1-year clinical outcome of elective percutaneous coronary intervention with drug-eluting or bare-metal stents. J Am Coll Cardiol 2008;51:1925–34.

22. Mega JL, Close SL, Wiviott SD, et al. Cytochrome P450 genetic polymorphisms and the response to prasugrel: relationship to pharmacokinetic, pharmacodynamic, and clinical outcomes. Circulation 2009;119:2553–60.

23. Shuldiner AR, O'Connell JR, Bliden KP, et al. Association of cytochrome P450 2C19 genotype with the antiplatelet effect and clinical efficacy of clopidogrel therapy. JAMA 2009;302:849–57.

24. Sibbing D, Stegherr J, Latz W, et al. Cytochrome P450 2C19 loss-of-function polymorphism and stent thrombosis following percutaneous coronary intervention. Eur Heart J 2009;30:916–22.

25. Collet JP, Hulot JS, Pena A, et al. Cytochrome P450 2C19 polymorphism in young patients treated with clopidogrel after myocardial infarction: a cohort study. Lancet 2009;373:309–17.

26. Hulot JS, Bura A, Villard E, et al. Cytochrome P450 2C19 loss-of-function polymorphism is a major determinant of clopidogrel responsiveness in healthy subjects. Blood 2006;108:2244–7.

27. Scott SA, Sangkuhl K, Shuldiner AR, et al. PharmGKB summary: very important pharmacogene information for cytochrome P450, family 2, subfamily C, polypeptide 19. Pharmacogenet Genomics 2012;22:159–65.

28. Jeong YH, Bliden KP, Park Y, et al. Pharmacogenetic guidance for antiplatelet treatment. Lancet 2012;380:725 [author reply: 725–6].

29. Scott SA, Sangkuhl K, Stein CM, et al, Clinical Pharmacogenetics Implementation Consortium. Clinical Pharmacogenetics Implementation Consortium guidelines for CYP2C19 genotype and clopidogrel therapy: 2013 update. Clin Pharmacol Ther 2013;94:317–23.

30. Sibbing D, Gebhard D, Koch W, et al. Isolated and interactive impact of common CYP2C19 genetic variants on the antiplatelet effect of chronic clopidogrel therapy. J Thromb Haemost 2010;8:1685–93.

31. Tiroch KA, Sibbing D, Koch W, et al. Protective effect of the CYP2C19 *17 polymorphism with increased activation of clopidogrel on cardiovascular events. Am Heart J 2010;160:506–12.

32. Pare G, Mehta SR, Yusuf S, et al. Effects of CYP2C19 genotype on outcomes of clopidogrel treatment. N Engl J Med 2010;363:1704–14.

33. Mega JL, Close SL, Wiviott SD, et al. Cytochrome p-450 polymorphisms and response to clopidogrel. N Engl J Med 2009;360:354–62.

34. Palmerini T, Calabro P, Piscione F, et al. Impact of gene polymorphisms, platelet reactivity, and the SYNTAX score on 1-year clinical outcomes in patients with non-ST-segment elevation acute coronary syndrome undergoing percutaneous coronary intervention: the GEPRESS study. JACC Cardiovasc Interv 2014;7:1117–27.

35. Mega JL, Simon T, Collet JP, et al. Reduced-function CYP2C19 genotype and risk of adverse clinical outcomes among patients treated with clopidogrel predominantly for PCI: a meta-analysis. JAMA 2010;304:1821–30.

36. Doll JA, Neely ML, Roe MT, et al, TRILOGY ACS Investigators. Impact of CYP2C19 metabolizer status on patients with ACS treated with prasugrel versus clopidogrel. J Am Coll Cardiol 2016;67:936–47.

37. Holmes MV, Perel P, Shah T, et al. CYP2C19 genotype, clopidogrel metabolism, platelet function, and cardiovascular events: a systematic review and meta-analysis. JAMA 2011;306:2704–14.

38. Sorich MJ, Rowland A, McKinnon RA, et al. CYP2C19 genotype has a greater effect on adverse cardiovascular outcomes following percutaneous coronary intervention and in Asian populations treated with clopidogrel: a meta-analysis. Circ Cardiovasc Genet 2014;7:895–902.

39. Mega JL, Close SL, Wiviott SD, et al. Genetic variants in ABCB1 and CYP2C19 and cardiovascular outcomes after treatment with clopidogrel and prasugrel in the TRITON-TIMI 38 trial: a pharmacogenetic analysis. Lancet 2010;376:1312–9.

40. Lewis JP, Horenstein RB, Ryan K, et al. The functional G143E variant of carboxylesterase 1 is associated with increased clopidogrel active metabolite levels and greater clopidogrel response. Pharmacogenet Genomics 2013;23:1–8.

41. Brandt JT, Close SL, Iturria SJ, et al. Common polymorphisms of CYP2C19 and CYP2C9 affect the pharmacokinetic and pharmacodynamic response to clopidogrel but not prasugrel. J Thromb Haemost 2007;5:2429–36.

42. Harmsze A, van Werkum JW, Bouman HJ, et al. Besides CYP2C19*2, the variant allele CYP2C9*3 is associated with higher on-clopidogrel platelet reactivity in patients on dual antiplatelet therapy undergoing elective coronary stent implantation. Pharmacogenet Genomics 2010;20:18–25.

43. Malek LA, Kisiel B, Spiewak M, et al. Coexisting polymorphisms of P2Y12 and CYP2C19 genes as a risk factor for persistent platelet activation with clopidogrel. Circ J 2008;72:1165–9.

44. Horenstein RB, Madabushi R, Zineh I, et al. Effectiveness of clopidogrel dose escalation to normalize active metabolite exposure and antiplatelet effects in CYP2C19 poor metabolizers. J Clin Pharmacol 2014;54:865–73.

45. Mega JL, Hochholzer W, Frelinger AL 3rd, et al. Dosing clopidogrel based on CYP2C19 genotype and the effect on platelet reactivity in patients with stable cardiovascular disease. JAMA 2011; 306:2221–8.

46. Carreras ET, Hochholzer W, Frelinger AL, et al. Diabetes mellitus, CYP2C19 genotype, and response to escalating doses of clopidogrel. Insights form the ELEVATE-TIMIT 56 Trial. Thromb Haemost 2016;116:69–77.

47. Rehmel JL, Eckstein JA, Farid NA, et al. Interactions of two major metabolites of prasugrel, a thienopyridine antiplatelet agent, with the cytochromes P450. Drug Metab Dispos 2006;34:600–7.

48. Wallentin L, James S, Storey RF, et al, PLATO investigators. Effect of CYP2C19 and ABCB1 single nucleotide polymorphisms on outcomes of treatment with ticagrelor versus clopidogrel for acute coronary syndromes: a genetic substudy of the PLATO trial. Lancet 2010;376:1320–8.

49. Sorich MJ, Vitry A, Ward MB, et al. Prasugrel vs. clopidogrel for cytochrome P450 2C19-genotyped subgroups: integration of the TRITON-TIMI 38 trial data. J Thromb Haemost 2010;8: 1678–84.

50. Society for Cardiovascular Angiography and Interventions, Society of Thoracic Surgeons, Writing Committee Members, et al. ACCF/AHA Clopidogrel clinical alert: approaches to the FDA "boxed warning": a report of the American College of Cardiology Foundation Task Force on clinical expert consensus documents and the American Heart Association. Circulation 2010;122:537–57.

51. Peterson JF, Field JR, Unertl K, et al. Physician response to implementation of genotype-tailored antiplatelet therapy. Clin Pharmacol Ther 2016; 100(1):67–74.

52. Shuldiner AR, Palmer K, Pakyz RE, et al. Implementation of pharmacogenetics: the University of Maryland Personalized Anti-platelet Pharmacogenetics Program. Am J Med Genet C Semin Med Genet 2014;166C:76–84.

53. Weitzel KW, Elsey AR, Langaee TY, et al. Clinical pharmacogenetics implementation: approaches, successes, and challenges. Am J Med Genet C Semin Med Genet 2014;166C:56–67.

54. Lee JA, Lee CR, Reed BN, et al. Implementation and evaluation of a CYP2C19 genotype-guided antiplatelet therapy algorithm in high-risk coronary artery disease patients. Pharmacogenomics 2015; 16:303–13.

55. Cavallari LH, Magvanjav O, Anderson RD, et al. Clinical implementation of CYP2C19 genotype guided antiplatelet therapy reduces cardiovascular events after PCI. Circulation 2015;132: A11802.

56. Franken CC, Kaiser AF, Kruger JC, et al. Cytochrome P450 2B6 and 2C9 genotype polymorphism–a possible cause of prasugrel low responsiveness. Thromb Haemost 2013;110: 131–40.

57. Varenhorst C, Eriksson N, Johansson A, et al, PLATO Investigators. Effect of genetic variations on ticagrelor plasma levels and clinical outcomes. Eur Heart J 2015;36:1901–12.

Current Role of Platelet Function Testing in Percutaneous Coronary Intervention and Coronary Artery Bypass Grafting

Lisa Gross, MD[a],
Dirk Sibbing, MD, MHBA, FESC[a,b],*

KEYWORDS

- Platelet function testing • Platelet reactivity • PCI • Risk prediction
- Tailored antiplatelet therapy • Guidance of treatment • CABG • Transfusion algorithm

---

KEY POINTS

- There is substantial evidence for the value of $P2Y_{12}$ receptor-directed platelet function testing for the prediction of thrombotic events in patients having undergone percutaneous coronary interventions.
- There seems to be an "optimal" level of platelet reactivity during treatment with $P2Y_{12}$ inhibitors within which both thrombotic and bleeding complications are the lowest.
- The society of thoracic surgeons guidelines and the 2014 ESC/EACTS guidelines on myocardial revascularization provide a class IIa recommendation for the use of platelet function testing to time surgical procedures.

INTRODUCTION

Guidelines provide a class IA recommendation for the use of dual antiplatelet therapy in patients undergoing percutaneous coronary intervention (PCI).[1] However, multiple studies, mostly focusing on $P2Y_{12}$-receptor directed treatment, have shown that there is great inter-individual variability in the pharmacodynamic response to standard doses of antiplatelet medications.[2–6] Several studies have demonstrated a strong association between high on-treatment platelet reactivity (HPR) on clopidogrel therapy, reflecting a failure to achieve adequate platelet inhibition, and post-PCI ischemic events, such as stent thrombosis, myocardial infarction, or cardiovascular death.[2,4,7,8] Recently, evidence has also emerged supporting the association between low on-treatment platelet reactivity (LPR) and bleeding events.[8,9]

This review presents the current evidence regarding platelet function testing in patients undergoing PCI and coronary artery bypass grafting (CABG). The possible role of platelet function testing for individualized antiplatelet treatment regimens in high-risk PCI patients and for guidance of surgical timing and transfusion management algorithms in CABG patients will also be highlighted.

Disclosure Statement: D. Sibbing reports having received speaker fees and honoraria for consulting from Eli Lilly, MSD, Daiichi-Sankyo, Bayer Vital, AstraZeneca, Verum Diagnostica and Roche Diagnostics and research grants from Roche Diagnostics. L. Gross declares that she has no conflicts of interest.

[a] Department of Cardiology, Ludwig-Maximilians-Universität München (LMU Munich), Marchioninistr. 15, Munich 81377, Germany; [b] DZHK (German Center for Cardiovascular Research), Partner Site Munich Heart Alliance, Munich, Germany
* Corresponding author. Department of Cardiology, Ludwig-Maximilians-University, Marchioninistr. 15, Munich 81377, Germany.
E-mail address: dirk.sibbing@med.uni-muenchen.de

METHODS FOR PLATELET FUNCTION TESTING

There are numerous assays available for the assessment of the antiplatelet effect of $P2Y_{12}$ receptor blockers. There are pharmacodynamic assays measuring in vitro platelet reactivity that use different techniques, for example, platelet aggregometry (light transmission, impedance), flow cytometry, thromboelastography, or shear-dependent aggregation. Among the available methods, near-patient assays like the VerifyNow or the Multiplate analyzer are rapid, easy to perform, standardized, and highly reproducible. Table 1 summarizes the characteristics of the most commonly used platelet function testing assays in patients undergoing PCI and CABG as well as their key advantages and disadvantages. A detailed description on assessment methodology is beyond the scope of this review and is summarized elsewhere.[8,10]

PLATELET FUNCTION TESTING FOR PREDICTION OF ADVERSE EVENTS AFTER PERCUTANEOUS CORONARY INTERVENTION

There are numerous large prospective studies that provide significant evidence for the prognostic value of $P2Y_{12}$ receptor-directed platelet function testing for risk prediction of ischemic events after PCI (Table 2).[7,11–24] HPR as a marker of inadequate platelet inhibition by clopidogrel has been shown to be an independent and strong predictor of ischemic events after PCI (see Table 2).[9,12,15,20,25,26] A large and independent metaanalysis of 17 studies including overall more than 20,000 patients confirmed that thienopyridine-treated patients with HPR have a 2.7-fold higher risk for stent thrombosis (relative risk [RR], 2.73; 95% confidence interval [CI], 2.03–3.69; $P<.00001$) and a 1.5-fold higher risk for overall mortality ($P<.05$) compared with those with optimal platelet reactivity (OPR) after PCI.[9] Importantly, consensus cutoff values[8,27] for standardized platelet function tests (VerifyNow, Multiplate, vasodilator-stimulated phosphoprotein phosphorylation) have been established to allow for risk stratification regarding ischemic events[8] (Fig. 1). Small observational studies suggest that HPR is largely, but not completely, eliminated by the new $P2Y_{12}$ inhibitors prasugrel and ticagrelor compared with clopidogrel,[28–30] suggesting a less pronounced clinical importance for platelet function testing to identify HPR in patients treated with novel potent antiplatelet agents.

Although the relationship between platelet reactivity and ischemic events has been well-established, the link between platelet reactivity and bleeding events has emerged more recently. Several observational studies provide support for the existence of an association between enhanced platelet reactivity and bleeding risk (see Table 2).[12,15,29,31–38] The metaanalysis including 20,839 patients mentioned confirmed that patients with LPR have a significantly higher risk of bleeding in contrast with those with OPR (RR, 1.74; 95% CI, 1.47–2.06; $P<.00001$).[9] This relative risk increase translates into an absolute increase in major bleeding events of 2.6% in the LPR group (Fig. 2), suggesting that platelet function testing can identify patients at high risk of significant bleeding. Uniform cutoff values for LPR for risk stratification of significant bleeding events have been defined for the standardized platelet function assays[8] (see Fig. 1).

THERAPEUTIC WINDOW FOR PLATELET REACTIVITY AFTER PERCUTANEOUS CORONARY INTERVENTION

Because bleeding events after PCI are associated with worse outcomes, in the era of new and more potent antiplatelet medications, there is heightened importance to achieve maximum ischemic benefit while avoiding excessive bleeding. In this regard, evidence is accumulating that an OPR flanked by LPR and HPR cutoffs does indeed exist, within which the rates of both thrombotic and bleeding complications are the lowest.[3,14,17,18,29,39] Such a therapeutic window was first identified in an observational study including 2533 clopidogrel-treated patients undergoing PCI.[3] The metaanalysis introduced and summarizing all relevant studies in this field of research confirmed the existence of a therapeutic window and an OPR range for $P2Y_{12}$ treatment.[9] For this analysis, consensus-defined, uniform cutoff values for standardized platelet function assays were applied. LPR–OPR–HPR categories were defined as less than 95, 95 to 208, and greater than 208 P2Y12 reaction units for VerifyNow, less than 19, 19 to 46, greater than 46 units for the Multiplate analyzer (ADPtest), and less than 16, 16 to 50, and greater than 50% for vasodilator-stimulated phosphoprotein phosphorylation assay (see Fig. 1). When platelet reactivity levels were grouped only as low or high, the results suggested that a significant reduction in stent thrombosis in the non-HPR group could only be achieved at the price of a large increase in bleeding, and vice versa. However, when an

Table 1
Platelet function testing devices

Test	Medium	Method	Advantages	Limitations
VerifyNow P2Y$_{12}$	Whole blood	Light transmission	Easy to perform Rapid Standardized procedure Near-patient method Fully automated Small required sample volume	Very expensive Nonflexible Limited platelet count range Results affected by hematocrit level
VASP	Whole blood	Flow cytometry to quantify VASP phosphorylation	Longer sample storage possible P2Y$_{12}$ receptor specific Allows assessment of P2Y$_{12}$ receptor inhibition while on treatment with GPIIb/IIIa inhibitors High reproducibility in experienced hands	Time consuming Complex sample preparation Requires flow cytometry equipment Need for experienced technician
Multiplate electrode aggrometry	Whole blood	Electrical impedance	Easy to perform Rapid Standardized procedure No sample processing Different platelet pathways investigated Near-patient method Dual measurement as an internal control Good reproducibility Small required sample volume	Semiautomated Limited platelet count range
Light transmission aggregometry	Platelet-rich plasma	Light transmission	Instrument adjustment possible Long experience, well-studied Flexible Different platelet pathways investigated	Limited standardization Time consuming Complex sample preparation Variable reproducibility Large sample volumes required
Platelet function analyzer PFA-100	Whole blood	Closure time: time for platelet plug to stop blood flow across aperture	Easy to perform Rapid Standardized procedure Near-patient method	Rigid closed system Dependent on hematocrit, platelet count, and von Willebrand factor Limited experience and study results with P2Y$_{12}$ inhibitors Not sensitive to platelet secretion defects
Thrombelastography (platelet mapping)	Whole blood	Tensile strength of clot	Global hemostasis test	Expensive Complex and time consuming Low standardization Limited experience
Rotational thromboelastometry	Whole blood	Platelet contribution to clot strength	Whole blood assay	Not approved in the United States

Abbreviation: VASP, vasodilator stimulatory protein assay.

Table 2
Studies on platelet reactivity and outcomes for P2Y$_{12}$ inhibitors in PCI patients

Study	PCI Indication	No. of Patients	Platelet Function Test	Follow-Up	Outcome
			Studies on HPR and Ischemic Events		
Bonello et al,[11] 2007	Stable CAD, Unstable angina	144	VASP	6 mo	Increased rate of major adverse cardiovascular events
Breet et al,[12] 2010	Stable CAD, NSTE-ACS	1052	VerifyNow P2Y$_{12}$, LTA ADP	1 y	Increased rate of death, stent thrombosis, MI, stroke
Campo et al,[13] 2010	Stable CAD	468	VerifyNow P2Y$_{12}$	1 y	Increased rate of death, MI, stroke
Campo et al,[14] 2011	Stable CAD, NSTE-ACS	300	VerifyNow P2Y$_{12}$	1 y	Increased rate of death, MI, stroke
Cuisset et al,[15] 2009	NSTE-ACS	597	LTA ADP	30 d	Increased rate of stent thrombosis
Cuisset et al,[16] 2013	ACS	1542	VASP	6 mo	Increased rate of stent thrombosis
Gurbel et al,[17] 2010	Stable CAD	225	Thrombelastography ADP	3 y	Increased rate of composite endpoint (cardiac death, stent thrombosis, MI, stroke, unplanned revascularization)
Mangiacapra et al,[18] 2012	Stable CAD	732	VerifyNow P2Y$_{12}$	30 d	Increased rate of death, MI, TVR
Marcucci et al,[19] 2009	ACS	683	VerifyNow P2Y$_{12}$	1 y	Increased rate of CV death and nonfatal MI
Parodi et al,[20] 2011	ACS	1789	LTA ADP	2 y	Increased rate of cardiac death, MI, urgent revascularization, stroke
Price et al,[21] 2008	Stable CAD, NSTE-ACS	380	VerifyNow P2Y$_{12}$	6 mo	Increased rate of CV death, nonfatal MI, stent thrombosis
Price et al,[22] 2011	Stable CAD, NSTE-ACS	2796	VerifyNow P2Y$_{12}$	60 d	Increased rate of CV death, nonfatal MI, stent thrombosis
Sibbing et al,[7] 2009	Stable CAD, ACS	1608	Multiplate ADP	30 d	Increased rate of death and stent thrombosis
Sibbing et al,[23] 2012	Non–ST-segment elevation MI	564	Multiplate ADP	30 d	Increased rate of death, MI, urgent TVR
Stone et al,[24] 2013	Stable CAD, ACS	8449	VerifyNow P2Y$_{12}$	1 y	Increased rate of stent thrombosis and MI

Studies on Platelet Reactivity and Bleeding Events

Study	PCI Indication	No. of Patients	Platelet Function Test	Bleeding Criteria	Outcome
GRAVITAS Trial[31]	Stable CAD, NSTE-ACS	2214	VerifyNow P2Y$_{12}$	GUSTO	No association
ARCTIC Trial[32]	Stable CAD, NSTE-ACS	2440	VerifyNow P2Y$_{12}$	Major bleeding according to STEEPLE trial	No association
POPULAR Trial[12]	Stable CAD, NSTE-ACS	1052	VerifyNow P2Y$_{12}$, LTA ADP, PFA-100 Collagen/ADP	TIMI	No association
Bonello et al,[29] 2012	ACS	301	VASP	TIMI major and minor	VASP-PRI ≤16% associated with major bleeding
Cuisset et al,[64] 2009	NSTE-ACS	597	LTA ADP-induced aggregation, VASP	Non-CABG TIMI major and minor	<40% aggregation associated with higher risk of bleeding within 30 d after discharge
Michelson et al,[33] 2009	ACS	125	VASP	Hemorrhagic events >3 d after PCI	Lower platelet reactivity on prasugrel associated with bleeding
Mokhtar et al,[34] 2010	Stable CAD, ACS	346	VASP	In-hospital non-CABG-related TIMI major	Low platelet reactivity associated with bleeding
Parodi et al,[35] 2012	STEMI, Stent thrombosis, DES implantation in diabetics, left main coronary artery, patients with HPR on clopidogrel	298	LTA ADP	Entry side bleeding	Low platelet reactivity associated with bleeding
Patti et al,[36] 2011	Stable CAD	310	VerifyNow P2Y$_{12}$	TIMI major	≤189 PRU associated with bleeding
Sibbing et al,[37] 2010	Stable CAD	2533	Multiplate ADP	Procedure-related TIMI major	<188 AU associated with a 3.5-fold increase in bleeding
Tsukahara et al,[38] 2010	Stable CAD	184	LTA ADP	REPLACE 2	First quartile of ADP-induced aggregation associated with bleeding

Abbreviations: ACS, acute coronary syndrome; ADP, adenosine diphosphate; AU, arbitrary aggregation units; CABG, coronary artery bypass grafting; CAD, coronary artery disease; CV, cardiovascular; DES, drug eluting stent; GUSTO, Global Use of Strategies to Open Occluded Arteries; HPR, high on-treatment platelet reactivity; LTA, light transmission aggregometry; MI, myocardial infarction; NSTE-ACS, non–ST-segment elevation acute coronary syndrome; PCI, percutaneous coronary intervention; PRI, platelet reactivity index; PRU, P2Y$_{12}$ reaction units; REPLACE 2, Randomized Evaluations of PCI Linking Angiomax to Reduced Clinical Events Trial; STEEPLE, Safety and Efficacy of Enoxaparin in Percutaneous Coronary Intervention Patients trial; STEMI, ST-segment elevation myocardial infarction; TIMI, Thrombolysis in Myocardial Infarction; TVR, target vessel revascularization; VASP, vasodilator-stimulated phosphoprotein.

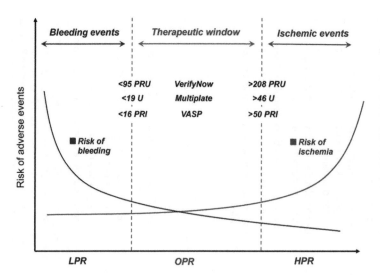

Fig. 1. The therapeutic window concept and summarizes the proposed cutoff values for different platelet function tests. HPR, high platelet reactivity; LPR, low platelet reactivity; OPR, optimal platelet reactivity; PRI, platelet reactivity index; PRU, P2Y$_{12}$ reaction units; U, units; VASP, vasodilator-stimulated phosphoprotein. (*Data from* Aradi D, Kirtane A, Bonello L, et al. Bleeding and stent thrombosis on P2Y12-inhibitors: collaborative analysis on the role of platelet reactivity for risk stratification after percutaneous coronary intervention. Eur Heart J 2015;36(27):1762–71.)

"optimal range of platelet reactivity" (OPR) was introduced, there was a large reduction in bleeding without any excess in stent thrombosis compared with LPR (see **Fig. 2**). These findings strengthen the importance of future randomized trials to test the benefit of tailoring treatment into this therapeutic window of platelet reactivity.

PLATELET FUNCTION TESTING FOR GUIDANCE OF TREATMENT IN PATIENTS UNDERGOING PERCUTANEOUS CORONARY INTERVENTION

Because there is significant evidence for the prognostic value of platelet function testing for risk prediction of both ischemic and bleeding events as well as mortality after PCI, a positive

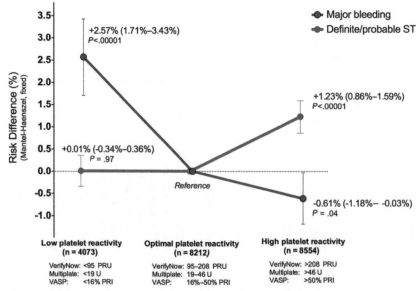

Fig. 2. Risk estimates when platelet reactivity is categorized as low, optimal, or high. HPR, high on-treatment platelet reactivity; LPR, low on-treatment platelet reactivity; OPR, optimal on-treatment platelet reactivity; PRI, platelet reactivity index; PRU, P2Y$_{12}$ reaction units; ST, stent thrombosis; U, units; VASP, vasodilator-stimulated phosphoprotein phosphorylation. (*From* Aradi D, Kirtane A, Bonello L, et al. Bleeding and stent thrombosis on P2Y12-inhibitors: collaborative analysis on the role of platelet reactivity for risk stratification after percutaneous coronary intervention. Eur Heart J 2015;36:1767; with permission.)

impact of treatment modifications based on platelet function testing seems reasonable. However, although a smaller randomized study[40] and some observational studies provided positive results,[41–43] the 3 large randomized clinical trials on the topic conducted so far (GRAVITAS [Gauging Responsiveness with a VerifyNow P2Y12 assay: Impact on Thrombosis and Safety],[31] TRIGGER-PCI [Testing Platelet Reactivity In Patients Undergoing Elective Stent Placement on Clopidogrel to Guide Alternative Therapy With Prasugrel],[44] and ARCTIC [Double Randomization of a Monitoring Adjusted Antiplatelet Treatment Versus a Common Antiplatelet Treatment for DES Implantation, and Interruption Versus Continuation of Double Antiplatelet Therapy][32]), were not been able to prove the value of platelet function testing for the guidance of treatment, because they detected no differences regarding hard clinical endpoints (for a summary of studies see Table 3). It should be acknowledged, however, that these 3 important randomized trials have limitations, such as the enrollment of mostly low-risk patients, which resulted in low event rates and lack of statistical power to detect differences in the primary endpoint, and the use of high-dose clopidogrel instead of the newer, more potent antiplatelet agents such as ticagrelor or prasugrel to overcome HPR on clopidogrel.

Thus, regarding the potential value of platelet function testing for guidance of treatment, there are several major knowledge gaps that need to be addressed in future studies. These include studies in patients with acute coronary syndrome and/or high-risk (eg, elderly) patients, studies evaluating the concept of a therapeutic window of platelet reactivity, large-scale randomized trials using standardized assays other than the VerifyNow device, and studies that investigate the approach of antiplatelet treatment deescalation with intensive platelet inhibition during the acute phase of acute coronary syndrome and moderate levels during chronic treatment.

The ongoing TROPICAL-ACS (Testing Responsiveness to Platelet Inhibition on Chronic Antiplatelet Treatment for Acute Coronary Syndromes, NCT01959451; see Table 3) trial aims at closing some of these knowledge gaps. Another important and on-going randomized trial, ANTARCTIC (Tailored Antiplatelet Therapy Versus Recommended Dose of Prasugrel, NCT01538446), will also provide important new insights into the role of platelet function testing for guidance of antiplatelet therapy, especially in elderly patients (see Table 3).

ROLE OF PLATELET FUNCTION TESTING IN PATIENTS UNDERGOING CORONARY ARTERY BYPASS GRAFTING

Bleeding after cardiac surgery accounts for approximately 20% of all hospital blood transfusions[45] and is associated with significant morbidity and mortality.[46] Thus, development of strategies to reduce blood loss after cardiac surgery is crucial. There have been numerous observational studies demonstrating that platelet function testing can help to predict bleeding complications and transfusion requirements in patients undergoing CABG (Table 4).[47–52] However, the available studies are heterogeneous in design, as are the respective bleeding definitions used, thereby limiting their comparability.[8] It has been suggested that platelet reactivity assessed by point-of-care (POC) platelet function testing might be a more reliable predictor of bleeding and transfusion risk than the arbitrary use of a specified surgical delay.[47] The TARGET-CABG (Timing Based on Platelet Function Strategy to Reduce Clopidogrel-Associated Bleeding Related to CABG) study (see Table 4) showed that a strategy based on preoperative thromboelastography platelet mapping to determine the timing of CABG in clopidogrel-treated patients was associated with the same amount of bleeding as observed in clopidogrel-naïve patients, despite an approximately 50% shorter waiting time than that recommended by current guidelines.[48] Based on these data and other evidence, the Society of Thoracic Surgeons Guidelines and the 2014 European Society of Cardiology/European Association for Cardio-Thoracic Surgery guidelines on myocardial revascularization provide a class IIa recommendation for timing of operation based on the determination of platelet inhibition.[1,53]

There have been several smaller randomized trials of platelet function testing as part of a blood transfusion management algorithm in cardiac surgery patients (see Table 4).[54–62] A recent metaanalysis involving overall 1057 patients demonstrated that POC platelet function testing was associated with a statistically significant reduction in bleeding.[63] There was a greater effect size for bleeding reduction in trials using thromboelastography/ROTEM in combination with other POC platelet function tests ($P = .0005$), compared with thromboelastography/ROTEM alone ($P = .02$; Fig. 3). POC platelet function testing was associated with a significant reduction in the proportion of patients receiving packed red blood cells (RR, 0.86; 95%

Table 3
Studies on platelet function testing for guidance of treatment for P2Y$_{12}$ inhibitors in PCI patients

Study	Platelet Function Test	PCI Indication	No. of Patients	Intervention in HPR Patients	Outcome PFT-Guided Group vs Control
				Published Studies	
GRAVITAS Trial[31]	VerifyNow P2Y$_{12}$	Stable CAD NSTE-ACS	2214	Randomization to 75 mg clopidogrel MD vs extra 600 mg LD + 150 mg MD clopidogrel	MACE: 2.3% vs 2.3% (HR, 1.01; 95% CI, 0.58–1.76) Severe or moderate bleeding: 1.4% vs 2.3% (HR, 0.59; 95% CI, 0.31–1.11)
ARCTIC Trial[32]	VerifyNow P2Y$_{12}$	Stable CAD NSTE-ACS	2440	At baseline: extra 600 mg LD + 150 mg MD clopidogrel or extra 60 mg LD + 10 mg MD prasugrel or GPIIb/IIIa inhibitors At 14–30 d: increase in clopidogrel MD (+75 mg) or switch to prasugrel MD	MACE: 34.6% vs 31.1% (HR, 1.13; 95% CI, 0.98–1.29) Stent thrombosis: 1.0 vs 0.7% (HR, 1.34; 95% CI, 0.56–3.18) Major bleeding: 2.3% vs 3.3% (HR, 0.70; 95% CI, 0.43–1.14)
MADONNA study[43]	Multiplate ADP	Stable CAD	798	Randomization to repeated extra 600 mg LD clopidogrel or repeated extra 60 mg LD prasugrel vs no change in treatment	Stent thrombosis: 0.2% vs 1.9%; P = .027 ACS: 0% vs 2.5%; P = .001 Cardiac death: 2% vs 1.3%; P = .422 Major bleeding: 1% vs 0.3%; P = .186
ISAR-HPR registry[42]	Multiplate ADP	Stable CAD	999	Reloading with 600 mg LD clopidogrel, switch to 10 mg MD prasugrel vs no treatment modification	Death from any cause or stent thrombosis: 7 (1.2%) vs 16 (3.7%) events (HR, 0.32; 95% CI, 0.13–0.79; P = .009) Major bleeding: 1.9 vs 0.7%; P = .10
PECS registry[41]	Multiplate ADP	ACS	219	Switch to 10 mg MD prasugrel or 150 mg MD clopidogrel vs 75 mg MD clopidogrel	MACE: Similar outcomes for prasugrel MD compared with non-HPR patients (HR, 0.90; 95% CI, 0.44–1.81; P = .76). Higher risk of thrombotic and bleeding complications with high-dose clopidogrel

Study	Platelet Function Test	PCI Indication		Strategy	
Bonello et al,[40] 2009	VASP	Stable CAD NSTE-ACS	429	Randomization to no extra LDs vs up to 3 extra 600 mg LDs clopidogrel to achieve a VASP-PRI <50%	MACE: 0.5% vs 8.9%; $P<.001$; Major bleeding: 0.9% vs 0.9%
Wang et al,[65] 2011	VASP	Stable CAD NSTE-ACS	306	Randomization to no adjustment vs PFT-guided increases in MD clopidogrel (+75 mg) at 3, 6, 9 mo	MACE: 9.3% vs 20.4%, $P = .008$; Major bleeding: 0 vs 0
EFFICIENT Trial[66]	VerifyNow P2Y$_{12}$	Stable CAD	94	Randomization to 75 mg vs 150 mg MD clopidogrel for 1 mo	MACE: 4.3% vs 17%, $P = .02$; Major bleeding: 2.1% vs 0%, $P>.05$
Hazarbasanov et al,[67] 2012	Multiplate ADP	Stable CAD ACS	192	Extra 600 mg LD + 150 mg MD clopidogrel for 1 mo	MACE: 0% vs 2.6%, $P = .03$; Stent thrombosis: 0% vs 2.1%, $P = .06$; Major bleeding: 1 vs 0 event

Ongoing Randomized Trials

Study	Platelet Function Test	PCI Indication	Strategy
ANTARCTIC Trial NCT01538446	VerifyNow P2Y$_{12}$	ACS >74 y	Randomization to PFT-guided down-/up-adjustment of the prasugrel MD in high/low responders vs fixed dose of 5 mg prasugrel
TROPICAL-ACS Trial NCT01959451	Multiplate ADP	Troponin-positive ACS	Randomization to a PFT-guided approach with a short-term (1 wk) prasugrel treatment and a switch-over to clopidogrel treatment in adequate responders to clopidogrel vs standard prasugrel therapy

Abbreviations: ACS, acute coronary syndrome; ADP, adenosine diphosphate; CAD, coronary artery disease; DAPT, dual antiplatelet therapy; HPR, high on-treatment platelet reactivity; LD, loading dose; MD, maintenance dose; NSTE-ACS, non-ST-segment elevation acute coronary syndrome; PFT, platelet function testing; PRI, platelet reactivity index; STEMI, ST-segment elevation acute coronary syndrome; VASP, vasodilator-stimulated phosphoprotein.

Table 4
Selected studies on platelet function testing in CABG patients

	No. of Patients	Patient Population	Observational Studies Platelet Function Assay	Timing of PFT	Key Findings
Kwak et al,[47] 2010	100	Off pump CABG patients on DAPT	TEG Platelet Mapping Assay	Preoperative	Platelet inhibition associated with postoperative transfusion requirement (P<.001)
Mahla et al,[48] 2012	180	CABG patients on/not on clopidogrel	TEG Platelet Mapping Assay	Preoperative	Similar perioperative bleeding as compared with clopidogrel-naïve patients and approximately 50% shorter waiting time than recommended
Schimmer et al,[49] 2013	223	Mixed cardiac surgery patients	Multiplate ADP/ASPI/TRAPtest	Preoperative and postoperative	ADPtest and TRAPtest predicted perioperative transfusion requirement
Ranucci et al,[50] 2014	435	Cardiac surgery patients exposed to P2Y$_{12}$ inhibitors	Multiplate ADP/TRAPtest	Preoperative	ADPtest and TRAPtest results associated with postoperative bleeding (P = .001)
Mannacio et al,[51] 2014	300	Off-pump CABG for ACS patients	PFA-100	Preoperative	Similar perioperative bleeding as compared with clopidogrel-naïve patients and shorter waiting time (3.6 ± 1.7 d) than recommended.
Reed et al,[52] 2015	39	CABG patients on clopidogrel	VerifyNowP2Y12	Preoperative	PRU ≤207 predicted major bleeding during surgery (P = .018)

	No. of Patients	Type of Procedure	Randomized Controlled Trials Platelet Function Test	Study Design	Key Findings
Shore-Lesserson et al,[54] 1999	105	High-risk cardiac surgery	TEG	Randomization to TEG-guided transfusion algorithm vs routine transfusion therapy	Fewer transfusions in the TEG group (P<.002 for FFP, P<.05 for platelets)
Royston et al,[55] 2001	60	High risk cardiac surgery	TEG	Randomization to TEG-guided transfusion algorithm vs routine transfusion therapy	Less transfusion in the guided group (P<.05)

Study	N	Procedure	Test	Study design	Results
Nuttall et al,[56] 2011	92	Mixed CABG + valvular heart surgery	TEG + Coaguchek Plus and Coulter-MD II	Randomization to a transfusion algorithm guided by coagulation tests vs routine transfusion therapy	Less transfusion in the guided group (P = .0002 for FFP, P = .0001 for platelets)
Avidan et al,[57] 2004	102	Elective CABG	TEG + PFA-100	Randomization to POC vs laboratory test group and comparison to retrospective group with management left to the clinician's discretion	Transfusion of PRBCs and blood components greater in the clinician discretion group (P<.05)
Ak et al,[58] 2009	224	Elective CABG	TEG	Randomization to TEG-guided group vs routine transfusion therapy	Significantly fewer units of FFP and platelets (P = .001) and total allogeneic units (P = .001) and diminished need for tranexamic acid in the TEG group (P = .007).
Westbrook et al,[59] 2009	69	Mixed cardiac procedures	TEG + platelet mapping	Randomization to strict TEG-guided protocol vs physician directed product administration with reference to APTT, INR, fibrinogen and platelet count	Reduction of total product usage by 58.8% in the study group, not statistically significant.
Girdauskas et al,[60] 2010	56	High-risk aortic surgery with deep hypothermic circulatory arrest	ROTEM	Randomization to ROTEM-guided algorithm vs routine transfusion practices (clinical judgment-guided transfusion followed by transfusion according to coagulation test results)	Transfusion significantly reduced (P = .02).
Weber et al,[61] 2012	100	Complex cardiac surgery	ROTEM + Multiplate	Randomization to POC (ROTEM + Multiplate-guided) group vs routine transfusion group	Lower erythrocyte transfusion rate for the POC group (P<.001)
Agarwal et al,[62] 2015	249	CABG	TEG + Multiplate and TEG + platelet mapping	Randomization to PFT preoperatively with multiple electrode aggregometry (A) vs TEG + platelet mapping (B) vs none (C)	Significant reduction in transfusion for A and B (P = .02). For A and B, significant cost saving (P = .006).

Abbreviations: APTT, activated partial thromboplastin time; CABG, coronary artery bypass grafting; FFP, fresh frozen plasma; ICU, intensive care unit; INR, International Normalized Ratio; PFT, platelet function testing; POC, point of care; PRBCs, packed red blood cells; ROTEM, rotational thromboelastometry; TEG, thromboelastography.

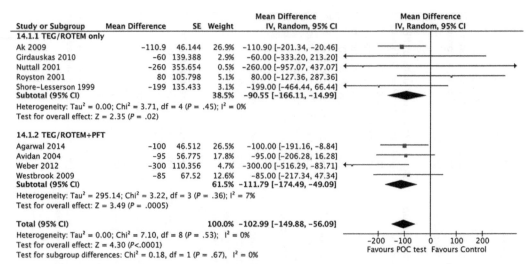

Fig. 3. Studies are grouped by studies using thromboelastography/rotational thromboelastometry (TEG/ROTEM) alone and TEG/ROTEM plus other point-of-care platelet function test. CI, confidence interval; PFT, platelet function testing; POC, point of care. (*From* Corredor C, Wasowicz M, Karkouti K, et al. The role of point-of-care platelet function testing in predicting postoperative bleeding following cardiac surgery: a systematic review and meta-analysis. Anaesthesia 2015;70:725; with permission.)

CI, 0.78–0.94; $P = .001$) and fresh frozen plasma (RR, 0.42; 95% CI, 0.30–0.59; $P<.00001$).[63] There was no mortality benefit at longest follow-up favoring a POC platelet function testing-guided transfusion algorithm (RR, 0.66; 95% CI, 0.31–1.39; $P = .27$). POC platelet function testing did not confer statistically significant benefit in terms of need for surgical reexploration (RR, 0.68; 95% CI, 0.36–1.26; $P = .22$) or duration of hospital stay (mean difference, -2.1 days; 95% CI, -4.3 to 0.2 days; $P = .08$). Thus, in CABG, platelet function testing can predict perioperative blood loss and can be used to guide the administration of blood products and reduce postoperative bleeding. Multiple transfusion algorithms implementing platelet function testing have been proposed; however, none of them has been accepted universally or is endorsed in guidelines. However, further and larger randomized studies are warranted on guidance of transfusion management and surgical procedure timing based on preoperative platelet function testing results.

SUMMARY

There is significant evidence for the prognostic value of $P2Y_{12}$ receptor directed platelet function testing in PCI-treated patients for the prediction of thrombotic events, including cardiovascular death and stent thrombosis. Data are accumulating that an optimal window of platelet reactivity level may exist during treatment with $P2Y_{12}$ inhibitors, within which both

thrombotic and bleeding complications are the lowest and the "net clinical benefit" is the highest. Transfusion management algorithms that use POC platelet function testing lead to a significant reduction in the proportion of patients receiving packed red blood cells and fresh frozen plasma. The Society of Thoracic Surgeons guidelines and the 2014 European Society of Cardiology/European Association for Cardio-Thoracic Surgery guidelines on myocardial revascularization provide a class II recommendation for timing of operation based on determination of platelet inhibition. However, there are several major knowledge gaps that need to be addressed regarding the potential value of platelet function testing for guidance of treatment after PCI, which must be answered in large prospective randomized studies that are adequately powered and focus on high-risk populations.

REFERENCES

1. Authors/Task Force members, Windecker S, Kolh P, et al. 2014 ESC/EACTS Guidelines on myocardial revascularization: The Task Force on Myocardial Revascularization of the European Society of Cardiology (ESC) and the European Association for Cardio-Thoracic Surgery (EACTS) Developed with the special contribution of the European Association of Percutaneous Cardiovascular Interventions (EAPCI). Eur Heart J 2014;35(37): 2541–619.

2. Angiolillo DJ, Fernandez-Ortiz A, Bernardo E, et al. Variability in individual responsiveness to clopidogrel: clinical implications, management, and future perspectives. J Am Coll Cardiol 2007; 49(14):1505–16.

3. Sibbing D, Steinhubl SR, Schulz S, et al. Platelet aggregation and its association with stent thrombosis and bleeding in clopidogrel-treated patients: initial evidence of a therapeutic window. J Am Coll Cardiol 2010;56(4):317–8.

4. Serebruany VL, Steinhubl SR, Berger PB, et al. Variability in platelet responsiveness to clopidogrel among 544 individuals. J Am Coll Cardiol 2005; 45(2):246–51.

5. Mega JL, Simon T, Collet JP, et al. Reduced-function CYP2C19 genotype and risk of adverse clinical outcomes among patients treated with clopidogrel predominantly for PCI: a meta-analysis. JAMA 2010;304(16):1821–30.

6. Frelinger AL 3rd, Bhatt DL, Lee RD, et al. Clopidogrel pharmacokinetics and pharmacodynamics vary widely despite exclusion or control of polymorphisms (CYP2C19, ABCB1, PON1), noncompliance, diet, smoking, co-medications (including proton pump inhibitors), and pre-existent variability in platelet function. J Am Coll Cardiol 2013;61(8): 872–9.

7. Sibbing D, Braun S, Morath T, et al. Platelet reactivity after clopidogrel treatment assessed with point-of-care analysis and early drug-eluting stent thrombosis. J Am Coll Cardiol 2009;53(10):849–56.

8. Tantry US, Bonello L, Aradi D, et al. Consensus and update on the definition of on-treatment platelet reactivity to adenosine diphosphate associated with ischemia and bleeding. J Am Coll Cardiol 2013;62(24):2261–73.

9. Aradi D, Kirtane A, Bonello L, et al. Bleeding and stent thrombosis on P2Y12-inhibitors: collaborative analysis on the role of platelet reactivity for risk stratification after percutaneous coronary intervention. Eur Heart J 2015;36(27):1762–71.

10. Lordkipanidze M. Platelet function tests. Semin Thromb Hemost 2016;42(3):258–67.

11. Bonello L, Paganelli F, Arpin-Bornet M, et al. Vasodilator-stimulated phosphoprotein phosphorylation analysis prior to percutaneous coronary intervention for exclusion of postprocedural major adverse cardiovascular events. J Thromb Haemost 2007;5(8):1630–6.

12. Breet NJ, van Werkum JW, Bouman HJ, et al. Comparison of platelet function tests in predicting clinical outcome in patients undergoing coronary stent implantation. JAMA 2010;303(8):754–62.

13. Campo G, Fileti L, de Cesare N, et al. Long-term clinical outcome based on aspirin and clopidogrel responsiveness status after elective percutaneous coronary intervention: a 3T/2R (tailoring treatment with tirofiban in patients showing resistance to aspirin and/or resistance to clopidogrel) trial substudy. J Am Coll Cardiol 2010;56(18):1447–55.

14. Campo G, Parrinello G, Ferraresi P, et al. Prospective evaluation of on-clopidogrel platelet reactivity over time in patients treated with percutaneous coronary intervention relationship with gene polymorphisms and clinical outcome. J Am Coll Cardiol 2011;57(25):2474–83.

15. Cuisset T, Frere C, Quilici J, et al. Predictive values of post-treatment adenosine diphosphate-induced aggregation and vasodilator-stimulated phosphoprotein index for stent thrombosis after acute coronary syndrome in clopidogrel-treated patients. Am J Cardiol 2009;104(8):1078–82.

16. Cuisset T, Grosdidier C, Loundou AD, et al. Clinical implications of very low on-treatment platelet reactivity in patients treated with thienopyridine: the POBA study (predictor of bleedings with antiplatelet drugs). JACC Cardiovasc Interv 2013;6(8): 854–63.

17. Gurbel PA, Bliden KP, Navickas IA, et al. Adenosine diphosphate-induced platelet-fibrin clot strength: a new thrombelastographic indicator of long-term poststenting ischemic events. Am Heart J 2010; 160(2):346–54.

18. Mangiacapra F, Patti G, Barbato E, et al. A therapeutic window for platelet reactivity for patients undergoing elective percutaneous coronary intervention: results of the ARMYDA-PROVE (Antiplatelet therapy for Reduction of MYocardial Damage during Angioplasty-Platelet Reactivity for Outcome Validation Effort) study. JACC Cardiovasc Interv 2012;5(3):281–9.

19. Marcucci R, Gori AM, Paniccia R, et al. Cardiovascular death and nonfatal myocardial infarction in acute coronary syndrome patients receiving coronary stenting are predicted by residual platelet reactivity to ADP detected by a point-of-care assay: a 12-month follow-up. Circulation 2009;119(2):237–42.

20. Parodi G, Marcucci R, Valenti R, et al. High residual platelet reactivity after clopidogrel loading and long-term cardiovascular events among patients with acute coronary syndromes undergoing PCI. JAMA 2011;306(11):1215–23.

21. Price MJ, Endemann S, Gollapudi RR, et al. Prognostic significance of post-clopidogrel platelet reactivity assessed by a point-of-care assay on thrombotic events after drug-eluting stent implantation. Eur Heart J 2008;29(8):992–1000.

22. Price MJ, Angiolillo DJ, Teirstein PS, et al. Platelet reactivity and cardiovascular outcomes after percutaneous coronary intervention: a time-dependent analysis of the Gauging Responsiveness with a VerifyNow P2Y12 assay: Impact on Thrombosis and Safety (GRAVITAS) trial. Circulation 2011;124(10): 1132–7.

23. Sibbing D, Bernlochner I, Schulz S, et al. Prognostic value of a high on-clopidogrel treatment platelet reactivity in bivalirudin versus abciximab treated non-ST-segment elevation myocardial infarction patients. ISAR-REACT 4 (Intracoronary Stenting and Antithrombotic Regimen: Rapid Early Action for Coronary Treatment-4) platelet substudy. J Am Coll Cardiol 2012;60(5):369–77.

24. Stone GW, Witzenbichler B, Weisz G, et al. Platelet reactivity and clinical outcomes after coronary artery implantation of drug-eluting stents (ADAPT-DES): a prospective multicentre registry study. Lancet 2013; 382(9892):614–23.

25. Geisler T, Langer H, Wydymus M, et al. Low response to clopidogrel is associated with cardiovascular outcome after coronary stent implantation. Eur Heart J 2006;27(20):2420–5.

26. Hochholzer W, Trenk D, Bestehorn HP, et al. Impact of the degree of peri-interventional platelet inhibition after loading with clopidogrel on early clinical outcome of elective coronary stent placement. J Am Coll Cardiol 2006;48(9):1742–50.

27. Bonello L, Tantry US, Marcucci R, et al. Consensus and future directions on the definition of high on-treatment platelet reactivity to adenosine diphosphate. J Am Coll Cardiol 2010;56(12):919–33.

28. Alexopoulos D, Galati A, Xanthopoulou I, et al. Ticagrelor versus prasugrel in acute coronary syndrome patients with high on-clopidogrel platelet reactivity following percutaneous coronary intervention: a pharmacodynamic study. J Am Coll Cardiol 2012;60(3):193–9.

29. Bonello L, Mancini J, Pansieri M, et al. Relationship between post-treatment platelet reactivity and ischemic and bleeding events at 1-year follow-up in patients receiving prasugrel. J Thromb Haemost 2012;10(10):1999–2005.

30. Parodi G, Valenti R, Bellandi B, et al. Comparison of prasugrel and ticagrelor loading doses in ST-segment elevation myocardial infarction patients: RAPID (Rapid Activity of Platelet Inhibitor Drugs) primary PCI study. J Am Coll Cardiol 2013;61(15): 1601–6.

31. Price MJ, Berger PB, Teirstein PS, et al. Standard- vs high-dose clopidogrel based on platelet function testing after percutaneous coronary intervention: the GRAVITAS randomized trial. JAMA 2011; 305(11):1097–105.

32. Collet JP, Cuisset T, Range G, et al. Bedside monitoring to adjust antiplatelet therapy for coronary stenting. N Engl J Med 2012;367(22):2100–9.

33. Michelson AD, Frelinger AL 3rd, Braunwald E, et al. Pharmacodynamic assessment of platelet inhibition by prasugrel vs. clopidogrel in the TRITON-TIMI 38 trial. Eur Heart J 2009;30(14):1753–63.

34. Mokhtar OA, Lemesle G, Armero S, et al. Relationship between platelet reactivity inhibition and non-CABG related major bleeding in patients undergoing percutaneous coronary intervention. Thromb Res 2010;126(2):e147–9.

35. Parodi G, Bellandi B, Venditti F, et al. Residual platelet reactivity, bleedings, and adherence to treatment in patients having coronary stent implantation treated with prasugrel. Am J Cardiol 2012; 109(2):214–8.

36. Patti G, Pasceri V, Vizzi V, et al. Usefulness of platelet response to clopidogrel by point-of-care testing to predict bleeding outcomes in patients undergoing percutaneous coronary intervention (from the Antiplatelet Therapy for Reduction of Myocardial Damage During Angioplasty-Bleeding Study). Am J Cardiol 2011;107(7):995–1000.

37. Sibbing D, Schulz S, Braun S, et al. Antiplatelet effects of clopidogrel and bleeding in patients undergoing coronary stent placement. J Thromb Haemost 2010;8(2):250–6.

38. Tsukahara K, Kimura K, Morita S, et al. Impact of high-responsiveness to dual antiplatelet therapy on bleeding complications in patients receiving drug-eluting stents. Circ J 2010;74(4):679–85.

39. Kirtane AJ, Parikh PB, Stuckey TD, et al. Is There an Ideal Level of Platelet P2Y12-Receptor Inhibition in Patients Undergoing Percutaneous Coronary Intervention?: "Window" Analysis From the ADAPT-DES Study (Assessment of Dual AntiPlatelet Therapy With Drug-Eluting Stents). JACC Cardiovasc Interv 2015;8(15):1978–87.

40. Bonello L, Camoin-Jau L, Armero S, et al. Tailored clopidogrel loading dose according to platelet reactivity monitoring to prevent acute and sub-acute stent thrombosis. Am J Cardiol 2009; 103(1):5–10.

41. Aradi D, Tornyos A, Pinter T, et al. Optimizing P2Y12 receptor inhibition in patients with acute coronary syndrome on the basis of platelet function testing: impact of prasugrel and high-dose clopidogrel. J Am Coll Cardiol 2014;63(11): 1061–70.

42. Mayer K, Schulz S, Bernlochner I, et al. A comparative cohort study on personalised antiplatelet therapy in PCI-treated patients with high on-clopidogrel platelet reactivity. Results of the ISAR-HPR registry. Thromb Haemost 2014;112(2): 342–51.

43. Siller-Matula JM, Francesconi M, Dechant C, et al. Personalized antiplatelet treatment after percutaneous coronary intervention: the MADONNA study. Int J Cardiol 2013;167(5):2018–23.

44. Trenk D, Stone GW, Gawaz M, et al. A randomized trial of prasugrel versus clopidogrel in patients with high platelet reactivity on clopidogrel after elective percutaneous coronary intervention with implantation of drug-eluting stents: results of the TRIGGER-PCI (Testing Platelet Reactivity In

Patients Undergoing Elective Stent Placement on Clopidogrel to Guide Alternative Therapy With Prasugrel) study. J Am Coll Cardiol 2012;59(24): 2159–64.

45. Karkouti K, Wijeysundera DN, Yau TM, et al. The independent association of massive blood loss with mortality in cardiac surgery. Transfusion 2004; 44(10):1453–62.

46. Ranucci M, Baryshnikova E, Castelvecchio S, et al, Surgical and Clinical Outcome Research (SCORE) Group. Major bleeding, transfusions, and anemia: the deadly triad of cardiac surgery. Ann Thorac Surg 2013;96(2):478–85.

47. Kwak YL, Kim JC, Choi YS, et al. Clopidogrel responsiveness regardless of the discontinuation date predicts increased blood loss and transfusion requirement after off-pump coronary artery bypass graft surgery. J Am Coll Cardiol 2010;56(24): 1994–2002.

48. Mahla E, Suarez TA, Bliden KP, et al. Platelet function measurement-based strategy to reduce bleeding and waiting time in clopidogrel-treated patients undergoing coronary artery bypass graft surgery: the timing based on platelet function strategy to reduce clopidogrel-associated bleeding related to CABG (TARGET-CABG) study. Circ Cardiovasc Interv 2012;5(2): 261–9.

49. Schimmer C, Hamouda K, Sommer SP, et al. The predictive value of multiple electrode platelet aggregometry (multiplate) in adult cardiac surgery. Thorac Cardiovasc Surg 2013;61(8):733–43.

50. Ranucci M, Colella D, Baryshnikova E, et al. Surgical, Clinical Outcome Research G. Effect of preoperative P2Y12 and thrombin platelet receptor inhibition on bleeding after cardiac surgery. Br J Anaesth 2014;113(6):970–6.

51. Mannacio V, Meier P, Antignano A, et al. Individualized strategy for clopidogrel suspension in patients undergoing off-pump coronary surgery for acute coronary syndrome: a case-control study. J Thorac Cardiovasc Surg 2014;148(4): 1299–306.

52. Reed GW, Kumar A, Guo J, et al. Point-of-care platelet function testing predicts bleeding in patients exposed to clopidogrel undergoing coronary artery bypass grafting: Verify pre-op TIMI 45–a pilot study. Clin Cardiol 2015;38(2):92–8.

53. Ferraris VA, Saha SP, Oestreich JH, et al. 2012 update to the Society of Thoracic Surgeons guideline on use of antiplatelet drugs in patients having cardiac and noncardiac operations. Ann Thorac Surg 2012;94(5):1761–81.

54. Shore-Lesserson L, Manspeizer HE, DePerio M, et al. Thromboelastography-guided transfusion algorithm reduces transfusions in complex cardiac surgery. Anesth Analg 1999;88(2):312–9.

55. Royston D, von Kier S. Reduced haemostatic factor transfusion using heparinase-modified thrombelastography during cardiopulmonary bypass. Br J Anaesth 2001;86(4):575–8.

56. Nuttall GA, Oliver WC, Santrach PJ, et al. Efficacy of a simple intraoperative transfusion algorithm for nonerythrocyte component utilization after cardiopulmonary bypass. Anesthesiology 2001;94(5): 773–81 [discussion: 5A–6A].

57. Avidan MS, Alcock EL, Da Fonseca J, et al. Comparison of structured use of routine laboratory tests or near-patient assessment with clinical judgement in the management of bleeding after cardiac surgery. Br J Anaesth 2004;92(2):178–86.

58. Ak K, Isbir CS, Tetik S, et al. Thromboelastography-based transfusion algorithm reduces blood product use after elective CABG: a prospective randomized study. J Card Surg 2009;24(4): 404–10.

59. Westbrook AJ, Olsen J, Bailey M, et al. Protocol based on thromboelastograph (TEG) outperforms physician preference using laboratory coagulation tests to guide blood replacement during and after cardiac surgery: a pilot study. Heart Lung Circ 2009;18(4):277–88.

60. Girdauskas E, Kempfert J, Kuntze T, et al. Thromboelastometrically guided transfusion protocol during aortic surgery with circulatory arrest: a prospective, randomized trial. J Thorac Cardiovasc Surg 2010;140(5):1117–24.e2.

61. Weber CF, Gorlinger K, Meininger D, et al. Point-of-care testing: a prospective, randomized clinical trial of efficacy in coagulopathic cardiac surgery patients. Anesthesiology 2012;117(3):531–47.

62. Agarwal S, Johnson RI, Shaw M. Preoperative point-of-care platelet function testing in cardiac surgery. J Cardiothorac Vasc Anesth 2015;29(2): 333–41.

63. Corredor C, Wasowicz M, Karkouti K, et al. The role of point-of-care platelet function testing in predicting postoperative bleeding following cardiac surgery: a systematic review and meta-analysis. Anaesthesia 2015;70(6):715–31.

64. Cuisset T, Cayla G, Frere C, et al. Predictive value of post-treatment platelet reactivity for occurrence of post-discharge bleeding after non-ST elevation acute coronary syndrome. Shifting from antiplatelet resistance to bleeding risk assessment? EuroIntervention 2009;5(3):325–9.

65. Wang XD, Zhang DF, Zhuang SW, et al. Modifying clopidogrel maintenance doses according to vasodilator-stimulated phosphoprotein phosphorylation index improves clinical outcome in patients with clopidogrel resistance. Clin Cardiol 2011; 34(5):332–8.

66. Ari H, Ozkan H, Karacinar A, et al. The EFFect of hIgh-dose ClopIdogrel treatmENT in patients with

clopidogrel resistance (the EFFICIENT trial). Int J Cardiol 2012;157(3):374–80.

67. Hazarbasanov D, Velchev V, Finkov B, et al. Tailoring clopidogrel dose according to multiple electrode aggregometry decreases the rate of ischemic complications after percutaneous coronary intervention. J Thromb Thrombolysis 2012; 34(1):85–90.

Moving?

Make sure your subscription moves with you!

To notify us of your new address, find your **Clinics Account Number** (located on your mailing label above your name), and contact customer service at:

Email: journalscustomerservice-usa@elsevier.com

800-654-2452 (subscribers in the U.S. & Canada)
314-447-8871 (subscribers outside of the U.S. & Canada)

Fax number: 314-447-8029

Elsevier Health Sciences Division
Subscription Customer Service
3251 Riverport Lane
Maryland Heights, MO 63043

*To ensure uninterrupted delivery of your subscription, please notify us at least 4 weeks in advance of move.

Printed and bound by CPI Group (UK) Ltd, Croydon, CR0 4YY

03/10/2024

01040304-0011